Atlas of Tongue Diagnosis
for AIDS Patients

Supported by a grant from the national natural
Science Foundation of China (No.90409004) and
by a grant from the National Key Science and
Technology Program of China during the Tenth
Five-Year Plan Period (No.2004BA719A13)

CBS Publishers & Distributors Pvt Ltd
New Delhi • Bengaluru • Chennai • Kochi • Kolkata • Mumbai
Bhubaneswar • Hyderabad • Jharkhand • Nagpur • Patna • Pune • Uttarakhand

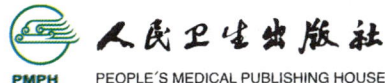
PEOPLE'S MEDICAL PUBLISHING HOUSE

Book Title: Atlas of Tongue Diagnosis for AIDS Patients
艾滋病舌诊图谱

ISBN: 978-93-86827-69-2

CBS Edition: 2019

This edition has been published by CBS Publishers & Distributors under arrangement with People's Medical Publishing House

First published: 2006

PMPH ISBN: 7-117-08042-6/R·8043

Not for sale outside India, Pakistan, Nepal, Bhutan and Sri Lanka.

Library of Congress Cataloguing in Publication Data:
A catalog record for this book is available from the Library of Congress.

Published by Satish Kumar Jain and produced by Varun Jain for

CBS Publishers & Distributors Pvt Ltd
4819/XI Prahlad Street, 24 Ansari Road, Daryaganj, New Delhi 110 002, India.
Ph: 23289259, 23266861, 23266867   Website: www.cbspd.com
Fax: 011-23243014   e-mail: delhi@cbspd.com; cbspubs@airtelmail.in.

Corporate Office: 204 FIE, Industrial Area, Patparganj, Delhi 110 092
Ph: 4934 4934   Fax: 4934 4935   e-mail: publishing@cbspd.com; publicity@cbspd.com

Branches

- **Bengaluru:** Seema House 2975, 17th Cross, K.R. Road, Banasankari 2nd Stage, Bengaluru 560 070, Karnataka, India
  Ph: +91-80-26771678/79   Fax: +91-80-26771680   e-mail: bangalore@cbspd.com
- **Chennai:** 7, Subbaraya Street, Shenoy Nagar, Chennai 600 030, Tamil Nadu, India.
  Ph: +91-44-26680620, 26681266 Fax: +91-44-42032115   e-mail: chennai@cbspd.com
- **Kochi:** 42/1325, 1326, Power House Road, Opposite KSEB Power House, Ernakulam 682 018, Kochi, Kerala, India.
  Ph: +91-484-4059061-65   Fax: +91-484-4059065   e-mail: kochi@cbspd.com
- **Kolkata:** 6/B, Ground Floor, Rameswar Shaw Road, Kolkata-700 014, West Bengal, India
  Ph: +91-33-22891126, 22891127, 22891128   e-mail: kolkata@cbspd.com
- **Mumbai:** 83-C, Dr E Moses Road, Worli, Mumbai-400018, Maharashtra, India
  Ph: +91-22-24902340/41   Fax: +91-22-24902342   e-mail: mumbai@cbspd.com

Representatives

| • **Bhubaneswar** | 0-9911037372 | • **Hyderabad** | 0-9885175004 | • **Jharkhand** | 0-9811541605 | • **Nagpur** | 0-9021734563 |
| • **Patna** | 0-9334159340 | • **Pune** | 0-9623451994 | • **Uttarakhand** | 0-9716462459 | | |

Printed at Nutech Print Services, Faridabad, India

Editorial Board

Project & Managing Editor:
Wang Li-zi

Book & Cover Designer:
Yin Yan

Typesetter:
Wei Hong-bo

PREFACE

Acquired Immunodeficiency Syndrome (AIDS) is a lethal, contagious disease identified approximately twenty years ago that is caused by the Human Immunodeficiency Virus (HIV), also known as the AIDS virus. In 2005, 2.8 million people worldwide died of AIDS, and 4.1 million were newly infected. Presently, the global population infected with HIV/AIDS is estimated to be 38.6 million, and $500 billion (USD) is spent annually to cover the expenditures arising from this disease. HIV/AIDS has become a public health problem and a growing global concern as it is greatly endangering the world population, and affecting economic development and social stability.

HIV/AIDS is transmitted from person to person, and HIV mainly exists in blood, semen, vaginal secretions, and breast milk of infected people. HIV/AIDS is passed by sexual contact, through blood or blood products, and from mother to child.

HIV belongs to a special class of retroviruses within the subgroup of human lentiviruses. Based on genetic diversity, HIV may be classified into two types; HIV-1 and HIV-2. Worldwide, the predominant virus is HIV-1, which may be further broken down into group M (major), group O (outlier) and group N (non-M & non-O / new). Within group M there are eleven genetically distinct subtypes of HIV-1. These are subtypes A, B, C, D, E, F, G, H, I, J and K. In recent years "circulating recombinant forms" (CRFs) of HIV-1 have been discovered. The predominant virus in China is HIV-1 with subtype A, B (Euro-American type), B' (Thai type), C, D, E, F, G and CRFs have been identified.

AIDS may involve multiple organ systems. Clinical pathological changes of AIDS include changes to the immune system, opportunistic infections of multiple systems, and malignant tumors arising from HIV infection. It is a prolonged and complicated disease progression from initial infection with HIV to the end of life, and the progression is generally divided into the stages of acute HIV infection, a clinically asymptomatic stage, and the AIDS stage. Biomedical medicine holds that special medical treatment is not necessary for the first two stages of infection. Rather, the focus is on work and rest, adequate nutrition, and minimizing the risk of transmission to others. As for AIDS patients, attention should be given mainly to the pathogenesis and treatment of various complications including supportive therapy, immune regulation/immunotherapy and psychological therapy. At present, highly active anti-retroviral therapy, which is also known as HAART, is commonly applied to inhibit HIV replication and help rebuild patient immune function.

Chinese Medicine is an ancient treasure in the world of medicine, and in recent years, it has received global attention and is playing an increasingly important role in the treatment of AIDS. Research on the treatment of AIDS with Chinese Medicine primarily focuses on the study of anti-viral or immune regulation effects of single herbal formulas or herbal components. Clinically, AIDS treatment is based on syndrome differentiation and clinical experiences that have shown positive benefits.

Syndrome differentiation is one of the foundations of Chinese Medicine which is based on the integrated application of the "four diagnostic methods": inspection/watching, auscultation/olfaction/hearing, inquiring, and pulse-taking/palpation. The *Huangdi Neijing (Yellow Emperor's Internal Classic, 黄帝内经)* states that "one who knows the patient's condition only by inspection is a master in Chinese Medicine". Inspection is the most important of the four methods, and tongue observation (also called "tongue diagnosis") is an essential part of inspection, and can be the primary basis for diagnosis and treatment.

Tongue diagnosis is a reflection of the features and experiences of Chinese Diagnostics, which refers to the understanding of physiological functions and pathological changes of the human body through observation of the tongue including the tongue body and tongue coating. Tongue diagnosis is a method of observing changes in the tongue to analyze and diagnose disease, and it is one of the main methods of diagnostic observation in Chinese medicine. Tongue diagnosis has a long history and it has been viewed as a critical diagnostic tool by physicians through the ages. Modern physicians have also proven its scientific validity. Chinese Medicine holds that the tongue is the external reflection or "mirror" of the *zang* and *fu* organs, and that it objectively reveals the true condition of the patient. Thus, it is highly significant in differential diagnosis, evaluation of disease, and prognosis. In the differential treatment of AIDS, tongue diagnosis also plays a unique and critical role.

In the past two years, pictures of 1284 AIDS patient's tongues were collected, of which 718 have been compiled into this volume. The authors hope that this valuable information will help human beings in their fight against AIDS, "the plague of the 21st century".

Bibliography

1. UNAIDS, UNAIDS 2006 Report on the Global AIDS Epidemic, May 30, 2006.

2. China State Bureau of Quality and Technical Supervision, National Standard of the People's Republic of China, 2001, HIV/AIDS Diagnostic Standard and Management Principle (For Trial Implementation).

3. Chinese Medical Association, A Guide to AIDS Diagnosis and Treatment (Draft), 2004.

4. ZHANG Xing-quan, FAN Jiang, HIV Infection and AIDS, People's Medical Publishing House, 1999.

5. YANG Shang-shan (Sui Dynasty), Huangdi Neijing Taisu, People's Medical Publishing House, 1965.

6. WANG Ji-li, YANG Shuan-cheng, Shezhen Yuanjian, 2001.

7. ZHU Wen-feng, Chinese Medicine Diagnostics, China Press of Traditional Chinese Medicine, 2005.

FOREWORD

This is a book about HIV/AIDS tongue manifestations based on clinical experience. This book not only carries on the tradition of tongue diagnosis that is based in Chinese Medicine theory, but also demonstrates its application to modern day contagious diseases.

This book is divided into three chapters. Chapter one outlines typical AIDS tongue manifestations from the perspective of color, shape, and coating. Chapter two examines common tongue manifestations in the asymptomatic stage of HIV infection and the AIDS stage. Chapter three gives a comprehensive analysis of the tongue manifestations of 1284 patients with HIV/AIDS, and helps readers with syndrome differentiation based on tongue manifestations. Although clinically complicated and highly variant, tongue manifestations must be viewed in terms of the appearance, color and shape of tongue as well as the quality and color of the coating. With a list of common tongue manifestations and an understanding of the essentials of tongue diagnosis, readers will be able to cope with complicated situations with much more flexibility. The pictures in this book were taken with a high-resolution digital camera by professional photographers in natural light, and they were categorized after colorimetric and comprehensive analysis by diagnostics experts. This book aims to offer clear pictures and accurate information about patient's conditions. It is well illustrated with outstanding focus, clear pictures, full and accurate content, and the cases are outlined in a succinct language making the information in this book simple and intelligible.

This book has been translated into the English language in the hope of benefiting health-care professionals engaged in the prevention, control, and research of AIDS. It is an excellent reference book for physicians, teachers and students at medical schools and hospitals, and it is hoped that it will help promote the international transmission of Traditional Chinese Medicine.

The Editorial Board

July 2006

TABLE OF CONTENTS

CHAPTER ONE
TYPICAL AIDS TONGUES

1. *Red Tongue*

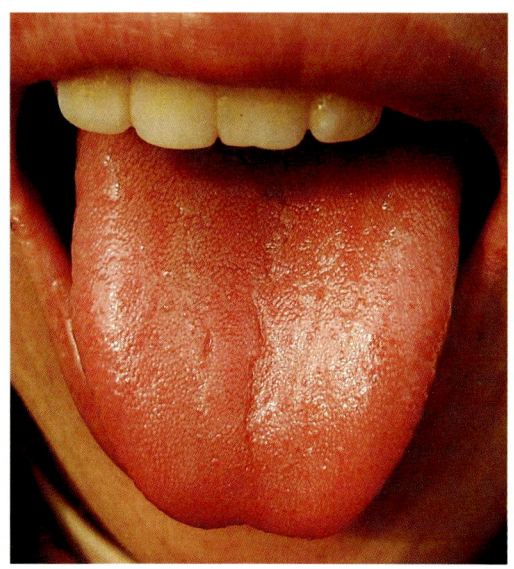

Fig 1.1-1

Tongue description:
red with thin yellow coating

Case No.:
W226 (female, 38years)

Clinical manifestations:
bitter taste, hypochondriac distention, depression, diarrhea, and borborygmus

Syndrome differentiation in CHINESE MEDICINE:
internal accumulation of damp-heat, stagnation of liver-qi with deficiency of the spleen

Stage:
AIDS

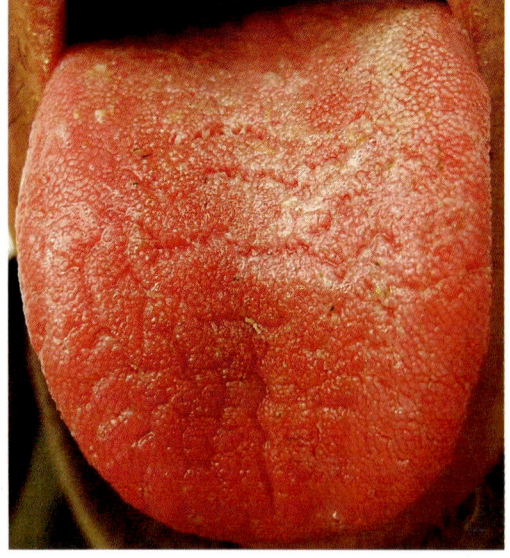

Fig 1.1-2

Tongue description:
red and cracked with thin, white and greasy coating

Case No.:
W362 (male, 37years)

Clinical manifestations:
lassitude, night sweat

Syndrome differentiation in CHINESE MEDICINE:
deficiency of both qi and yin

Stage:
infected with HIV yet clinically asymptomatic

Fig 1.1-3

Tongue description:
red with yellow, greasy and peeled coating

Case No.:
W186 (male, 55years)

Clinical manifestations:
lassitude, poor appetite, fullness and oppression in the epigastrium, diarrhea, restlessness and dry throat

Syndrome differentiation in Chinese medicine:
internal accumulation of damp-heat, deficiency of both qi and yin.

Stage:
AIDS

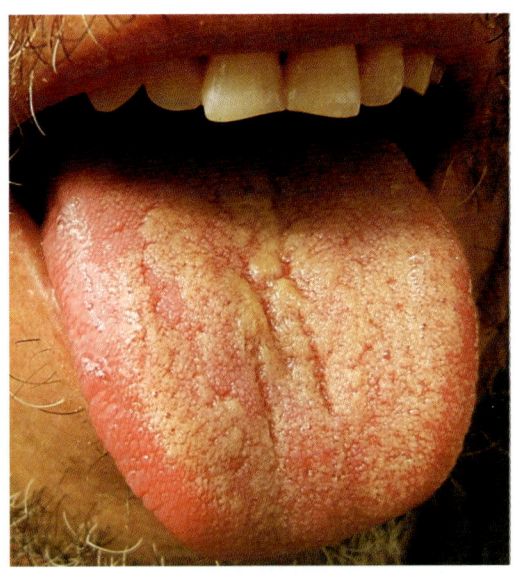

Fig 1.1-4

Tongue description:
red and cracked with yellow, thick and greasy coating at the root

Case No.:
W328 (male, 51years)

Clinical manifestations:
no discomfort

Syndrome differentiation in Chinese medicine:
internal accumulation of damp-heat

Stage:
infected with HIV yet clinically asymptomatic

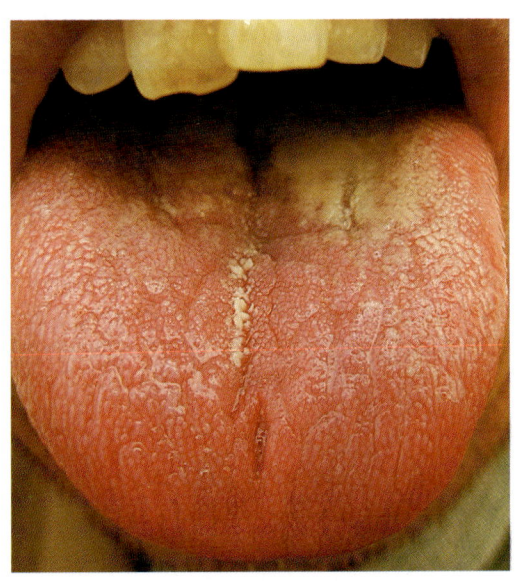

2. *Crimson Tongue*

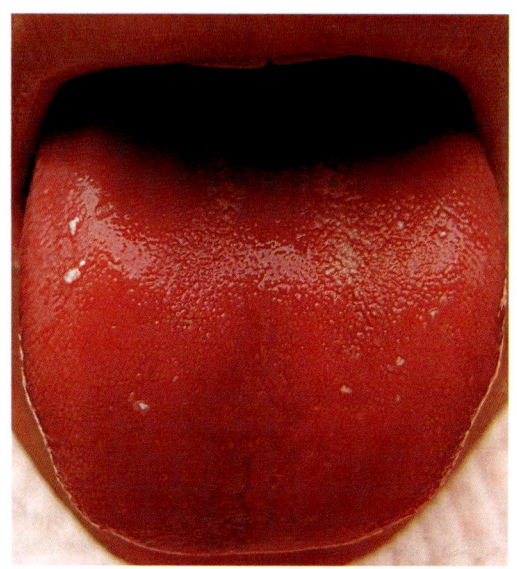

Fig 1.1-5

Tongue description:
crimson with scanty white coating

Case No.:
F6 (female, 49years)

Clinical manifestations:
feverish sensation in chest, palms and soles, night sweat, soreness and weakness of the waist and knees

Syndrome differentiation in Chinese medicine:
liver and kidney yin deficiency

Stage:
AIDS

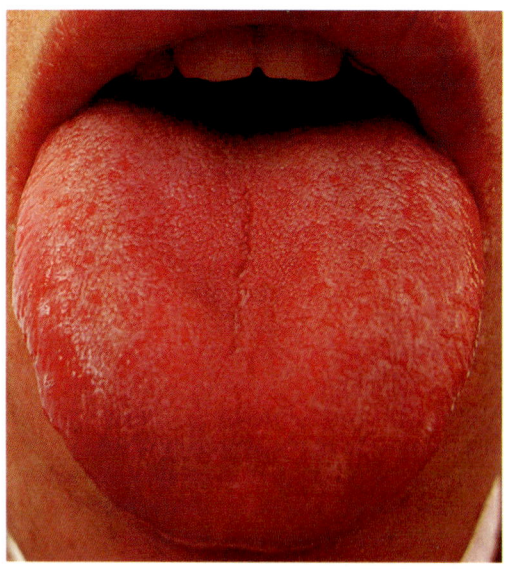

Fig 1.1-6

Tongue description:
crimson with thin yellow coating

Case No.:
W610 (female, 48years)

Clinical manifestations:
cough with sticky sputum, diarrhea with burning sensation over the anus, lumbago, vertigo

Syndrome differentiation in Chinese medicine:
internal accumulation of damp-heat, liver and kidney yin deficiency

Stage:
AIDS

Fig 1.1-7

Tongue description:
crimson

Case No.:
W595 (male, 58years)

Clinical manifestations:
night sweat, dizziness, dry and sore throat

Syndrome differentiation in Chinese medicine:
liver and kidney yin deficiency

Stage:
infected with HIV yet clinically asymptomatic

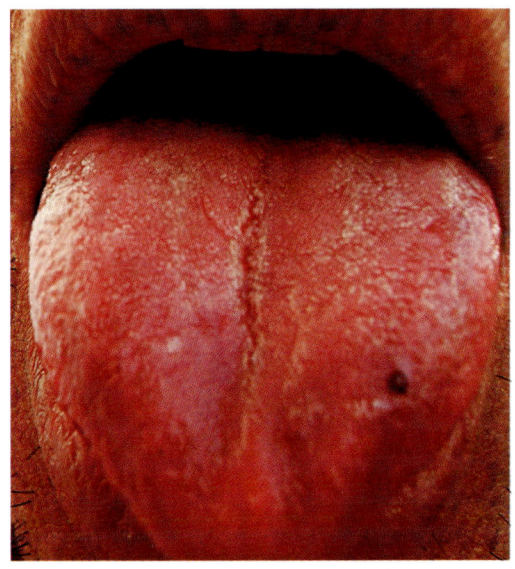

Fig 1.1-8

Tongue description:
crimson with thin and white coating

Case No.:
W621 (female, 45years)

Clinical manifestations:
oral anabrosis, lassitude, intermittent perspiration

Syndrome differentiation in Chinese medicine:
excessive accumulation of damp-heat evil, deficiency of spleen qi

Stage:
AIDS

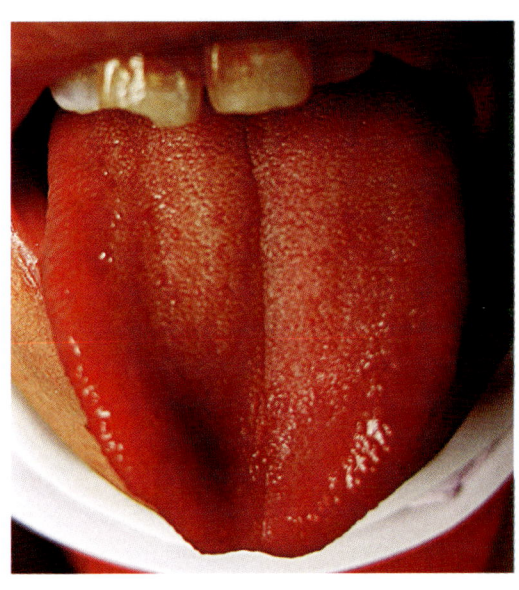

3. *Light Red Tongue*

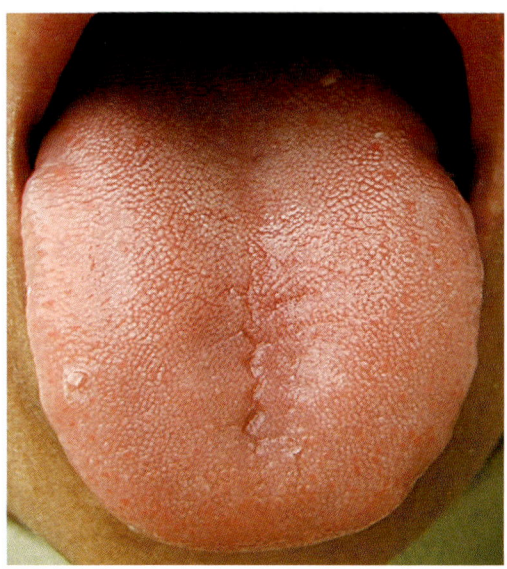

Fig 1.1-9

Tongue description:
reddish with thin white coating

Case No.:
W59 (female, 36years)

Clinical manifestations:
dysphoria, hypochondriac distention, epigastric distension, nausea, poor appetite

Syndrome differentiation in Chinese medicine:
stagnation of liver qi, deficiency of spleen qi

Stage:
AIDS

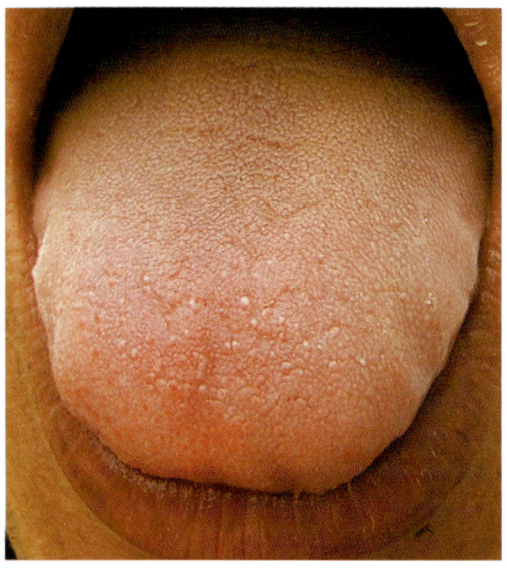

Fig 1.1-10

Tongue description:
reddish with teeth imprints

Case No.:
W90 (male, 31years)

Clinical manifestations:
lassitude, poor appetite

Syndrome differentiation in Chinese medicine:
deficiency of spleen qi

Stage:
infected with HIV yet clinically asymptomatic

Fig 1.1-11

Tongue description:
reddish and thin with thin white coating

Case No.:
W94 (male, 32 years)

Clinical manifestations:
fever, dry cough, spontaneous perspiration, night sweat

Syndrome differentiation in Chinese medicine:
wind-heat invasion, deficiency of both qi and yin

Stage:
AIDS

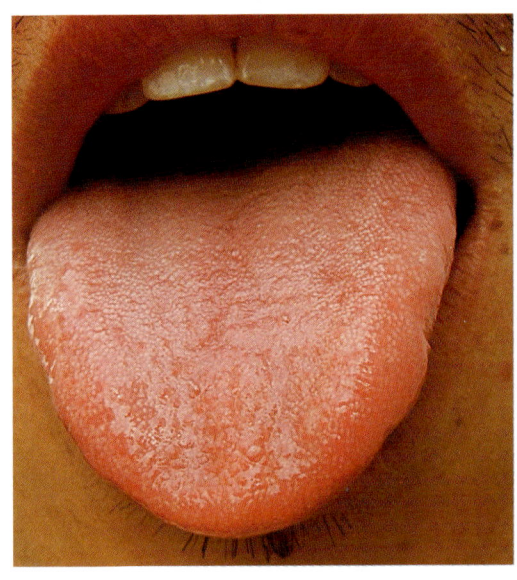

Fig 1.1-12

Tongue description:
reddish with thin white coating

Case No.:
W104 (male, 52years)

Clinical manifestations:
feverish sensation in chest, palms and soles, lassitude, fatigue, intermittent perspiration

Syndrome differentiation in Chinese medicine:
deficiency of both qi and yin

Stage:
AIDS

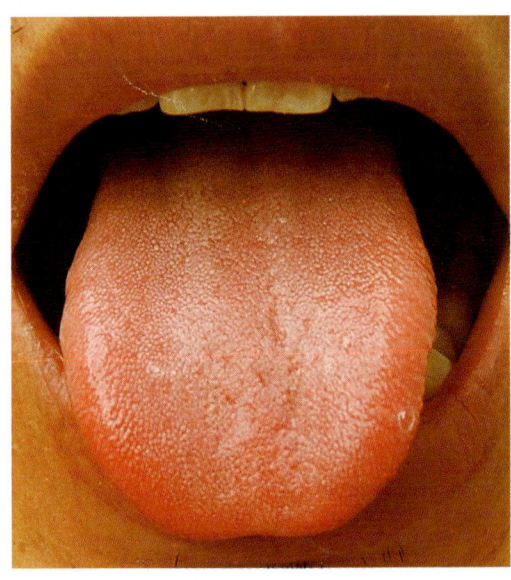

4. *Pale Tongue*

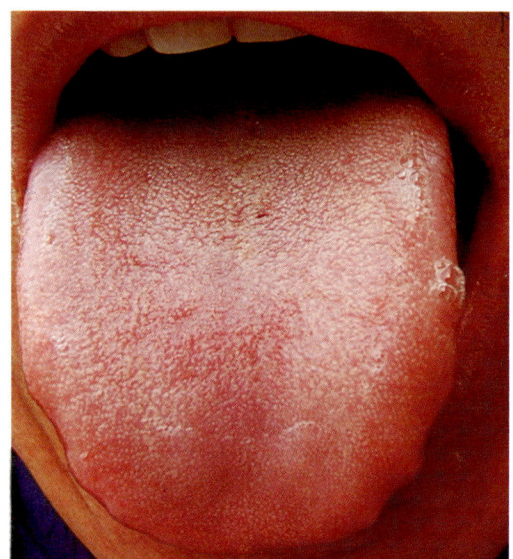

Fig 1.1-13

Tongue description:
pale with teeth imprints; thin, white, moist coating

Case No.:
W68 (male, 39years)

Clinical manifestations:
chest distress, short breath and lassitude

Syndrome differentiation in Chinese medicine:
deficiency of lung and spleen qi

Stage:
infected with HIV yet clinically asymptomatic

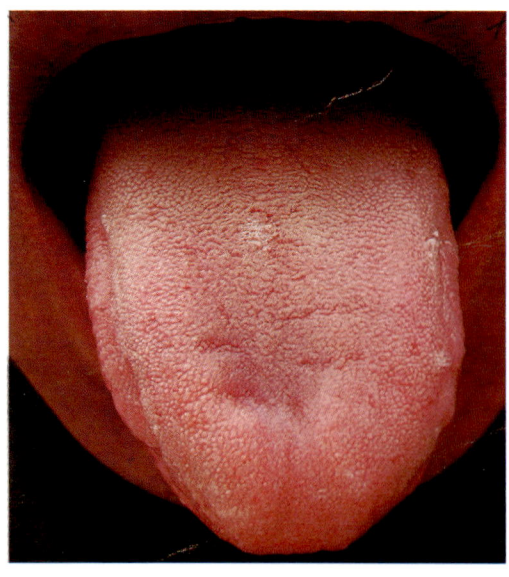

Fig 1.1-14

Tongue description:
pale and thin with teeth imprints; thin, white, moist coating

Case No.:
F137 (male, 41years)

Clinical manifestations:
lassitude, short breath, poor appetite and sallow complexion

Syndrome differentiation in Chinese medicine:
deficiency of qi and blood

Stage:
infected with HIV yet clinically asymptomatic

Fig 1.1-15

Tongue description:
pale with thin white coating

Case No.:
W303 (female, 53years)

Clinical manifestations:
soreness and weakness of the waist and knees, morning diarrhea, aversion to cold, lassitude

Syndrome differentiation in Chinese medicine:
deficiency of spleen and kidney yang

Stage:
AID

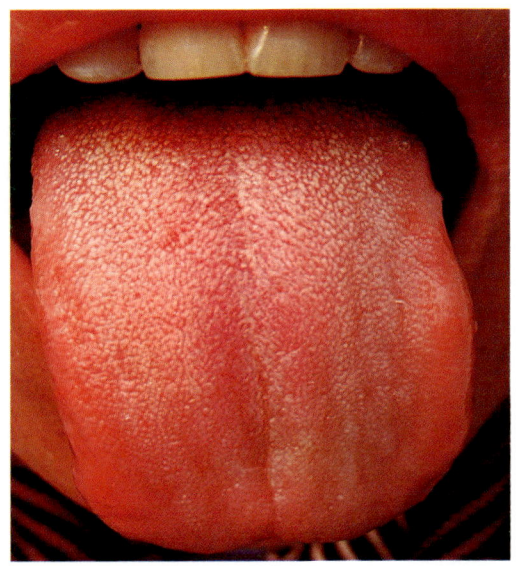

Fig 1.1-16

Tongue description:
pale with yellowish, thin and greasy coating

Case No.:
F178 (male, 46years)

Clinical manifestations:
fever, chest distress, short breath, diarrhea, lassitude

Syndrome differentiation in Chinese medicine:
internal accumulation of damp-heat, deficiency of lung and spleen qi

Stage:
AIDS

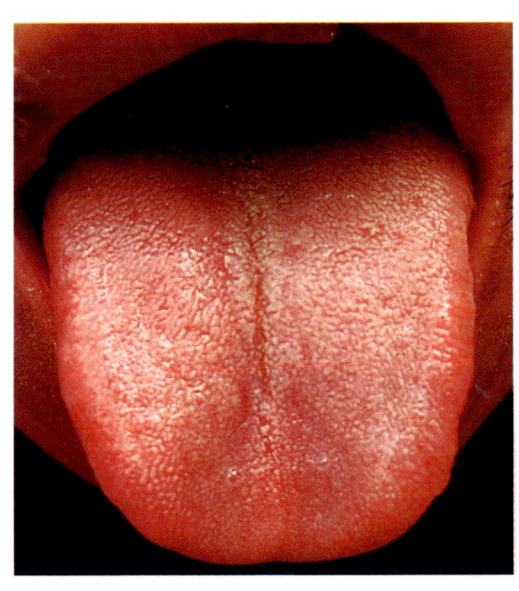

5. *Purple Tongue*

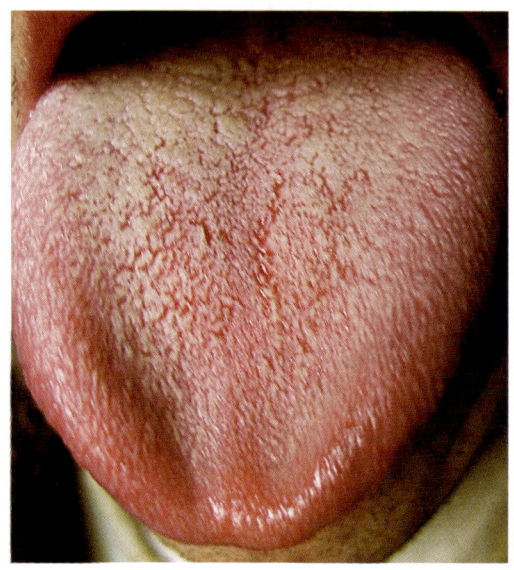

Fig 1.1-17

Tongue description:
purplish with yellow, thick and greasy coating at the root

Case No.:
W519 (male, 41years)

Clinical manifestations:
lymphadenectasis, yellow urine and dreaminess

Syndrome differentiation in Chinese medicine:
internal accumulation of damp-heat, combination of phlegm and blood stasis

Stage:
AIDS

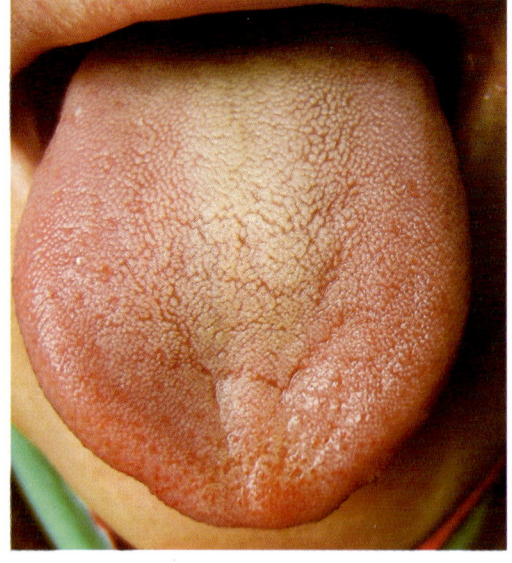

Fig 1.1-18

Tongue description:
purplish with thin, yellow and greasy coating in the central part

Case No.:
W521 (female, 53years)

Clinical manifestations:
bitter taste, epigastric distension, diarrhea, lassitude, and poor appetite

Syndrome differentiation in Chinese medicine:
internal accumulation of damp-heat, deficiency of spleen qi

Stage:
AIDS

6. *Petechial Tongue*

Fig 1.1-19

Tongue description:
red with petechia, thorny tip, white, thick and greasy coating in the central part

Case No.:
W101 (male, 39years)

Clinical manifestations:
herpes, lassitude

Syndrome differentiation in Chinese medicine:
excessive accumulation of damp-heat evil, deficiency of spleen qi

Stage:
AIDS

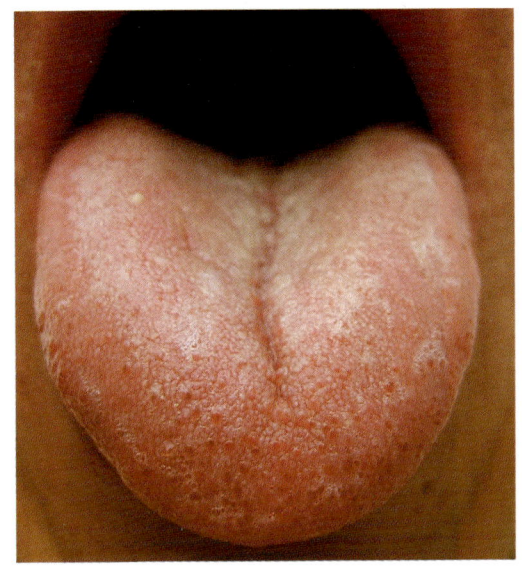

Fig 1.1-20

Tongue description:
red with petechia, scanty coating

Case No.:
F149 (female, 48years)

Clinical manifestations:
itchy skin, vertigo, dark, dry and cracked lips

Syndrome differentiation in Chinese medicine:
internal accumulation of damp-heat, deficiency of qi and blood with blood stasis

Stage:
AIDS

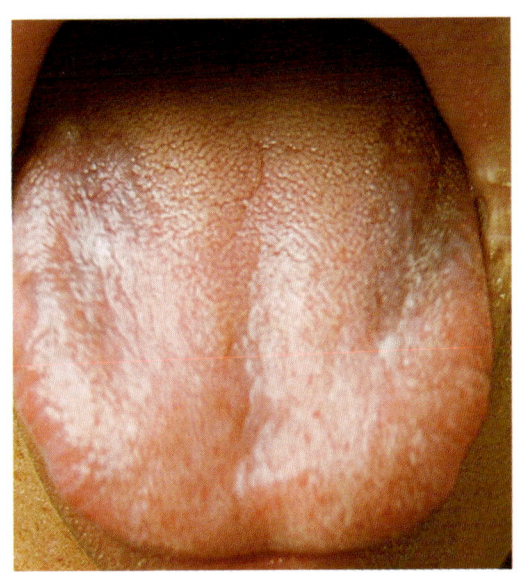

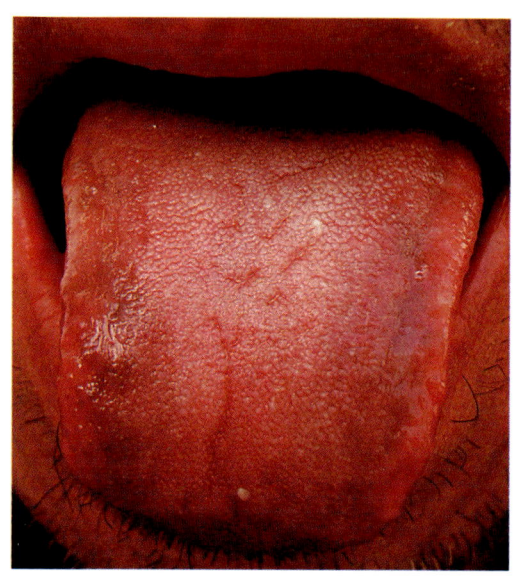

Fig 1.1-21

Tongue description:
reddish with petechia streaks on the border and tip of tongue, thin and white coating

Case No.:
F232 (male, 59years)

Clinical manifestations:
dry cough, itchy skin, morning diarrhea

Syndrome differentiation in Chinese medicine:
wind-heat invading lung, yang deficiency of spleen and kidney, blood stasis

Stage:
AIDS

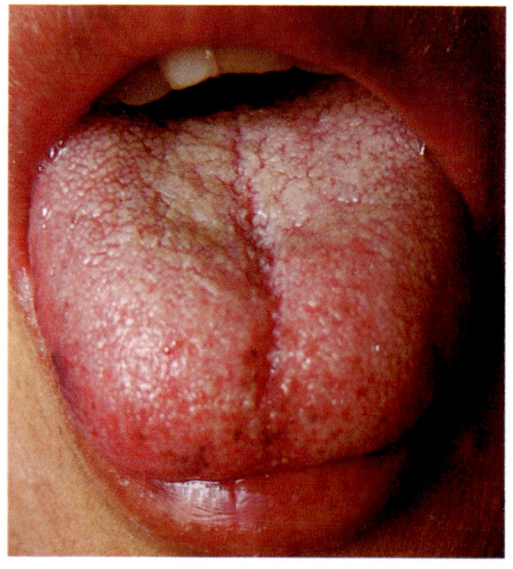

Fig 1.1-22

Tongue description:
red with petechia, white, yellow, thick and greasy coating

Case No.:
F210 (female, 54years)

Clinical manifestations:
fever, itchy skin with papules, lassitude

Syndrome differentiation in Chinese medicine:
excessive accumulation of damp-heat evil, deficiency of qi with blood stasis

Stage:
AIDS

1. *Swollen Tongue*

Fig 1.2-1

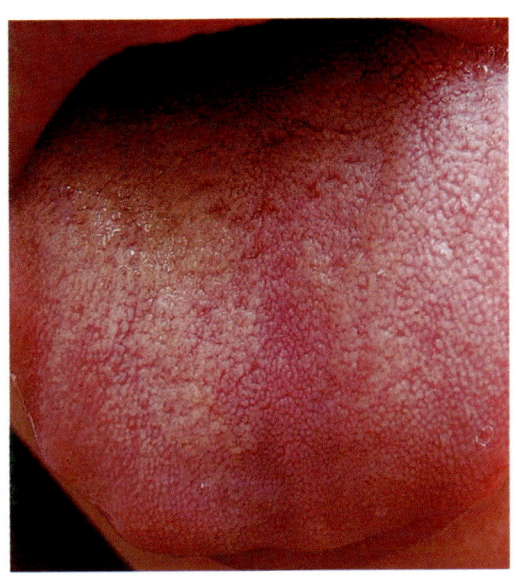

Tongue description:
reddish and swollen with teeth imprints, white, yellow, thick and greasy coating

Case No.:
F111 (female, 35years)

Clinical manifestations:
palpitation, vertigo, pale lips and lassitude

Syndrome differentiation in Chinese medicine:
deficiency of qi and blood, internal accumulation of damp-heat

Stage:
AIDS

Fig 1.2-2

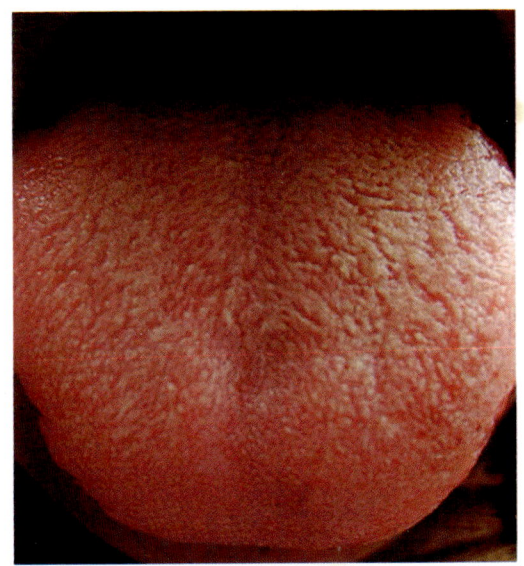

Tongue description:
pale and swollen with white, yellow and greasy coating

Case No.:
F269 (male, 43years)

Clinical manifestations:
aversion to cold, cold limbs, blackish complexion and fever with cold aversion

Syndrome differentiation in Chinese medicine:
yang deficiency of spleen and kidney, wind-heat invasion

Stage:
AIDS

Swollen tongue

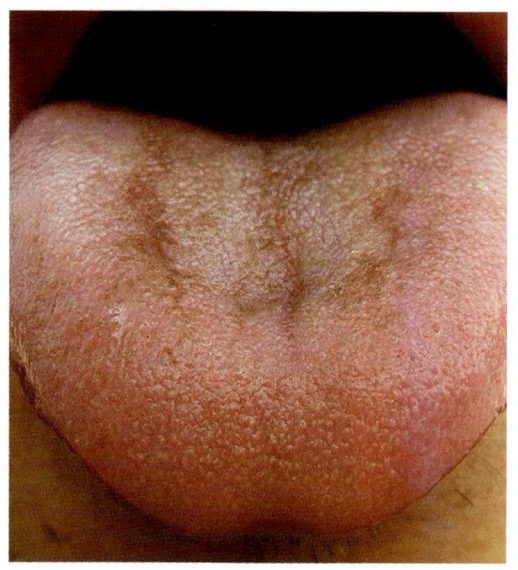

Fig 1.2-3

Tongue description:
dark and swollen with thin white coating

Case No.:
W675 (male, 42years)

Clinical manifestations:
constant low fever, chronic diarrhea, and constant fall in body weight

Syndrome differentiation in Chinese medicine:
qi deficiency of lung and spleen

Stage:
AIDS

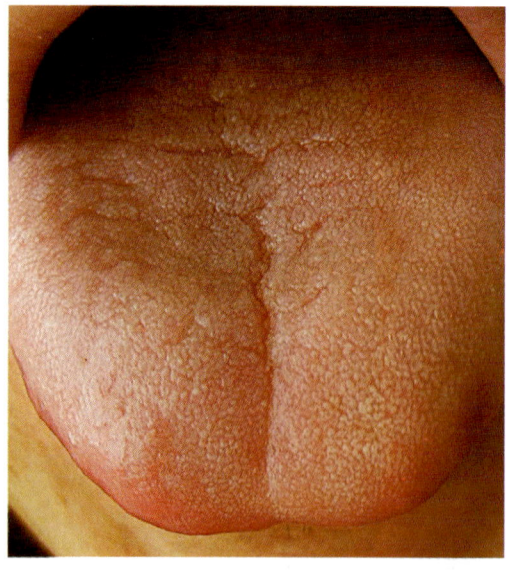

Fig 1.2-4

Tongue description:
reddish and swollen with crack, thin white and yellowish coating

Case No.:
F319 (male, 38years)

Clinical manifestations:
recurrent oral ulcer

Syndrome differentiation in Chinese medicine:
internal accumulation of damp-heat

Stage:
AIDS

2. *Tooth-marked Tongue*

Fig 1.2-5

Tongue description:
pale, dark and swollen with teeth imprints, yellowish coating

Case No.:
F104 (female, 50years)

Clinical manifestations:
chronic diarrhea and herpes

Syndrome differentiation in Chinese medicine:
deficiency of spleen-qi, excessive accumulation of damp heat evil

Stage:
AIDS

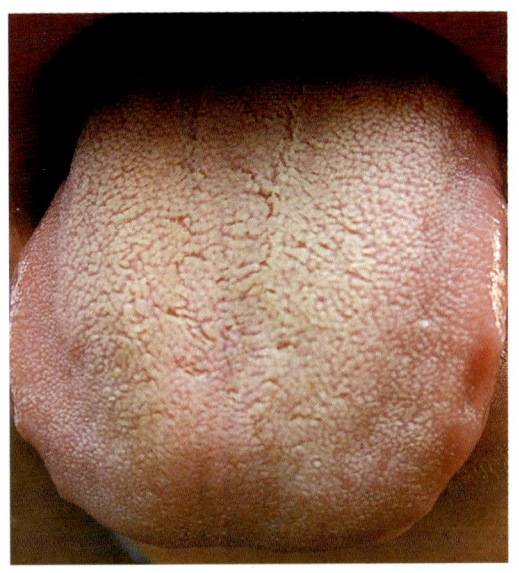

Fig 1.2-6

Tongue description:
pale and swollen with teeth imprints, white, yellow and thick coating

Case No.:
W523 (male, 40years)

Clinical manifestations:
lassitude, poor appetite, chest distress and short breath

Syndrome differentiation in Chinese medicine:
qi deficiency of lung and spleen, internal accumulation of damp-heat

Stage:
AIDS

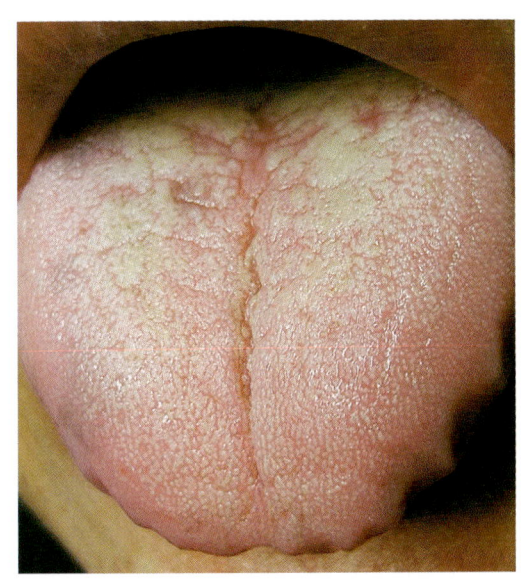

Tooth-markded tongue

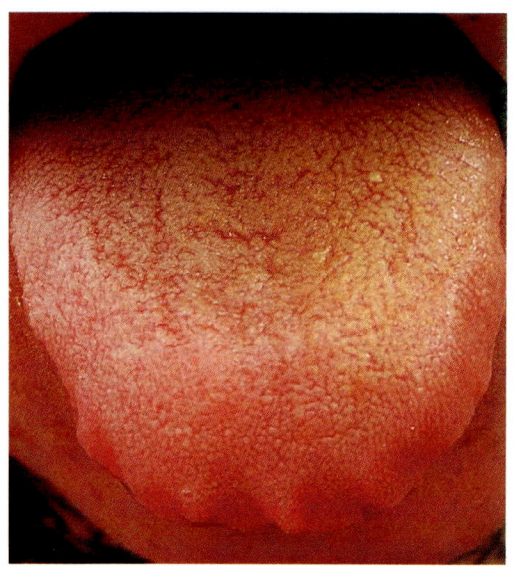

Fig 1.2-7

Tongue description:
reddish with teeth imprints, yellowish and slightly thick coating

Case No.:
W344 (female, 44years)

Clinical manifestations:
emaciation, lassitude, epigastric fullness, poor appetite, bitter taste, foul breath and hypochondriac distention

Syndrome differentiation in Chinese medicine:
deficiency of spleen-qi, internal accumulation of damp-heat

Stage:
AIDS

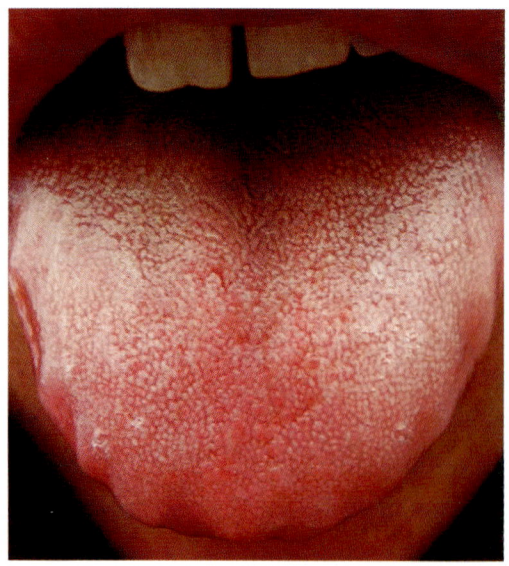

Fig 1.2-8

Tongue description:
purplish with teeth imprints, white, thick and greasy coating

Case No.:
F246 (female, 56years)

Clinical manifestations:
lassitude, low fever and limb numbness

Syndrome differentiation in Chinese medicine:
deficiency of both qi and yin, internal accumulation of damp-heat

Stage:
AIDS

3. *Thin Tongue*

Fig 1.2-9

Tongue description:
thin and reddish with yellow, thick and
greasy coating

Case No.:
292 (male, 39years)

Clinical manifestations:
sticky sputum, bitter taste, sticky mouth
and lassitude

**Syndrome differentiation in
Chinese medicine:**
internal accumulation of damp-heat,
deficiency of spleen-qi

Stage:
infected with HIV yet clinically asymptomatic

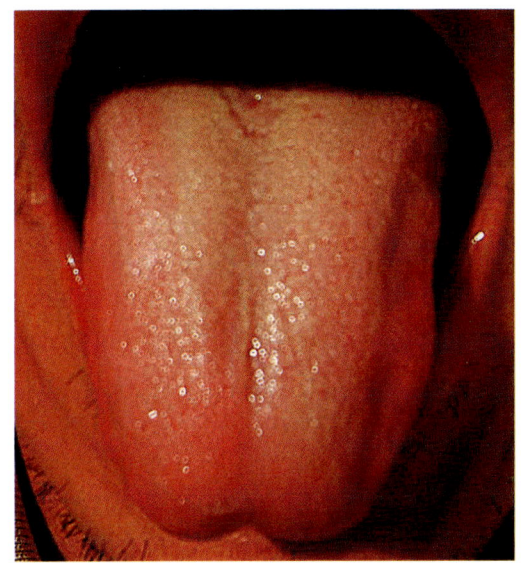

Fig 1.2-10

Tongue description:
reddish and thin with thin and white
coating

Case No.:
F204 (male, 42years)

Clinical manifestations:
chest distress, lassitude and gasp on
movement

**Syndrome differentiation in
Chinese medicine:**
qi deficiency of lung and spleen

Stage:
infected with HIV yet clinically asymptomatic

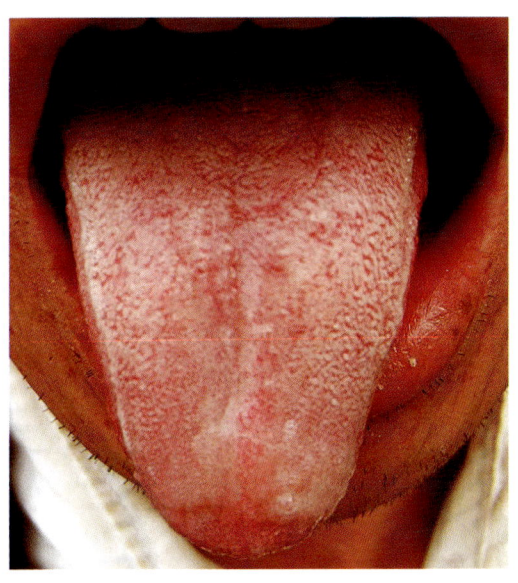

Thin tongue

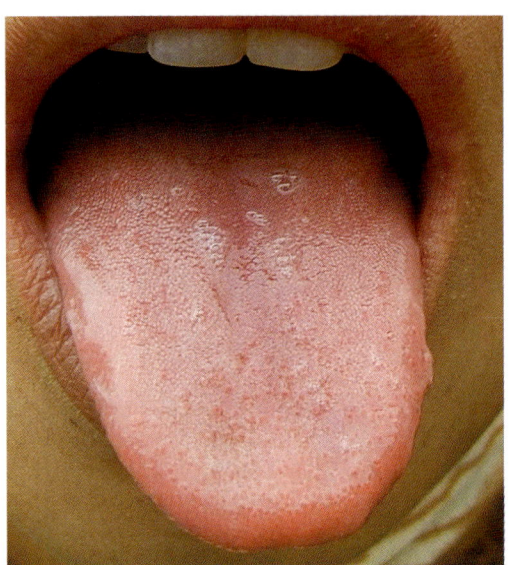

Fig 1.2-11

Tongue description:
red, thin and emaciated with thin and white coating

Case No.:
W26 (female, 30years)

Clinical manifestations:
itchy skin and dry cough

Syndrome differentiation in Chinese medicine:
wind-heat invasion

Stage:
infected with HIV yet clinically asymptomatic

4. *Cracked Tongue*

Fig 1.2-12

Tongue description:
red with crack, thin and white coating in the central part and root

Case No.:
F42 (male, 38years)

Clinical manifestations:
itchy skin, mucous stool, tenesmus and lassitude

Syndrome differentiation in Chinese medicine:
excessive accumulation of damp-heat evil, deficiency of spleen-qi

Stage:
AIDS

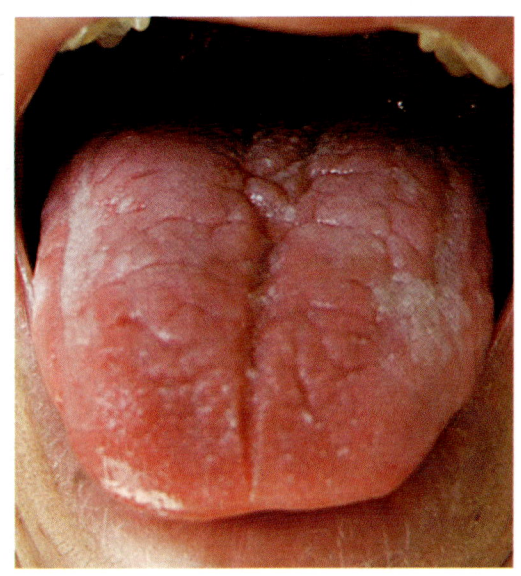

Fig 1.2-13

Tongue description:
pale and swollen with teeth imprints and crack, white and slightly thick coating

Case No.:
W340 (female, 44years)

Clinical manifestations:
sallow complexion, lassitude and emaciation

Syndrome differentiation in Chinese medicine:
deficiency of qi and blood

Stage:
AIDS

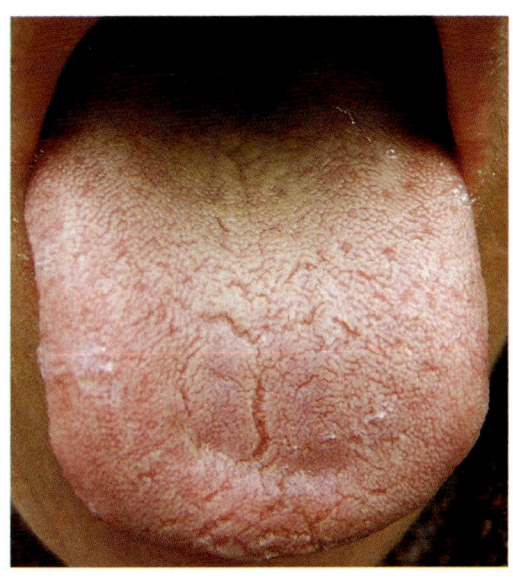

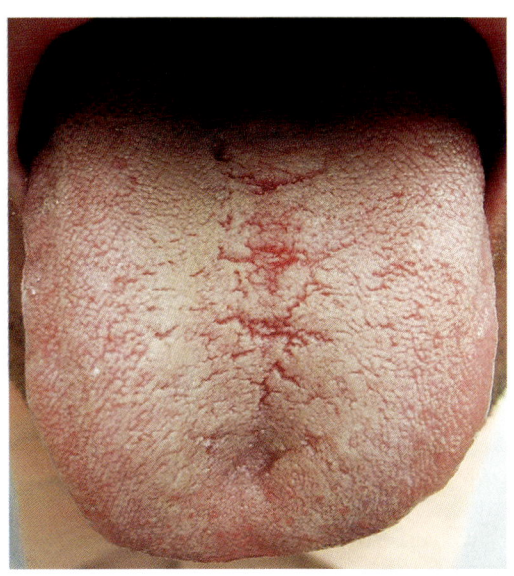

Fig 1.2-14

Tongue description:
red with crack, yellow and thick coating

Case No.:
W167 (male, 38years)

Clinical manifestations:
cough with yellow and sticky sputum

Syndrome differentiation in Chinese medicine:
pulmonary retention of phlegm-heat

Stage:
AIDS

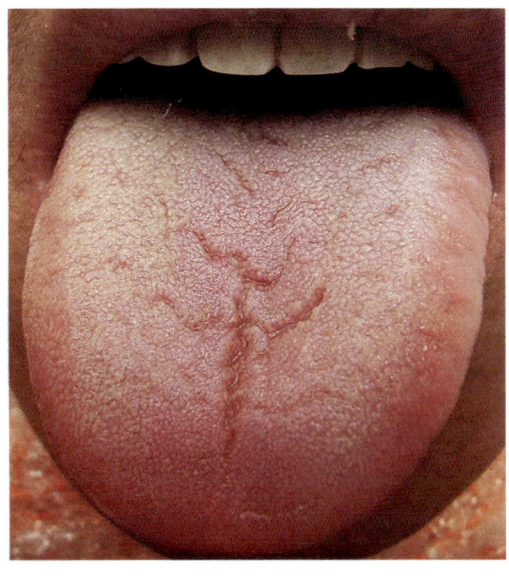

Fig 1.2-15

Tongue description:
red with crack, thin and yellow coating

Case No.:
W580 (female, 44years)

Clinical manifestations:
cough with yellow and sticky sputum, lassitude, short breath, epigastric fullness and poor appetite

Syndrome differentiation in Chinese medicine:
pulmonary retention of phlegm-heat, qi deficiency of lung and spleen

Stage:
AIDS

1. *Thick, White and Greasy Tongue Coating*

Fig 1.3-1

Tongue description:

reddish with white, thick and greasy coating

Case No.:

F74 (female, 36years)

Clinical manifestations:

lassitude, epigastric fullness and sticky leucorrhea

Syndrome differentiation in Chinese medicine:

deficiency of spleen-qi, internal accumulation of damp-heat

Stage:

infected with HIV yet clinically asymptomatic

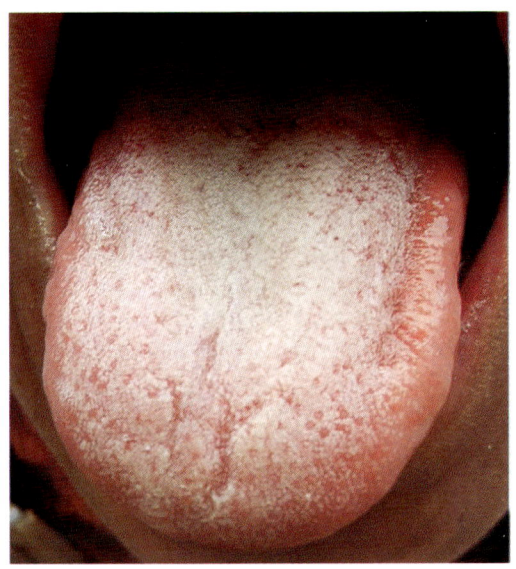

Fig 1.3-2

Tongue description:

pale with teeth imprints, white, thick and greasy coating

Case No.:

W548 (female, 39years)

Clinical manifestations:

gasp on movement, lassitude, poor appetite and loose stool

Syndrome differentiation in Chinese medicine:

qi deficiency of lung and spleen

Stage:

AIDS

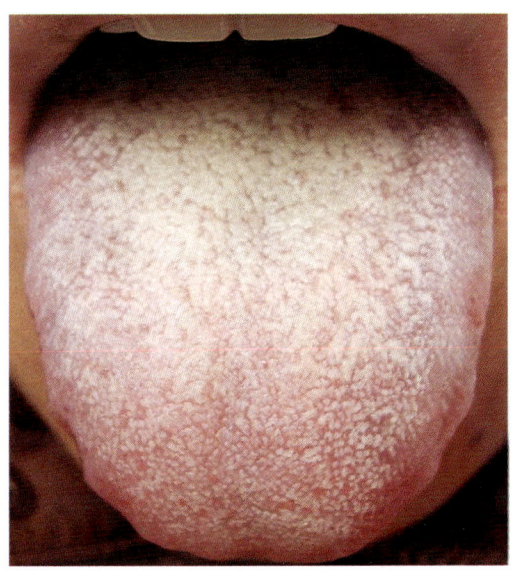

21

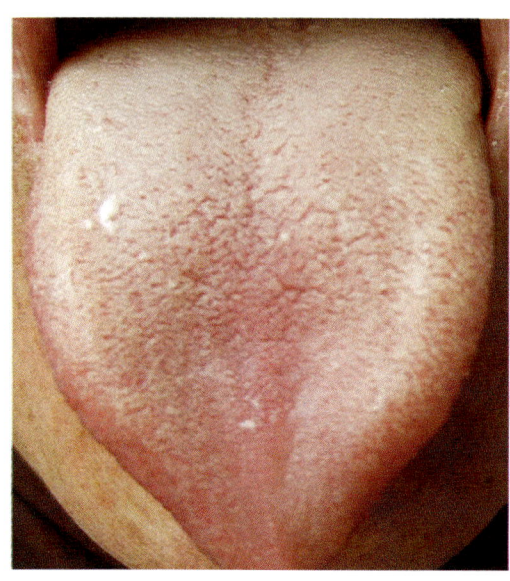

Fig 1.3-3

Tongue description:
red with white, thick and greasy coating

Case No.:
W415 (female, 49years)

Clinical manifestations:
lassitude, poor appetite, dysphoria, bitter taste and dry mouth without thirst for water

Syndrome differentiation in Chinese medicine:
deficiency of spleen-qi, internal accumulation of damp-heat

Stage:
AIDS

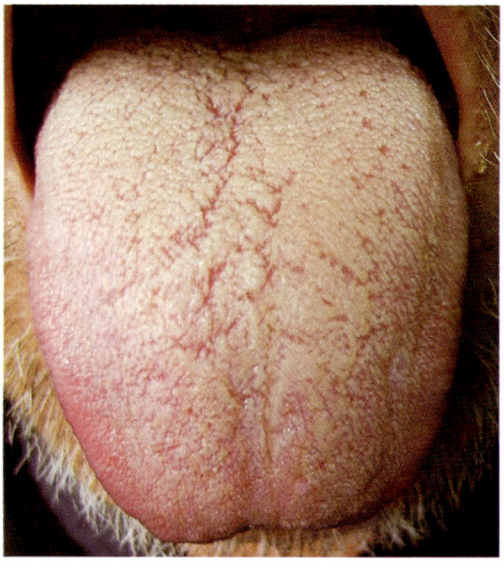

Fig 1.3-4

Tongue description:
red with white, thick and greasy coating

Case No.:
W524 (male, 53years)

Clinical manifestations:
chest distress, short breath, epigastric fullness, lassitude, diarrhea and brownish urine

Syndrome differentiation in Chinese medicine:
qi deficiency of lung and spleen, internal accumulation of damp-heat

Stage:
AIDS

2. *Thin-yellow Tongue Coating*

Fig 1.3-5

Tongue description:
dark red with thin, yellow and greasy coating

Case No.:
W255 (male, 47years)

Clinical manifestations:
fever, expectoration, chest distress, epigastric fullness and lassitude

Syndrome differentiation in Chinese medicine:
pulmonary retention of phlegm-heat, qi deficiency of lung and spleen

Stage:
AIDS

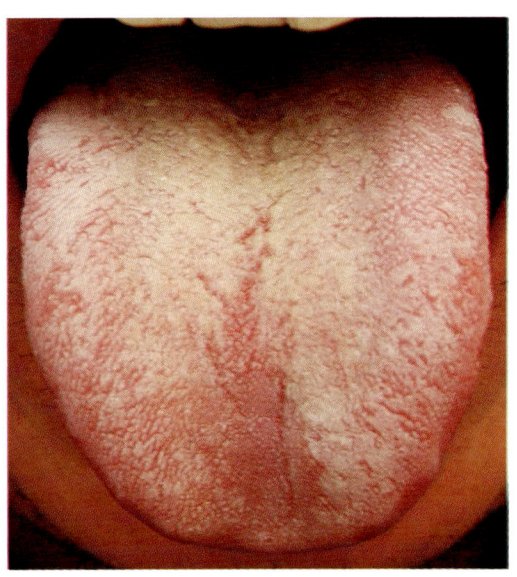

Fig 1.3-6

Tongue description:
red tongue with yellow and greasy coating at the root, brightly red and no coating tip

Case No.:
W672 (male, 36years)

Clinical manifestations:
lassitude, short breath, emaciation and dry pharynx

Syndrome differentiation in Chinese medicine:
deficiency of qi and yin

Stage:
infected with HIV yet clinically asymptomatic

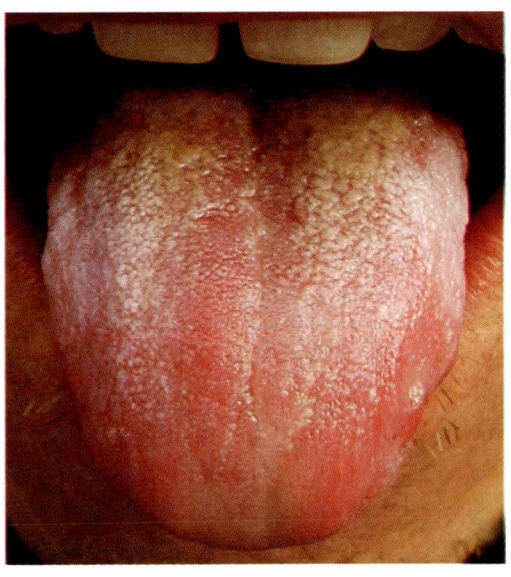

Thin-yellow tongue coating

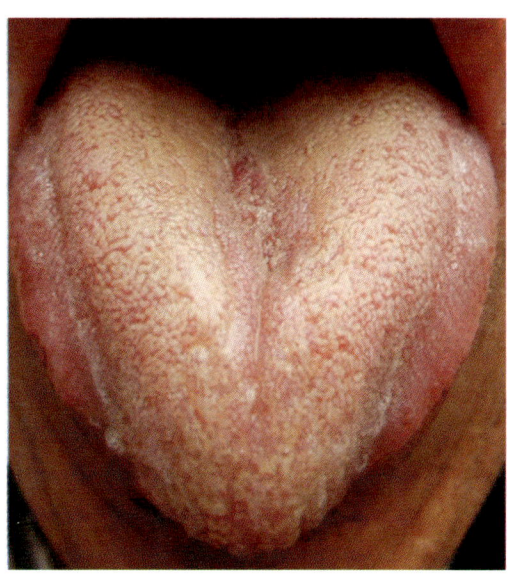

Fig 1.3-7

Tongue description:
dark red with yellow and greasy coating

Case No.:
F75 (male, 54years)

Clinical manifestations:
lassitude, poor appetite, foul breath and brownish urine

Syndrome differentiation in Chinese medicine:
internal accumulation of damp-heat, deficiency of spleen-qi

Stage:
AIDS

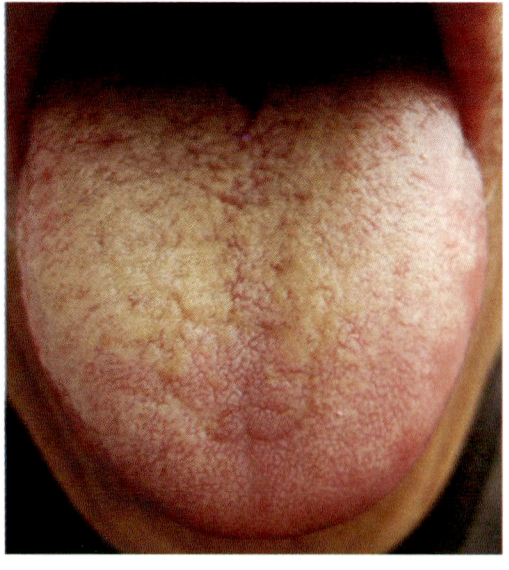

Fig 1.3-8

Tongue description:
red and swollen with teeth imprints, thin, yellow and greasy coating

Case No.:
F285 (male, 50years)

Clinical manifestations:
fever, sticky sputum, lassitude and short breath

Syndrome differentiation in Chinese medicine:
wind-heat invasion, weakness of the lung and wei-qi (defensive qi)

Stage:
AIDS

3. *Brown Tongue Coating*

Fig 1.3-9

Tongue description:
brown, thick, dry coating with cracks, ulcers on the tongue body

Case No.:
W639 (male, 60years)

Clinical manifestations:
extreme emaciation, yellow sputum, oral anabrosis and foul breath

Syndrome differentiation in
Chinese medicine:
qi and blood exhaustion of zang-fu organs, preponderance of heat evil

Stage:
AIDS

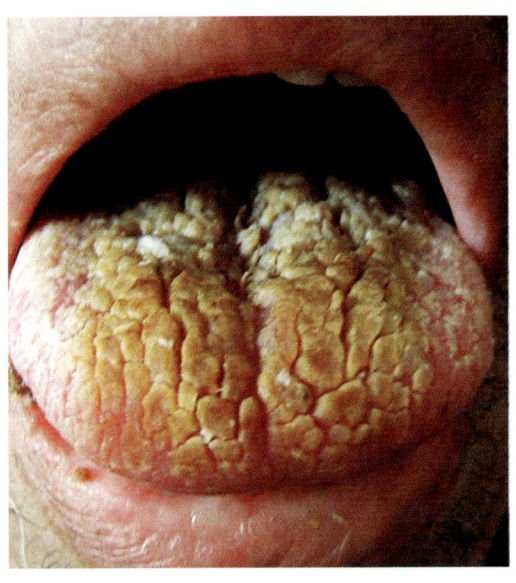

4. *Thin-white Tongue Coating*

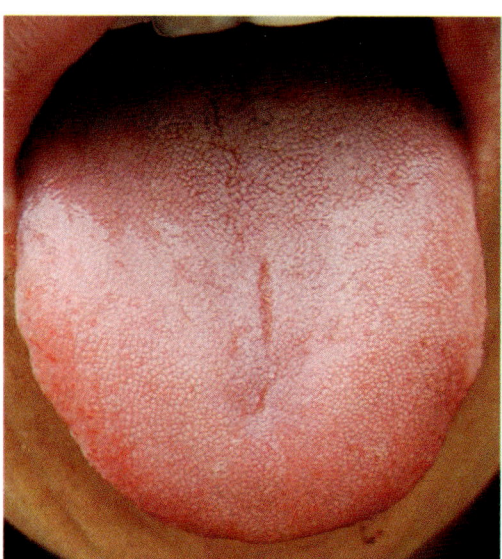

Fig 1.3-10

Tongue description:
reddish with thin and white coating

Case No.:
W28 (female, 43years)

Clinical manifestations:
emotional depression, lassitude and poor appetite

Syndrome differentiation in Chinese medicine:
stagnation of liver qi, deficiency of spleen-qi

Stage:
infected with HIV yet clinically asymptomatic

5. *Yellow, Greasy and Curd-like Tongue Coating*

Fig 1.3-11

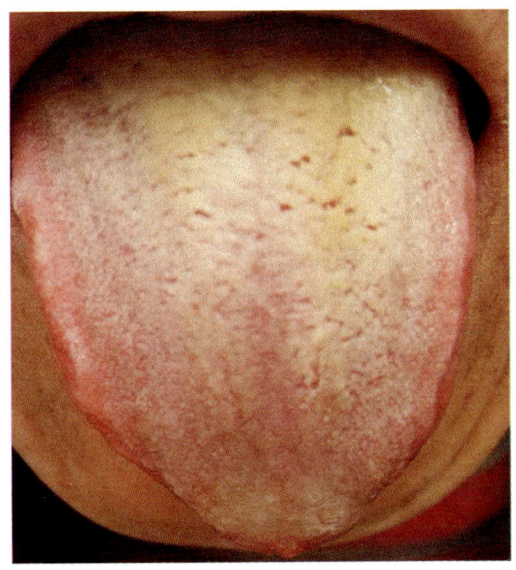

Tongue description:

reddish with yellow, thick, greasy and granular/curd-like coating

Case No.:

F173 (female, 45years)

Clinical manifestations:

fever, nausea, epigastric fullness, lassitude, short breath and sallow complexion

Syndrome differentiation in Chinese medicine:

excessive accumulation of damp-heat evil, deficiency of qi and blood

Stage:

AIDS

Fig 1.3-12

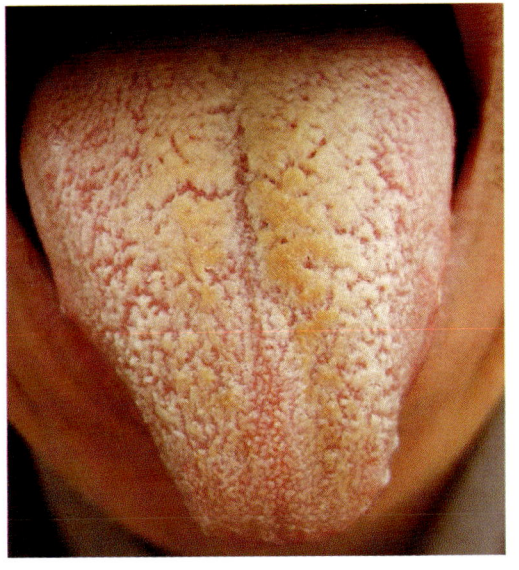

Tongue description:

red with yellow, thick, greasy and granular/curd-like coating

Case No.:

W542 (male, 35years)

Clinical manifestations:

loose stools, brownish urine, lassitude, dark lips and susceptibility to common colds

Syndrome differentiation in Chinese medicine:

internal accumulation of damp-heat, deficiency of qi and yin

Stage:

AIDS

6. *Thick-yellow Tongue Coating*

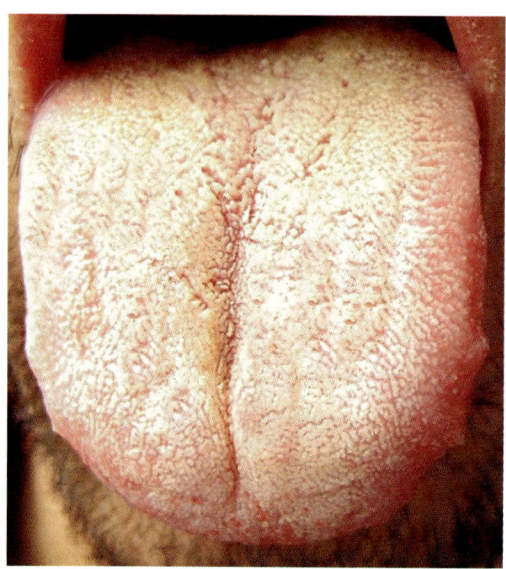

Fig 1.3-13

Tongue description:
reddish and swollen with teeth imprints, yellow and thick coating

Case No.:
W179 (male, 43years)

Clinical manifestations:
fever, mouth ulcers, epigastric fullness, lassitude and sallow complexion

Syndrome differentiation in Chinese medicine:
excessive accumulation of damp-heat evil, deficiency of qi and blood

Stage:
AIDS

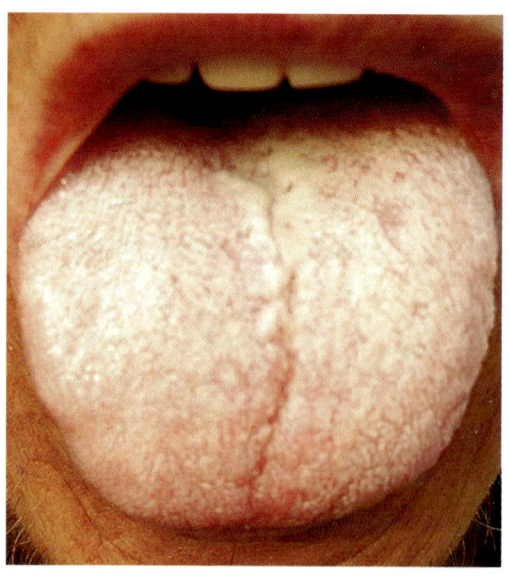

Fig 1.3-14

Tongue description:
pale, swollen and flaccid with yellow, thick and greasy coating

Case No.:
W231 (male, 58years)

Clinical manifestations:
fever, thirstiness, lassitude, poor appetite, vertigo and dryness of eyes

Syndrome differentiation in Chinese medicine:
excessive accumulation of damp-heat evil, deficiency of qi and blood

Stage:
AIDS

Fig 1.3-15

Tongue description:
reddish with yellowish and greasy coating

Case No.:
W227 (male, 38years)

Clinical manifestations:
aversion to cold and spontaneous perspiration, lassitude

Syndrome differentiation in Chinese medicine:
weakness of the lung and wei-qi (defensive qi).

Stage:
infected with HIV yet clinically asymptomatic

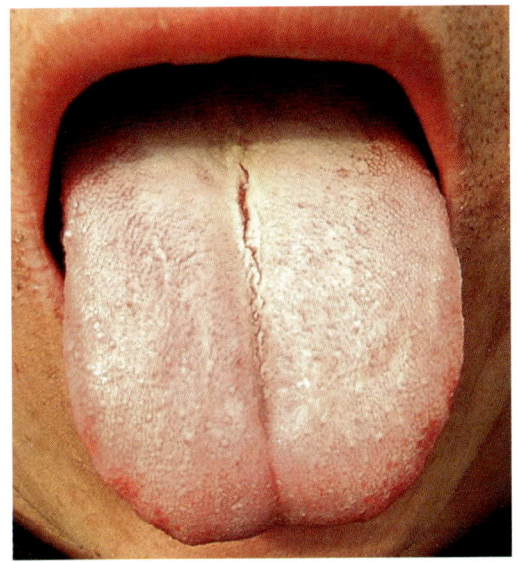

Fig 1.3-16

Tongue description:
reddish with yellow, thick and greasy coating

Case No.:
W302 (female, 45years)

Clinical manifestations:
bitter taste, dry mouth without thirst for water, lassitude and sallow complexion

Syndrome differentiation in Chinese medicine:
internal accumulation of damp-heat, deficiency of spleen-qi

Stage:
infected with HIV yet clinically asymptomatic

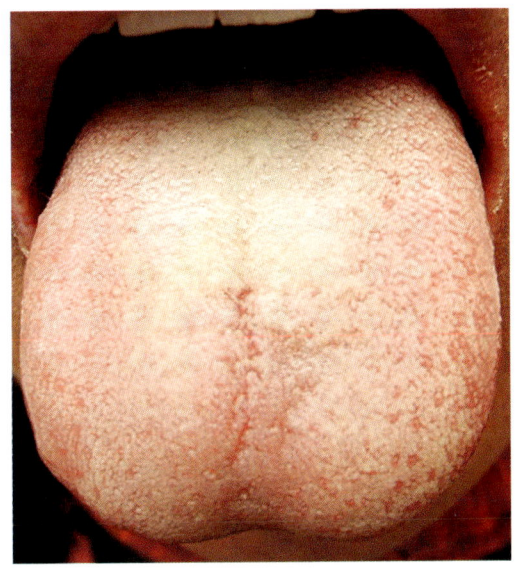

7. *Dry Tongue Coating*

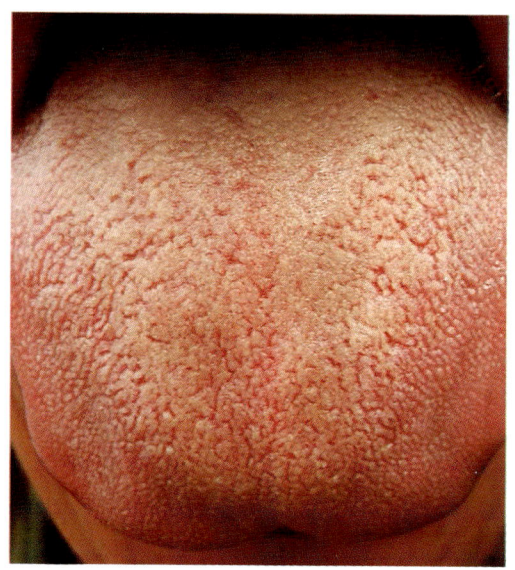

Fig 1.3-17

Tongue description:
dark red with yellow, thick and dry coating

Case No.:
F123 (male, 40years)

Clinical manifestations:
epigastric fullness, diarrhea, lassitude and poor appetite

Syndrome differentiation in Chinese medicine:
internal accumulation of damp-heat, deficiency of spleen-qi

Stage:
AIDS

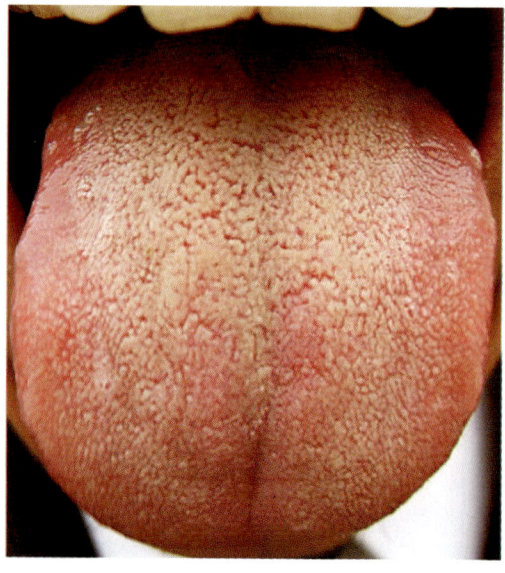

Fig 1.3-18

Tongue description:
dark red with white, thick and dry coating

Case No.:
w379 (male, 50years)

Clinical manifestations:
bitter taste, poor appetite and yellow urine

Syndrome differentiation in Chinese medicine:
internal accumulation of damp-heat

Stage:
infected with HIV yet clinically asymptomatic

Fig 1.3-19

Tongue description:
pale and dark with white, thick and dry coating

Case No.:
W680 (male, 45years)

Clinical manifestations:
yellow sputum, epigastric fullness, poor appetite, lassitude, short breath and sallow complexion

Syndrome differentiation in Chinese medicine:
internal accumulation of damp-heat, deficiency of qi and blood

Stage:
infected with HIV yet clinically asymptomatic

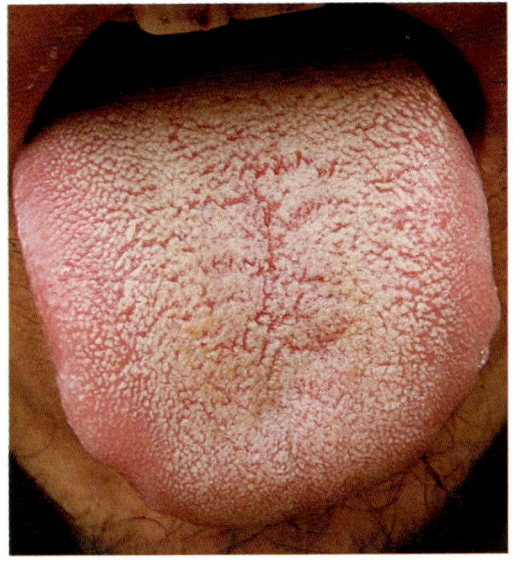

Fig 1.3-20

Tongue description:
pale, dark and swollen with white, thick and dry coating

Case No.:
F243 (male, 51years)

Clinical manifestations:
emotional depression, chest and hypochondriac fullness, lassitude and short breath

Syndrome differentiation in Chinese medicine:
stagnation of liver qi, deficiency of spleen-qi

Stage:
infected with HIV yet clinically asymptomatic

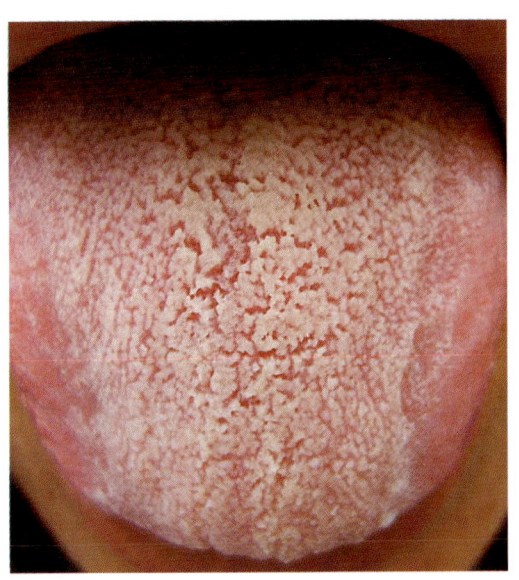

8. *Thick-white Tongue Coating*

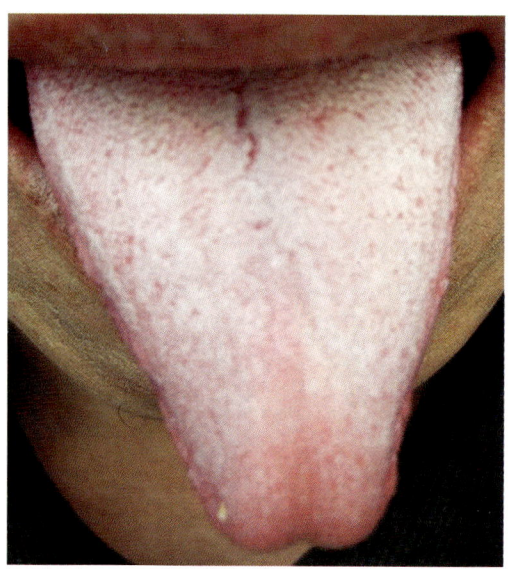

Fig 1.3-21

Tongue description:
reddish with white and thick coating

Case No.:
W251 (male, 40years)

Clinical manifestations:
chest distress, short breath, lassitude, poor appetite, dysphoria and epigastric fullness

Syndrome differentiation in Chinese medicine:
internal accumulation of damp-heat, qi deficiency of lung and spleen

Stage:
infected with HIV yet clinically asymptomatic

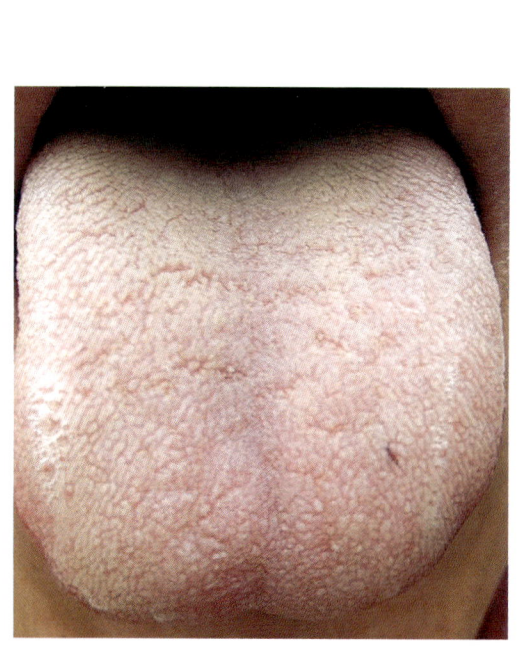

Fig 1.3-22

Tongue description:
reddish with white, thick and greasy coating

Case No.:
F136 (male, 39years)

Clinical manifestations:
ulcerous eruptions on the body, lassitude and poor appetite

Syndrome differentiation in Chinese medicine:
excessive accumulation of damp-heat evil, deficiency of spleen-qi

Stage:
infected with HIV yet clinically asymptomatic

Fig 1.3-23

Tongue description:
red with white, thick and greasy coating

Case No.:
W411 (female, 44years)

Clinical manifestations:
lassitude, poor appetite, epigastric fullness, diarrhea, oral ulcer and yellow urine

Syndrome differentiation in Chinese medicine:
deficiency of spleen-qi, excessive accumulation of damp-heat evil

Stage:
AIDS

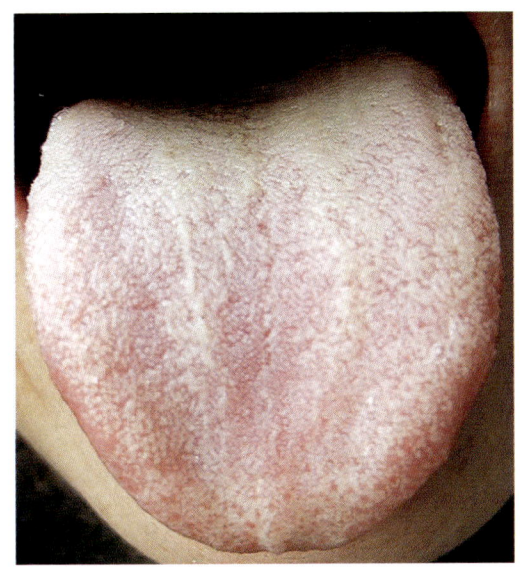

Fig 1.3-24

Tongue description:
red with white, thick and greasy coating

Case number:
F180 (male, 36years)
Clinical manifestations:
fever, insomnia, chest distress, short breath, white sputum, epigastric fullness and poor appetite

Syndrome differentiation in Chinese medicine:
internal accumulation of damp-heat, qi deficiency of lung and spleen

Stage:
AIDS

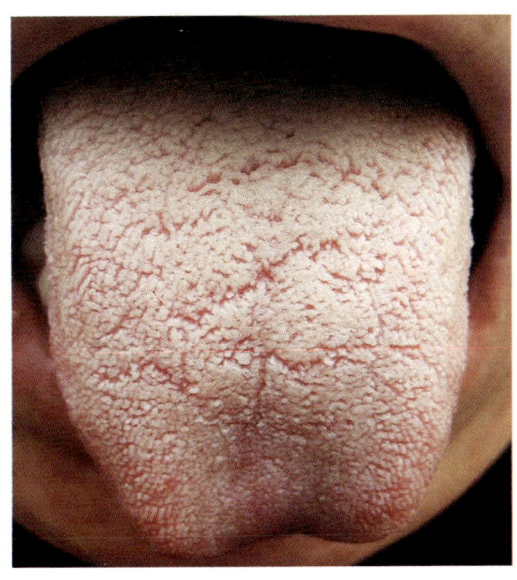

9. *Greasy Tongue Coating*

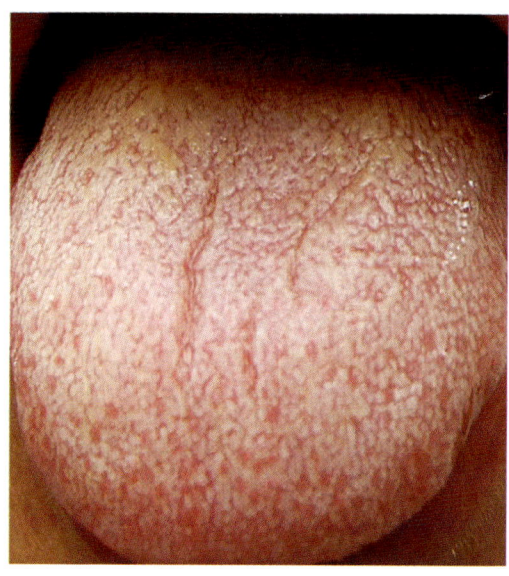

Fig 1.3-25

Tongue description:
reddish and swollen with yellowish and greasy coating

Case No.:
W131 (female, 43years)

Clinical manifestations:
bitter and sticky mouth, brownish scanty urine, lassitude

Syndrome differentiation in Chinese medicine:
internal accumulation of damp-heat, deficiency of spleen-qi

Stage:
infected with HIV yet clinically asymptomatic

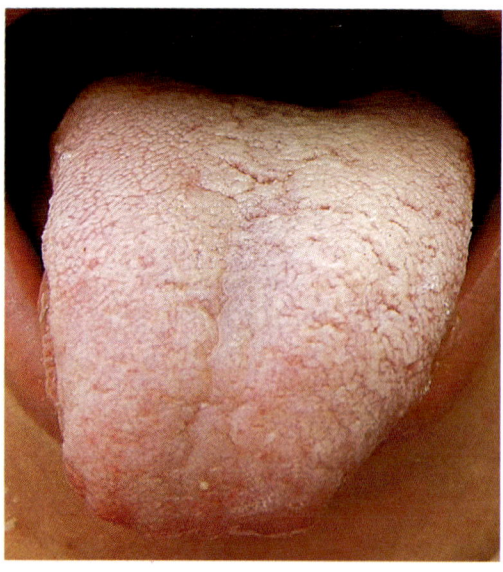

Fig 1.3-26

Tongue description:
reddish and thin with teeth imprints, white, thick and greasy coating

Case No.:
W107 (female, 45years)

Clinical manifestations:
lassitude and drowsiness aggravating with labor, itchy skin

Syndrome differentiation in Chinese medicine:
deficiency of spleen-qi, internal accumulation of damp-heat

Stage:
AIDS

Fig 1.3-27

Tongue description:
dark red with yellowish, thick and greasy coating

Case No.:
w677 (male, 36years)

Clinical manifestations:
no discomfort

Syndrome differentiation in Chinese medicine:
internal accumulation of damp-heat

Stage:
infected with HIV yet clinically asymptomatic

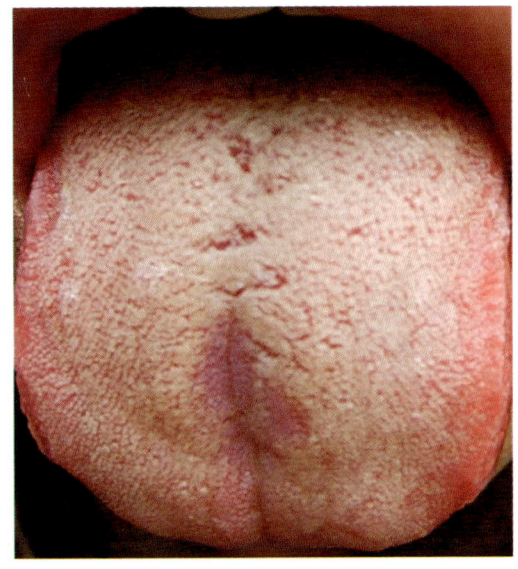

Fig 1.3-28

Tongue description:
dark and swollen with teeth imprints, yellowish, thick and greasy coating

Case No.:
F256 (male, 40years)

Clinical manifestations:
dry mouth without thirst for water, lassitude and short breath aggravating with labor

Syndrome differentiation in Chinese medicine:
internal accumulation of damp-heat, deficiency of spleen-qi

Stage:
infected with HIV yet clinically asymptomatic

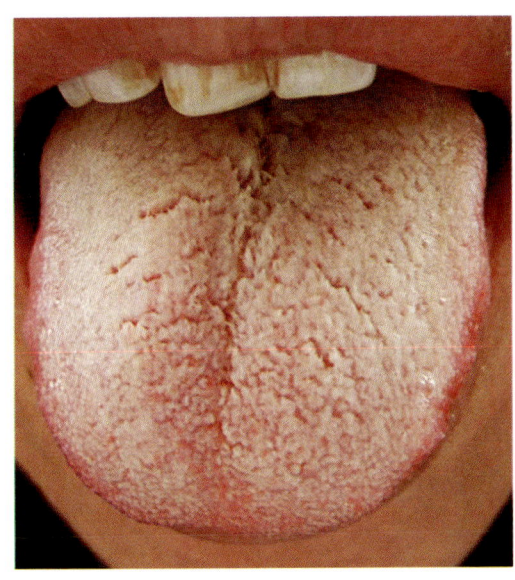

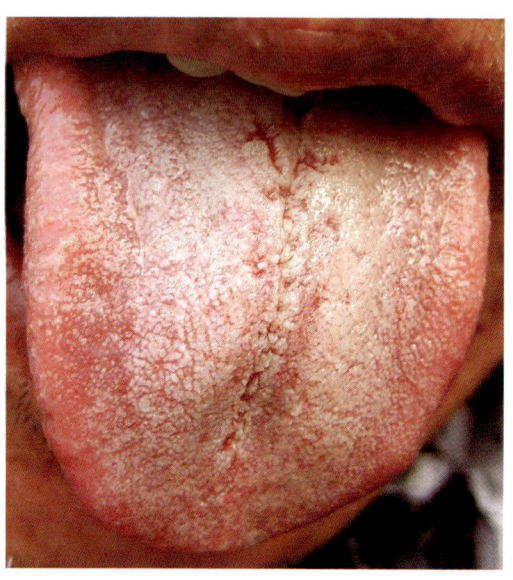

Fig 1.3-29

Tongue description:
red with yellowish, thick and greasy coating

Case No.:
W369 (male, 56years)

Clinical manifestations:
hypochondriac distention, lassitude and diarrhea

Syndrome differentiation in Chinese medicine:
internal accumulation of damp-heat, deficiency of spleen-qi

Stage:
AIDS

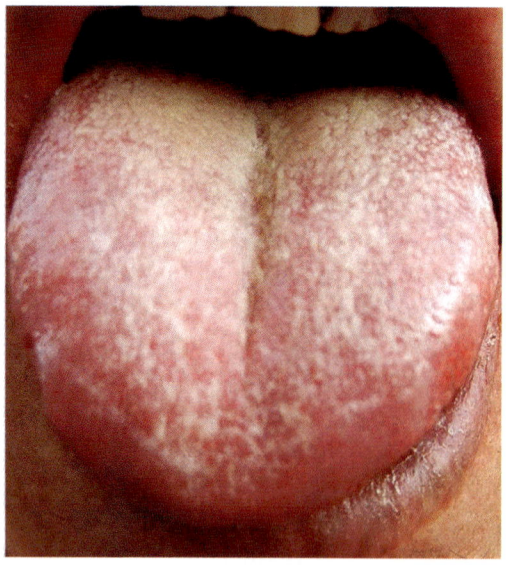

Fig 1.3-30

Tongue description:
red with yellow, thick and greasy coating at the root

Case No.:
W624 (male, 60years)

Clinical manifestations:
fever, brownish urine, nausea, epigastric fullness, chest distress and lassitude

Syndrome differentiation in Chinese medicine:
internal accumulation of damp-heat, qi deficiency of lung and spleen

Stage:
AIDS

10. *Slippery Tongue Coating*

Fig 1.3-31

Tongue description:
pale with white, moist and slippery coating

Case No.:
F148 (female, 43years)

Clinical manifestations:
lassitude, anorexia and aversion to cold

Syndrome differentiation in Chinese medicine:
deficiency of spleen-qi

Stage:
infected with HIV yet clinically asymptomatic

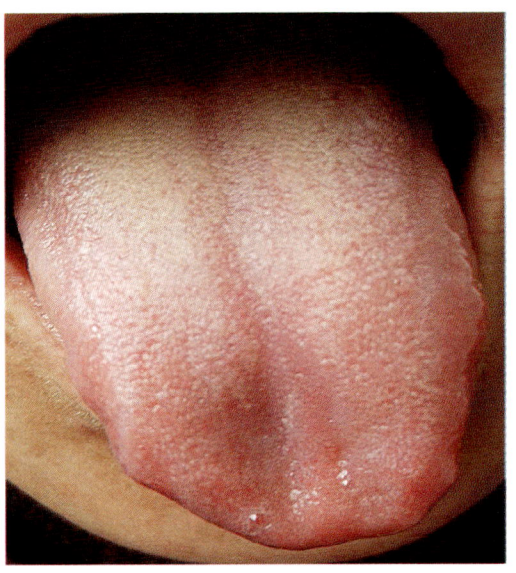

Fig 1.3-32

Tongue description:
pale with moist and slippery coating, but yellow, thick and greasy coating at the root

Case No.:
W510 (male, 50years)

Clinical manifestations:
cold body, diarrhea with the indigested, epigastric fullness, poor appetite, fever and painful urination

Syndrome differentiation in Chinese medicine:
yang deficiency of spleen and kidney, internal accumulation of damp-heat

Stage:
AIDS

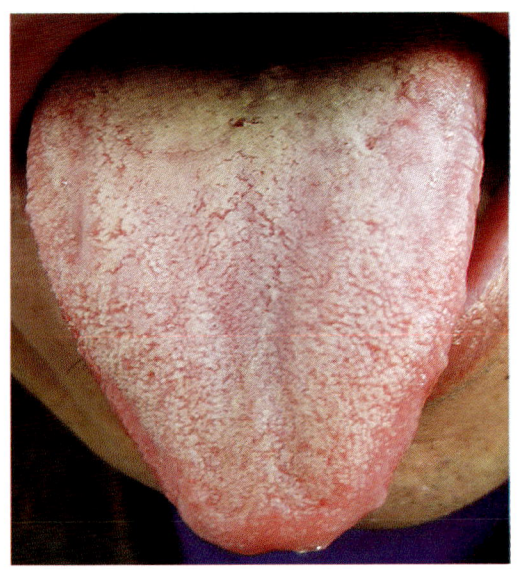

37

11. *Peeled Coating*

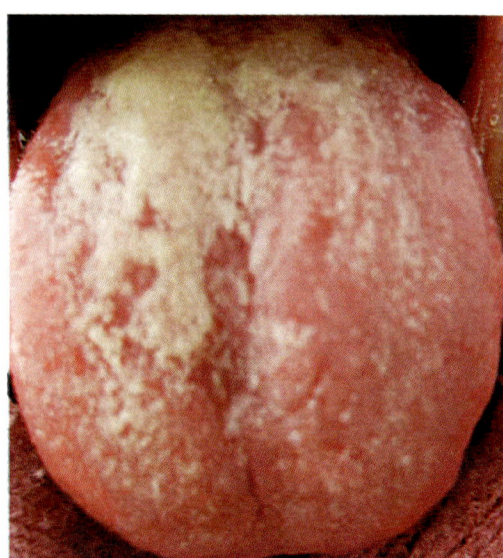

Fig 1.3-33

Tongue description:
red with peeled yellowish coating

Case No.:
F362 (female, 43years)

Clinical manifestations:
fever, night sweat, lassitude, oral anabrosis and herpes

Syndrome differentiation in Chinese medicine:
deficiency of qi and yin, excessive accumulation of damp-heat evil

Stage:
AIDS

CHAPTER TWO
COMMON AIDS TONGUES

1. *Tongue Color*

1.1 Pale tongue

Infected with HIV yet clinically asymptomatic

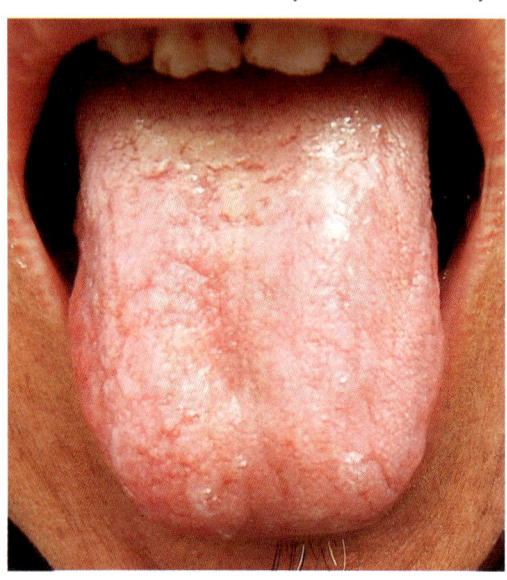

Fig 2.1-1

Patient, Male, 66years,

Case NO.: F116

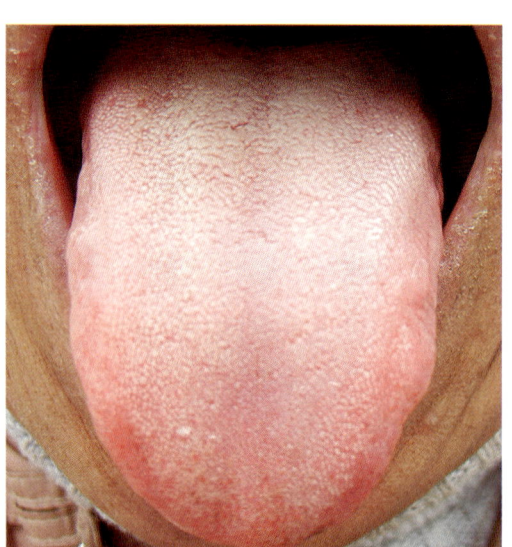

Fig 2.1-2

Patient, Female, 47years,

Case NO.: F112

Fig 2.1-3

Patient, Male, 43years,

Case NO.: F16

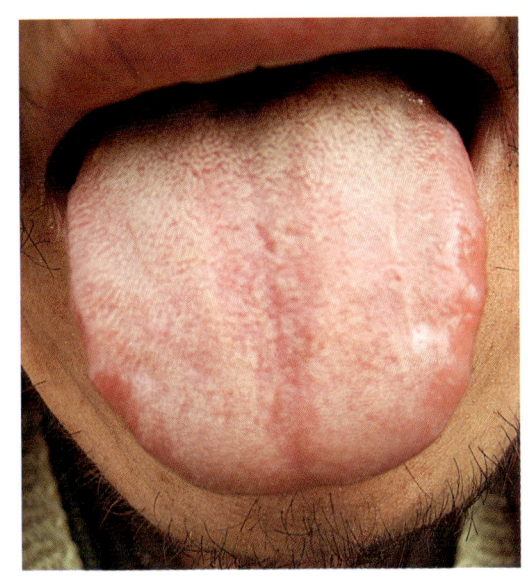

Fig 2.1-4

Patient, Female, 52years,

Case NO.: F288

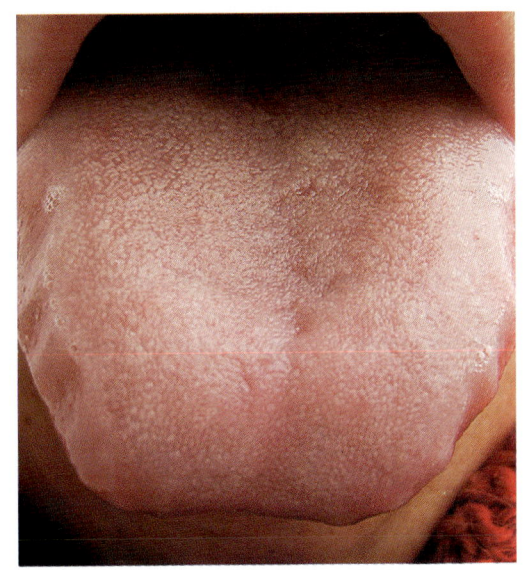

Pale tongue

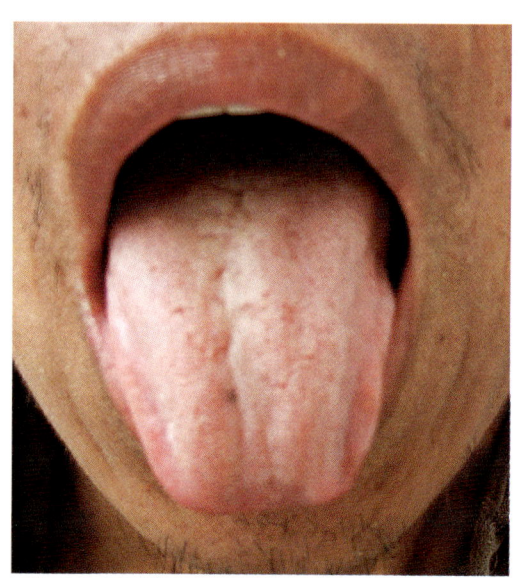

Fig 2.1-5

Patient, Male, 48years,

Case NO.: W12

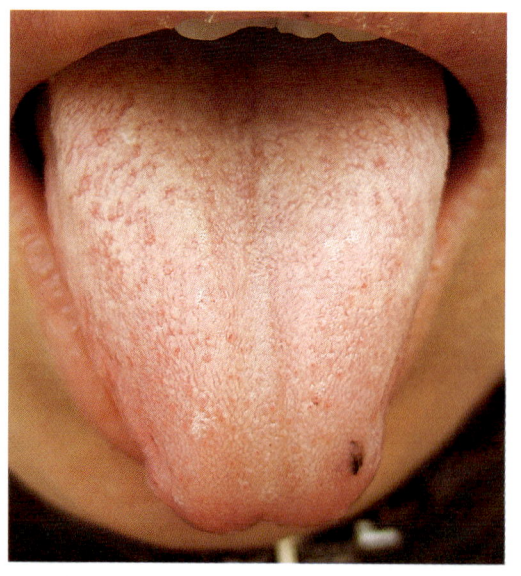

Fig 2.1-6

Patient, Female, 29years,

Case NO.: W310

Fig 2.1-7

Patient, Female, 49years,

Case NO.: W156

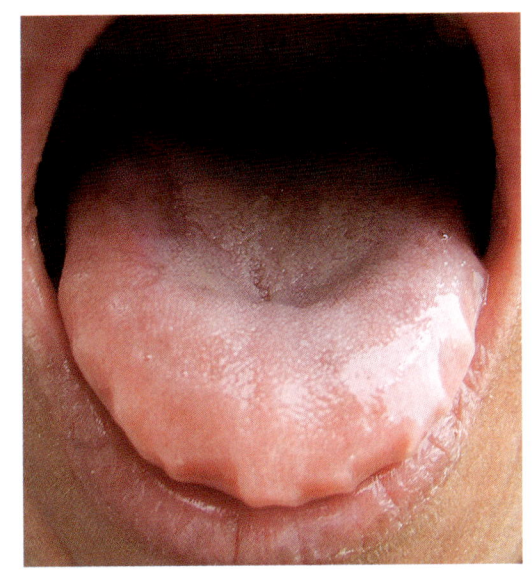

Fig 2.1-8

Patient, Female, 43years,

Case NO.: F329

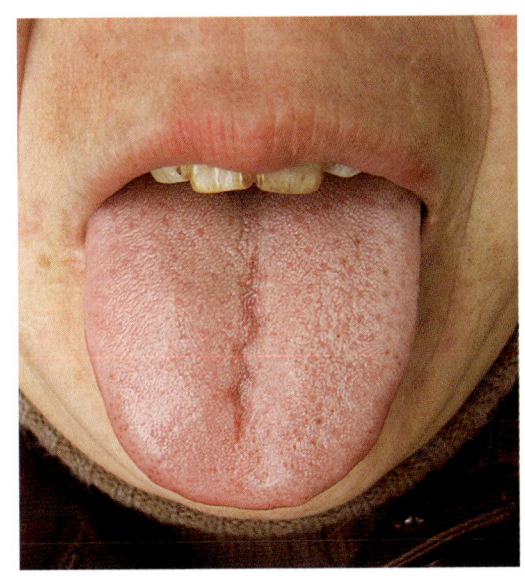

Pale tongue

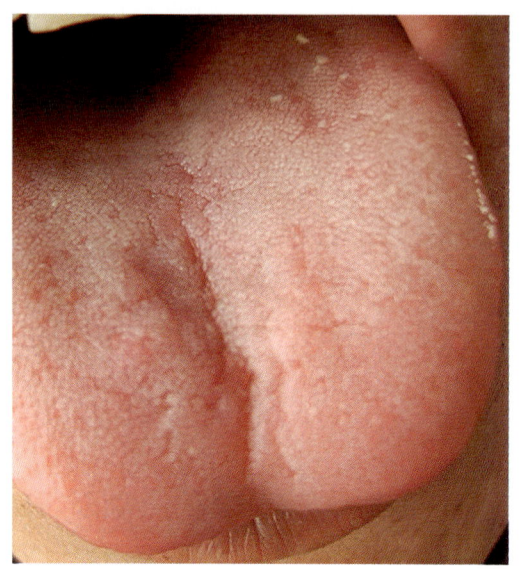

Fig 2.1-9

Patient, Female, 51years,

Case NO.: F311

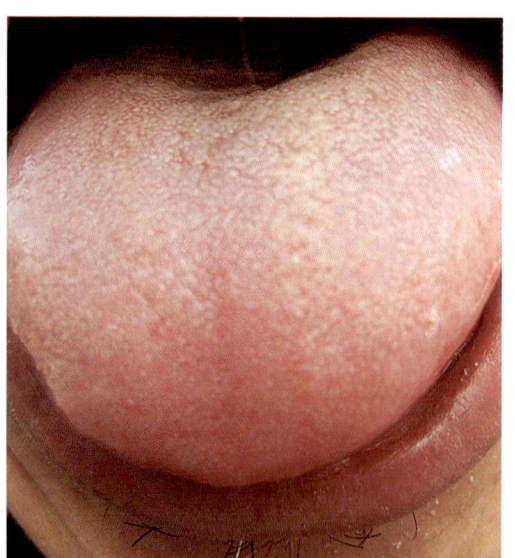

Fig 2.1-10

Patient, Male, 41years,

Case NO.: W630

Fig 2.1-11

Patient, Female, 39years,

Case NO.: W34

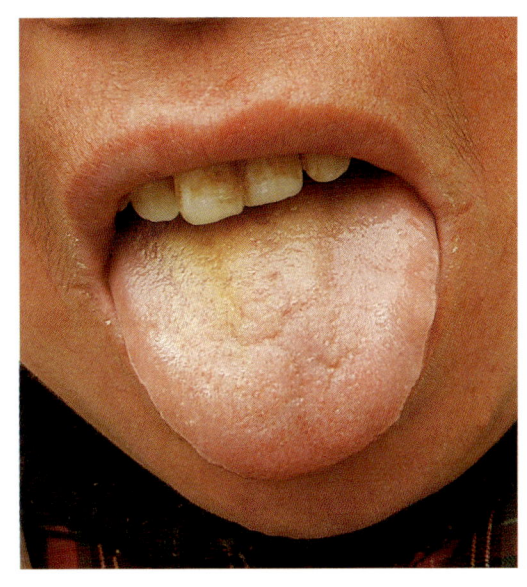

Fig 2.1-12

Patient, Female, 42years,

Case NO.: W58

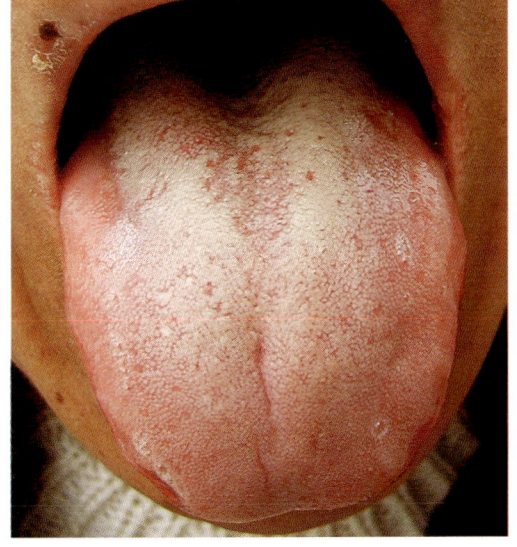

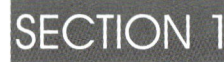

Pale tongue

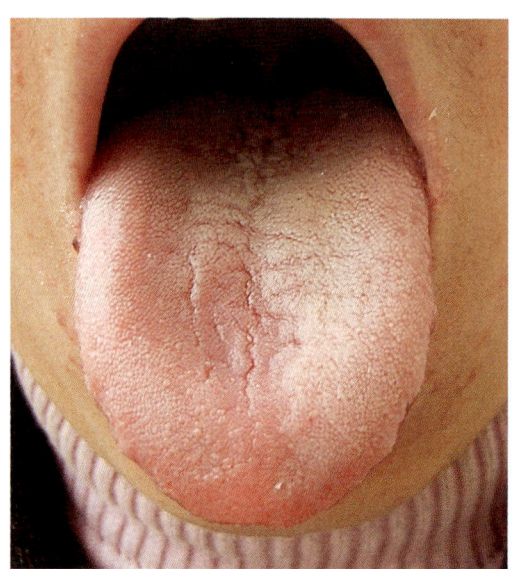

Fig 2.1-13

Patient, Female, 34years,

Case NO.: W7

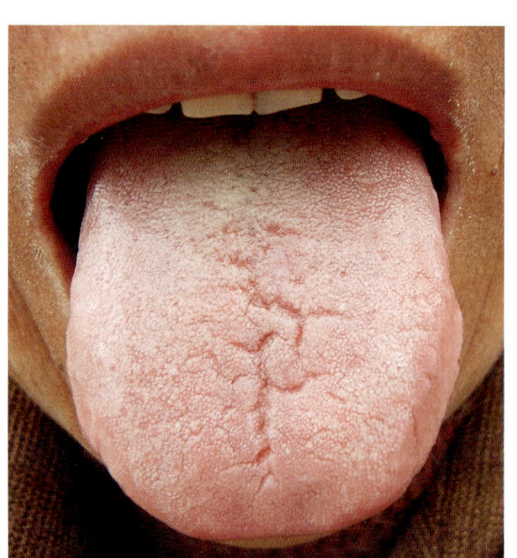

Fig 2.1-14

Patient, Female, 55years,

Case NO.: W41

Fig 2.1-15

Patient, Male, 54years,

Case NO.: F292

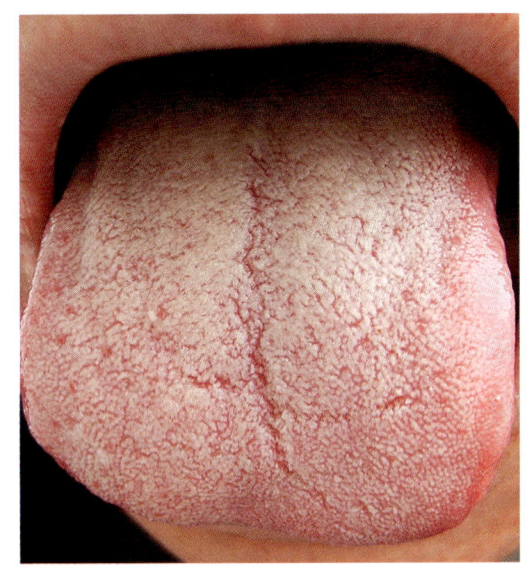

Fig 2.1-16

Patient, Female, 38years,

Case NO.: W567

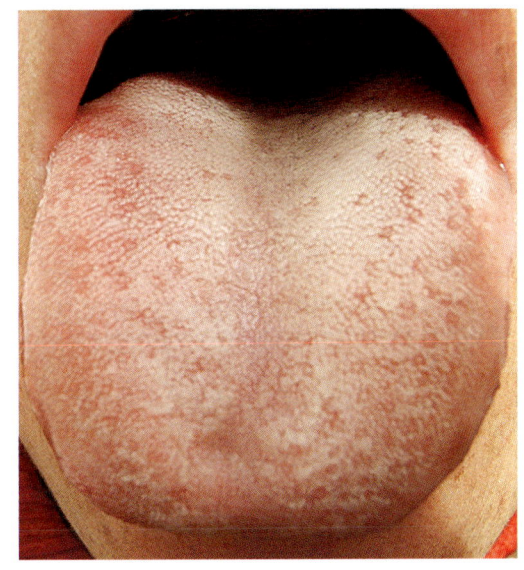

Pale tongue

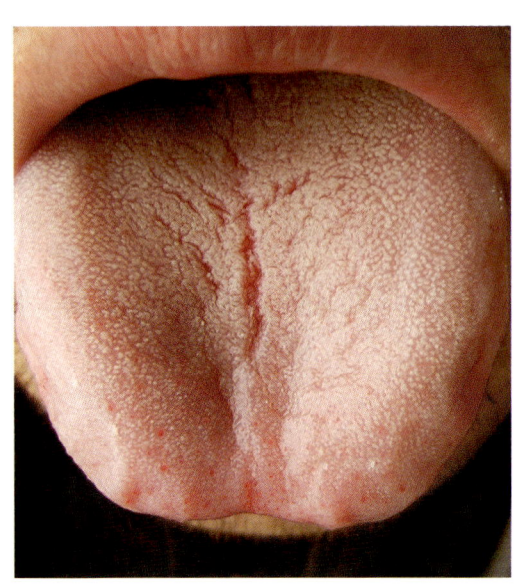

Fig 2.1-17

Patient, Male, 33years,

Case NO.: F313

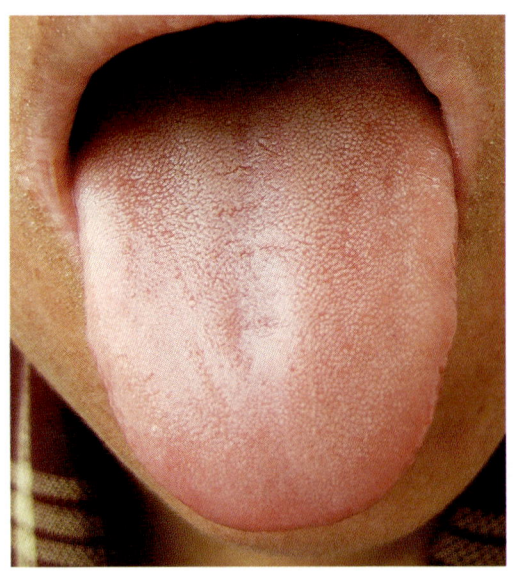

Fig 2.1-18

Patient, Female, 42years,

Case NO.: W18

Fig 2.1-19

Patient, Female, 39years,

Case NO.: F33

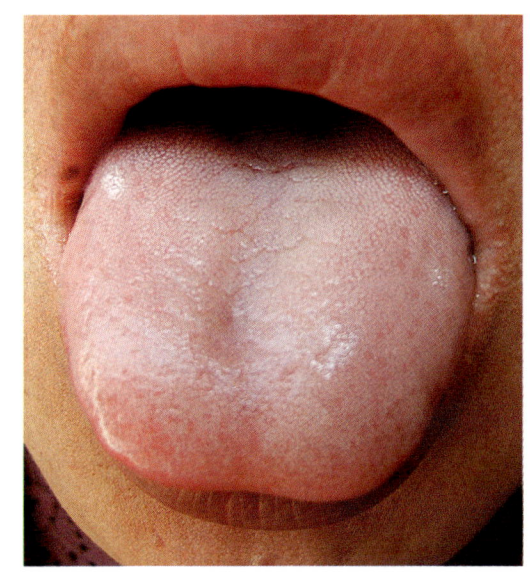

Fig 2.1-20

Patient, Female, 44years,

Case NO.: W298

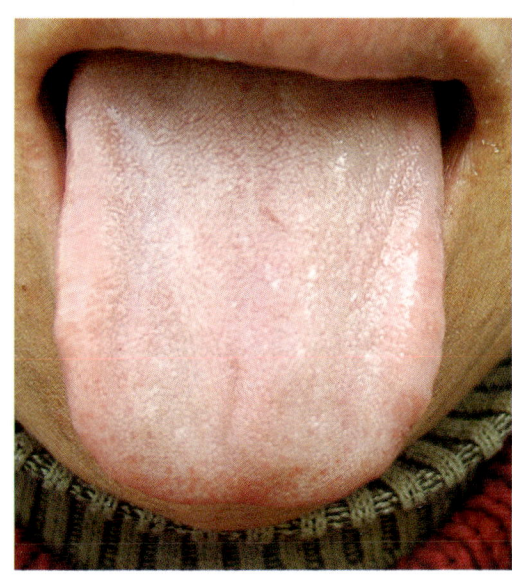

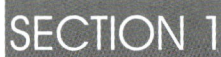

Pale tongue

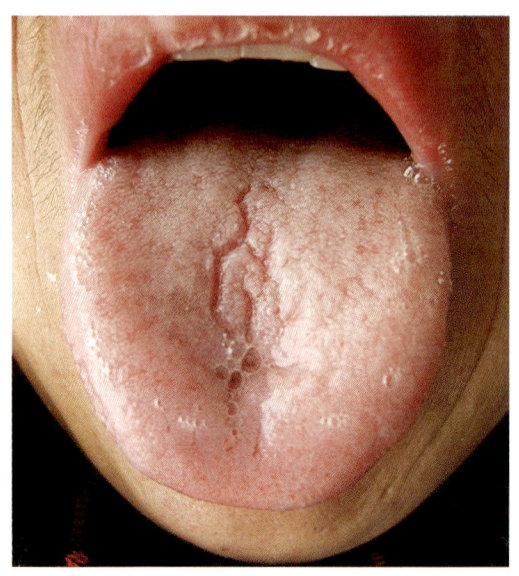

Fig 2.1-21

Patient, Female, 54years,

Case NO.: F344

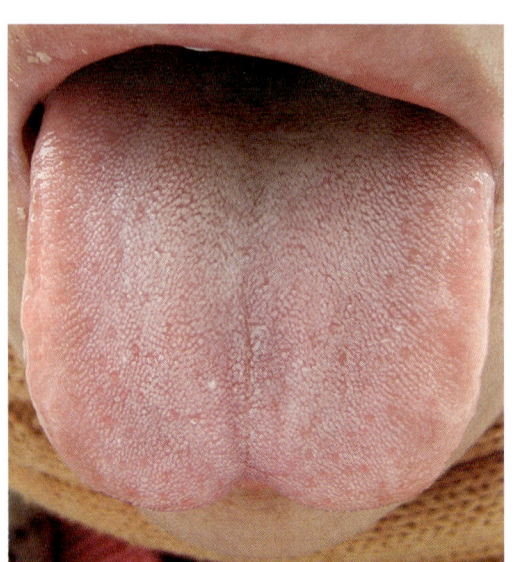

Fig 2.1-22

atient, Female, 33years,

Case NO.: F257

Fig 2.1-23

Patient, Male, 55years,

Case NO.: W112

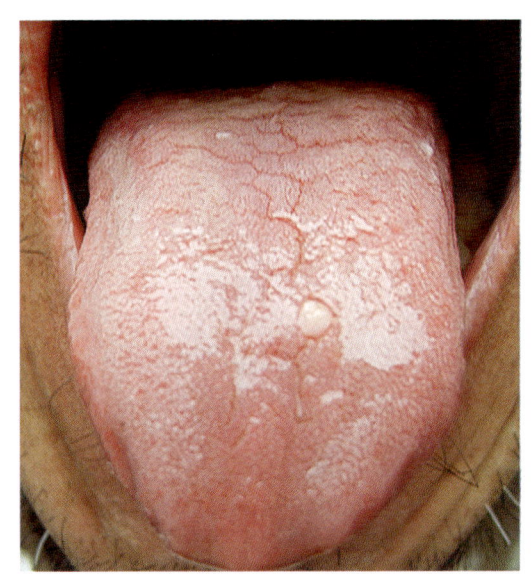

Fig 2.1-24

Patient, Female, 37years,

Case NO.: 681

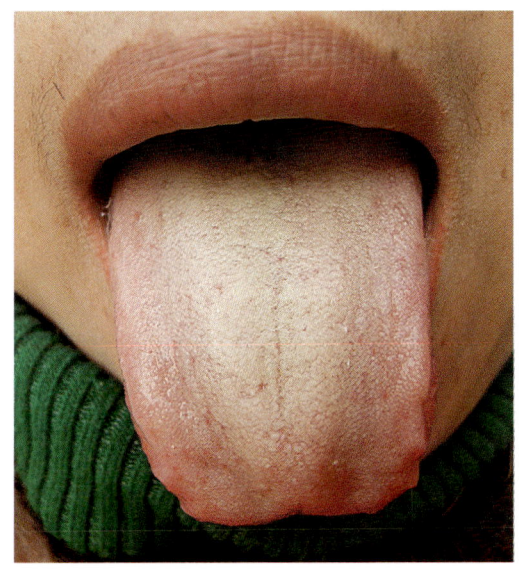

Pale tongue

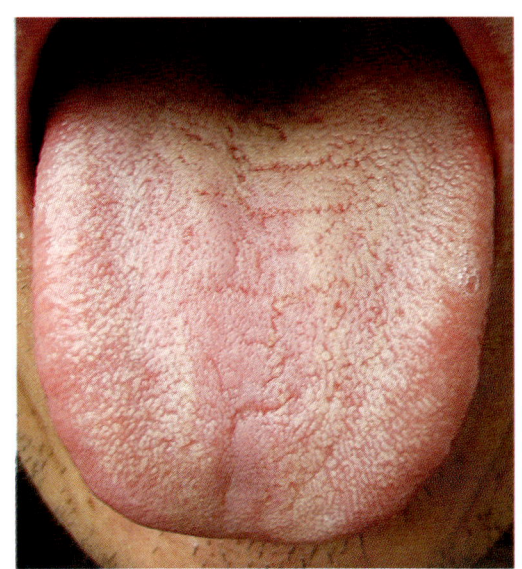

Fig 2.1-25

Patient, Male, 40years,

Case NO.: F146

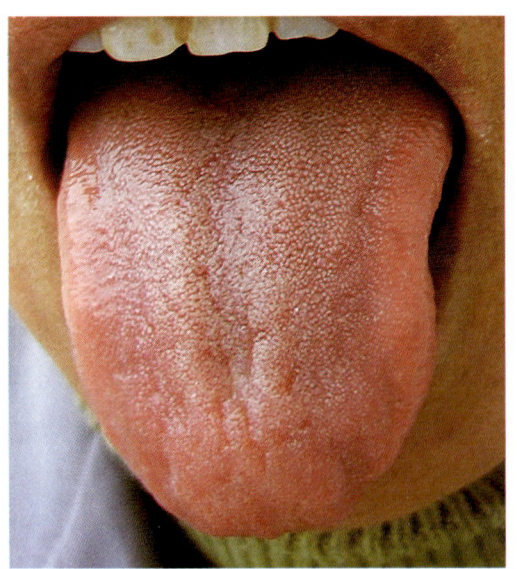

Fig 2.1-26

Patient, Female, 50years,

Case NO.: W13

1.2 Light red tongue

Infected with HIV yet clinically asymptomatic

Fig 2.1-27

Patient, Male, 57years,

Case NO.: W505

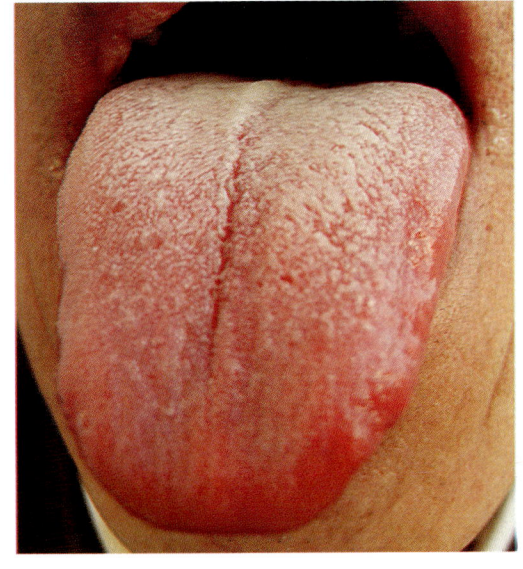

Fig 2.1-28

Patient, Male, 37years,

Case NO.: W371

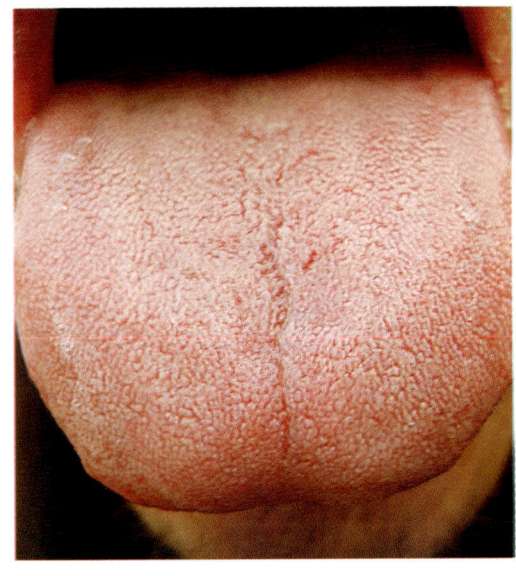

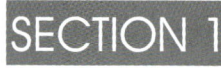
Light red tongue

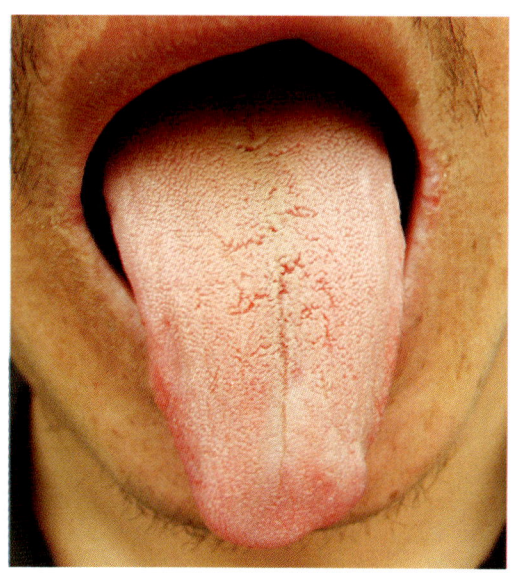

Fig 2.1-29

Patient, Male, 28years,

Case NO.: W287

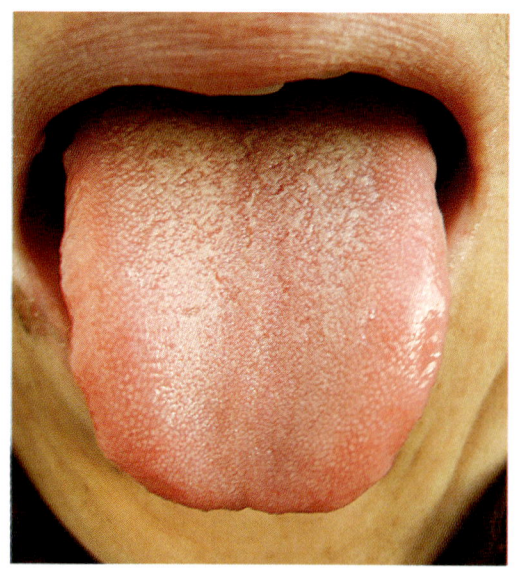

Fig 2.1-30

Patient, Female, 40years,

Case NO.: W497

Fig 2.1-31

Patient, Male, 42years,

Case NO.: W364

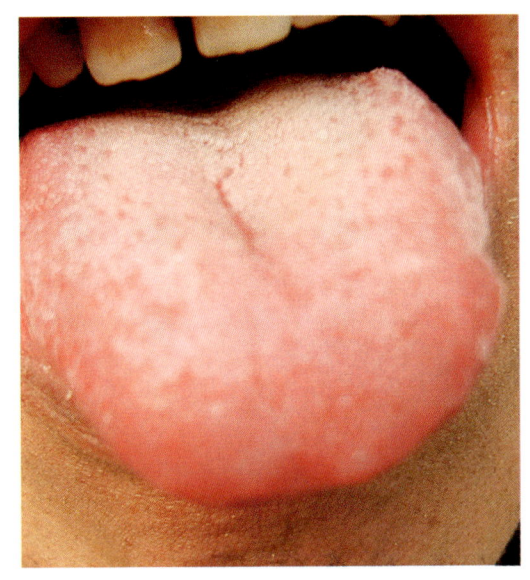

Fig 2.1-32

Patient, Female, 37years,

Case NO.: F356

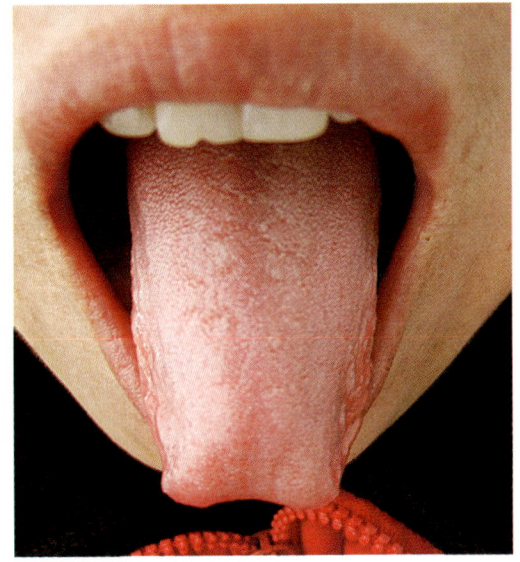

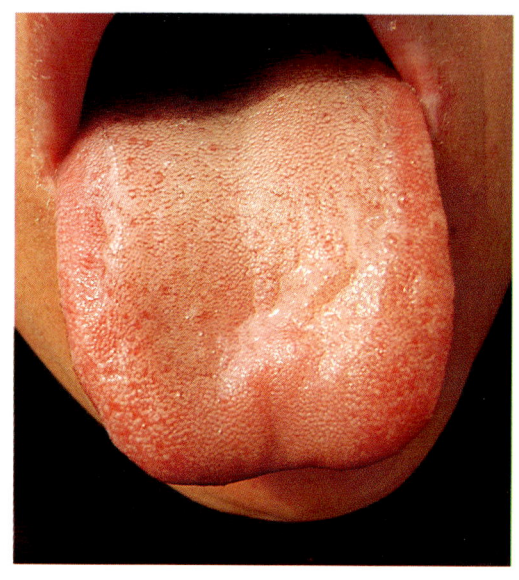

Fig 2.1-33

Patient, Female, 51years,

Case NO.: W92

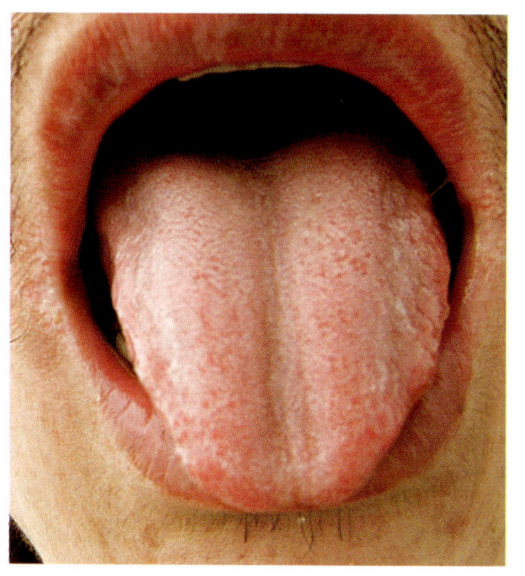

Fig 2.1-34

Patient, Male, 30years,

Case NO.: W751

Fig 2.1-35

Patient, Female, 37years,

Case NO.: W752

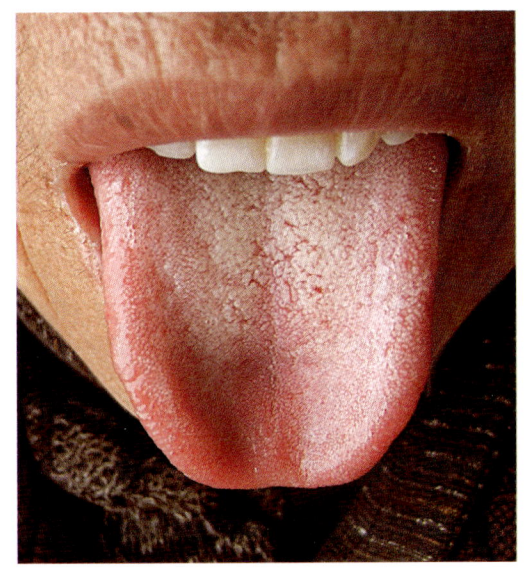

Fig 2.1-36

Patient, Male, 49years,

Case NO.: F369

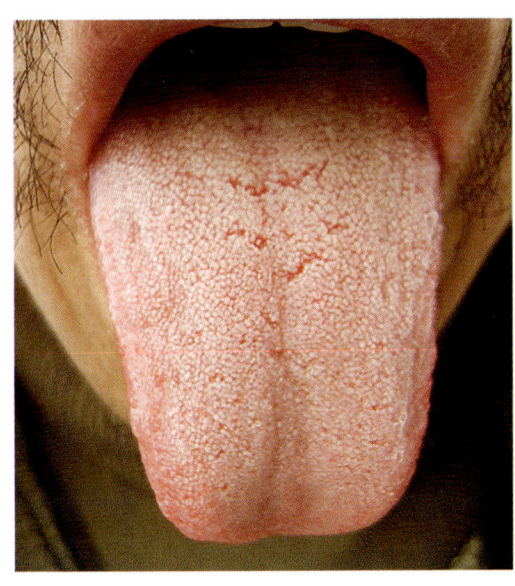

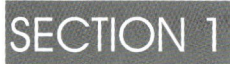

Light red tongue

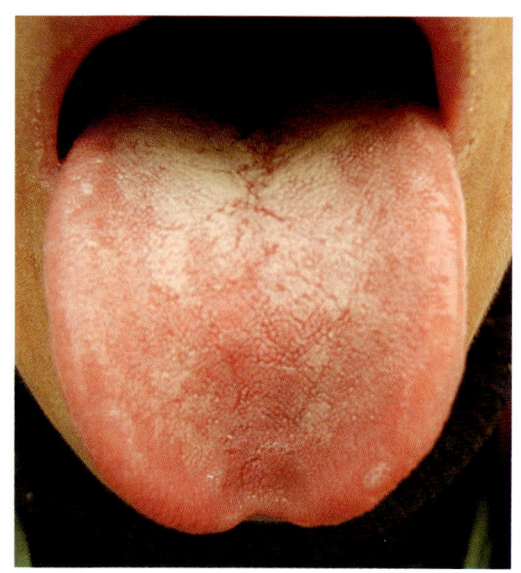

Fig 2.1-37

Patient, Female, 44years,

Case NO.: W234

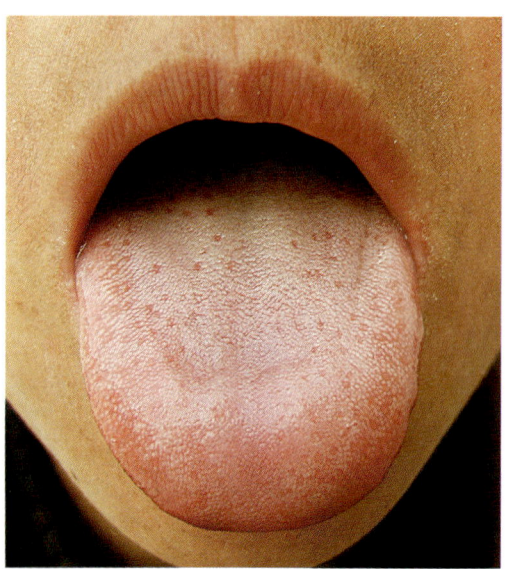

Fig 2.1-38

Patient, Female, 46years,

Case NO.: W71

Fig 2.1-39

Patient, Male, 40years,

Case NO.: W69

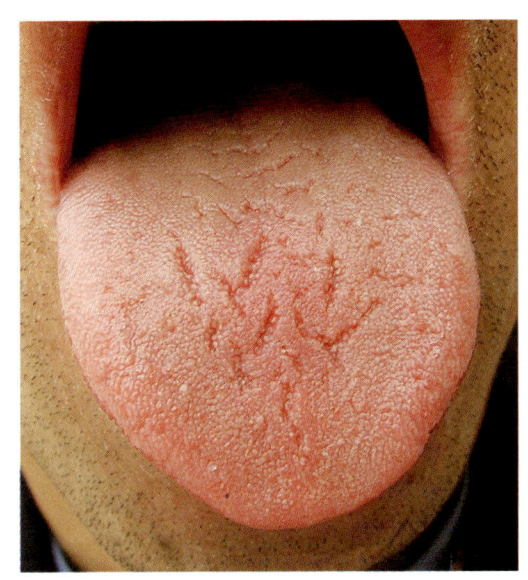

Fig 2.1-40

Patient, Male, 40years,

Case NO.: W381

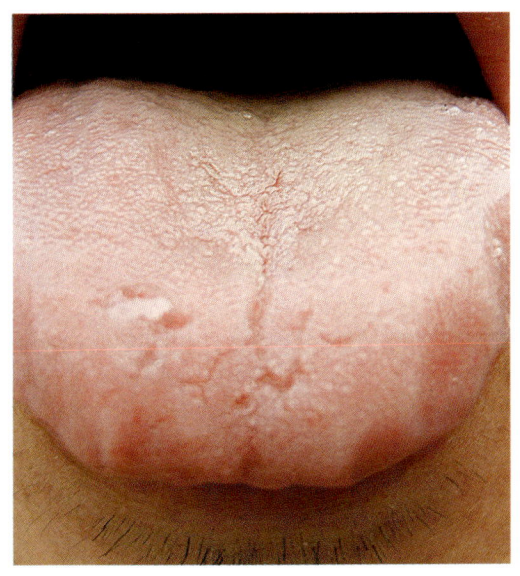

Light red tongue

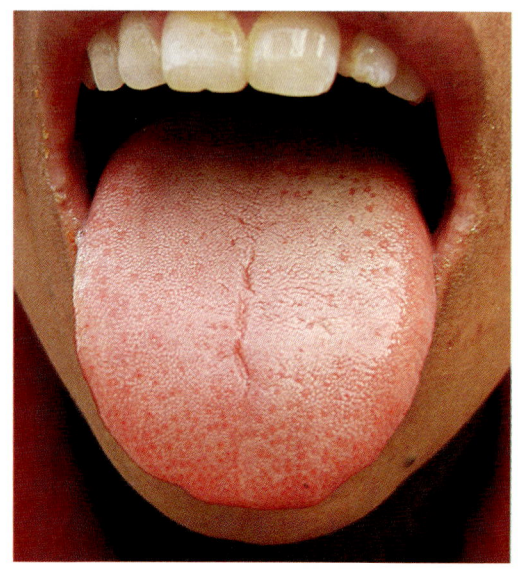

Fig 2.1-41

Patient, Female, 41years,

Case NO.: W346

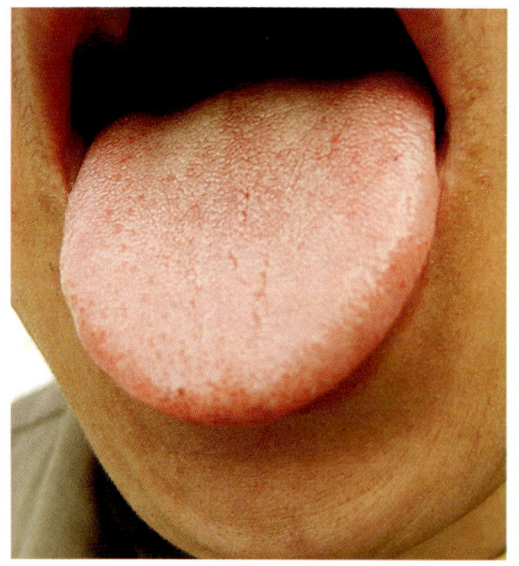

Fig 2.1-42

Patient, Female, 40years,

Case NO.: W337

Fig 2.1-43

Patient, Female, 43years,

Case NO.: W325

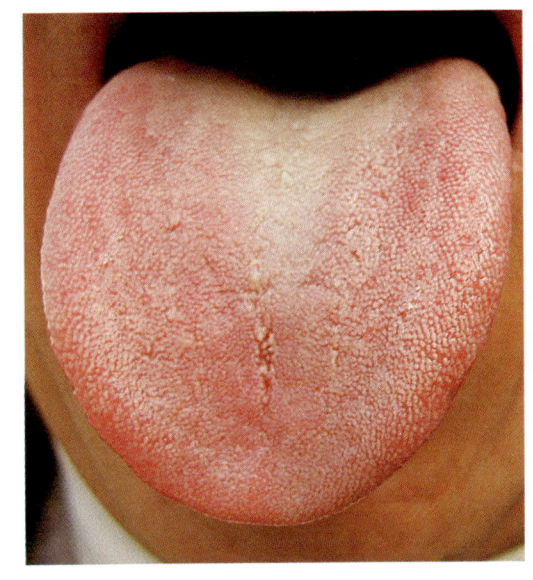

Fig 2.1-44

Patient, Female, 38years,

Case NO.: F57

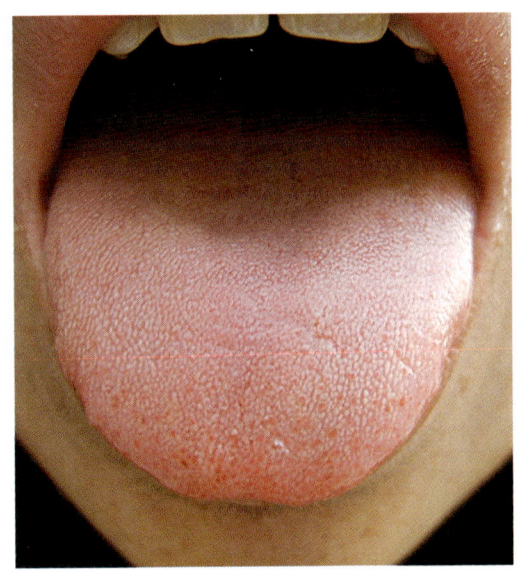

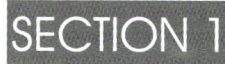

Light red tongue

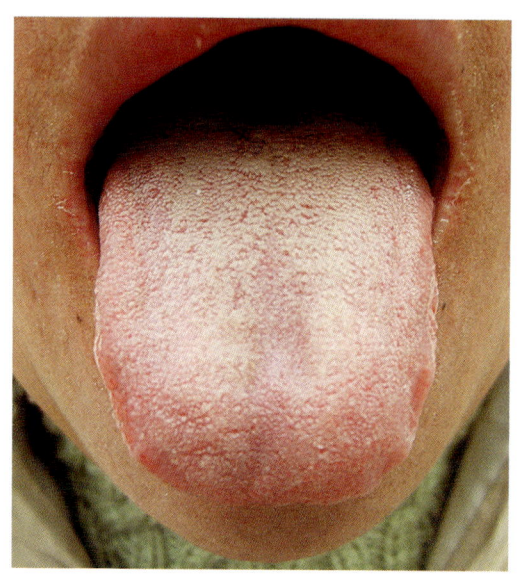

Fig 2.1-45

Patient, Female, 38years,

Case NO.: F138

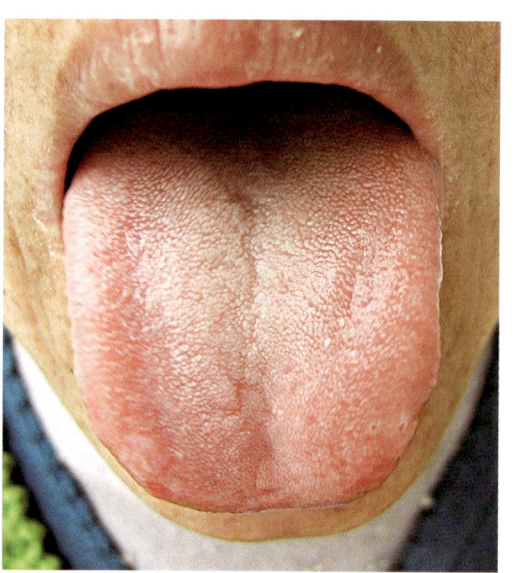

Fig 2.1-46

Patient, Female, 51years,

Case NO.: W409

Fig 2.1-47

Patient, Female, 49years,

Case NO.: F121

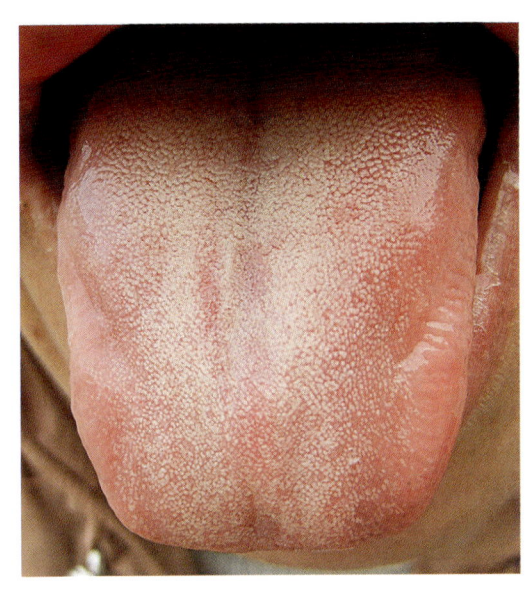

Fig 2.1-48

Patient, Female, 40years,

Case NO.: F140

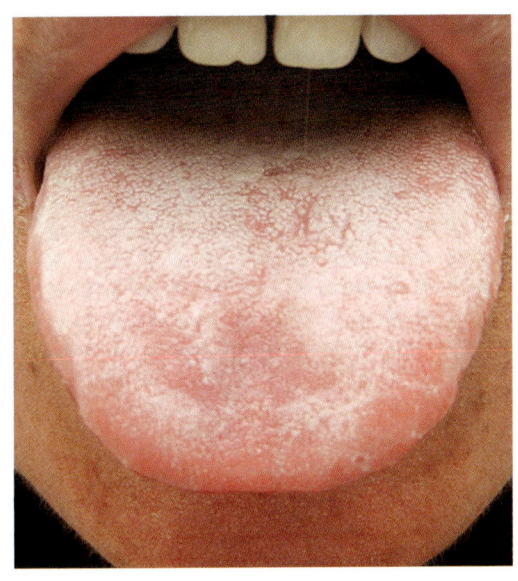

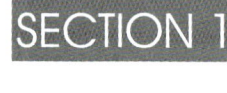

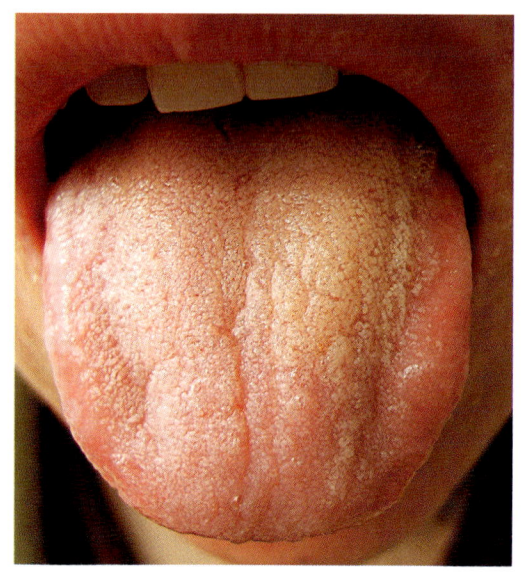

Fig 2.1-49

Patient, Female, 39years,

Case NO.: W243

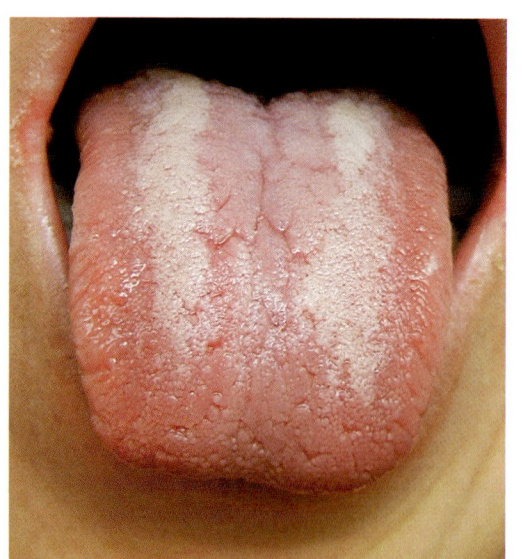

Fig 2.1-50

Patient, Female, 40years,

Case NO.: F43

Fig 2.1-51

Patient, Female, 50years,

Case NO.: F31

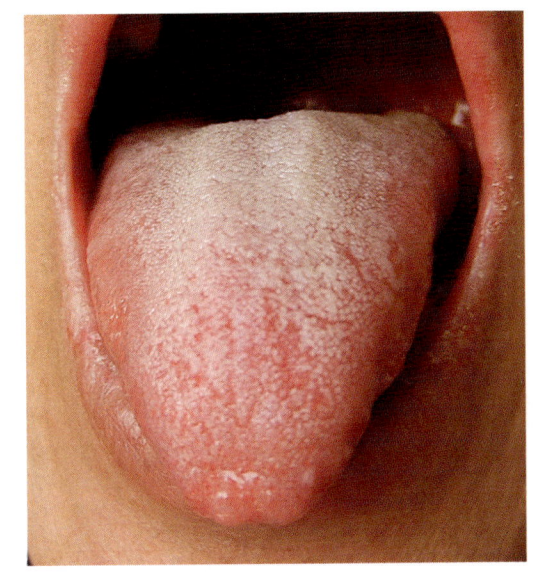

Fig 2.1-52

Patient, Male, 38years,

Case NO.: 250

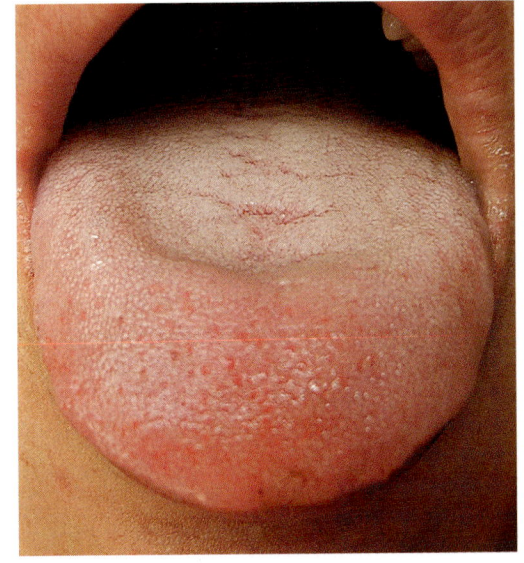

Light red tongue

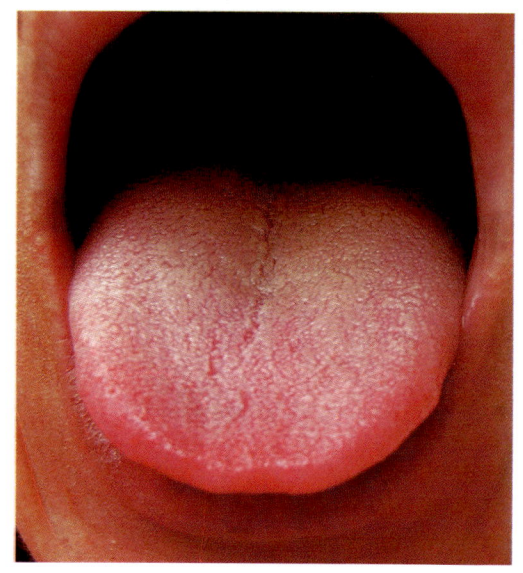

Fig 2.1-53

Patient, Female, 41years,

Case NO.: W121

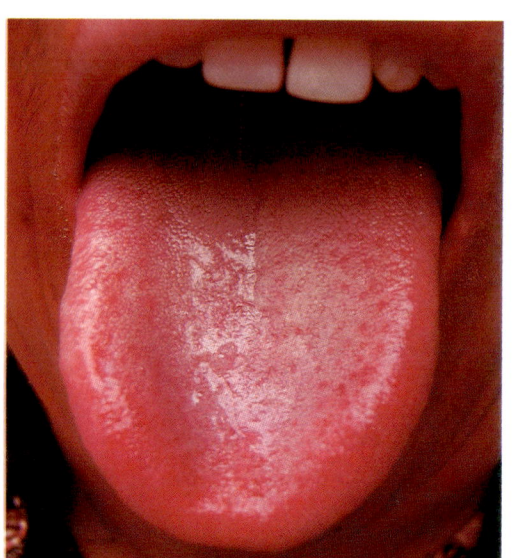

Fig 2.1-54

Patient, Female, 43years,

Case NO.: W120

Fig 2.1-55

Patient, Female, 44years,

Case NO.: W119

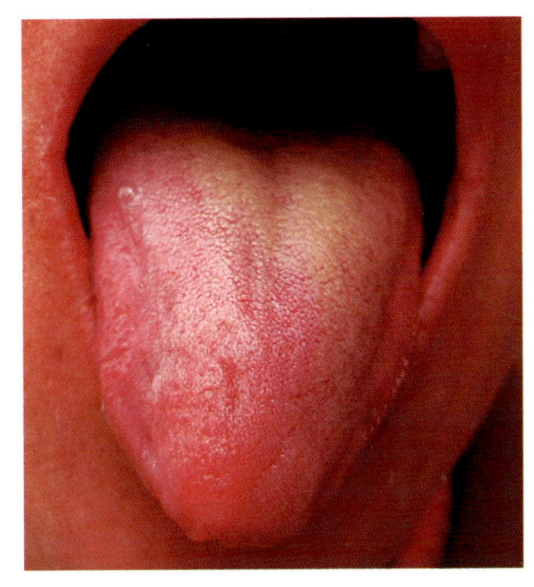

Fig 2.1-56

Patient, Female, 45years,

Case NO.: W217

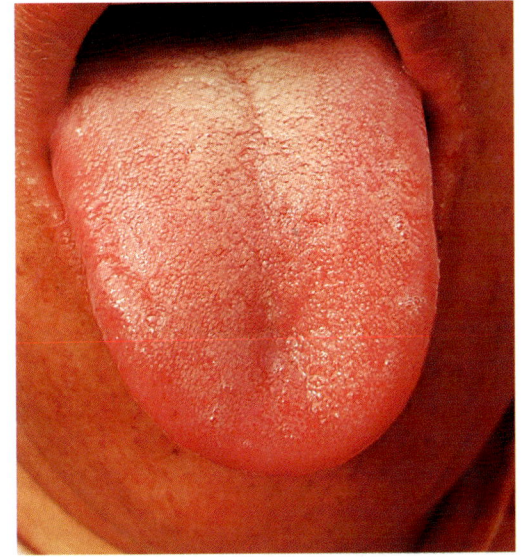

Light red tongue

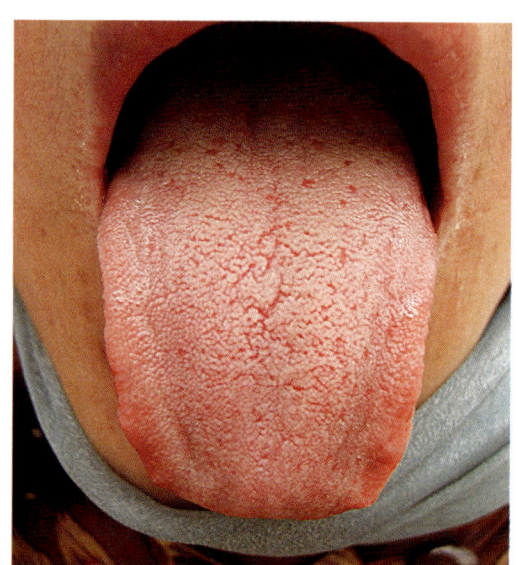

Fig 2.1-57

Patient, Female, 39years,

Case NO.: F231

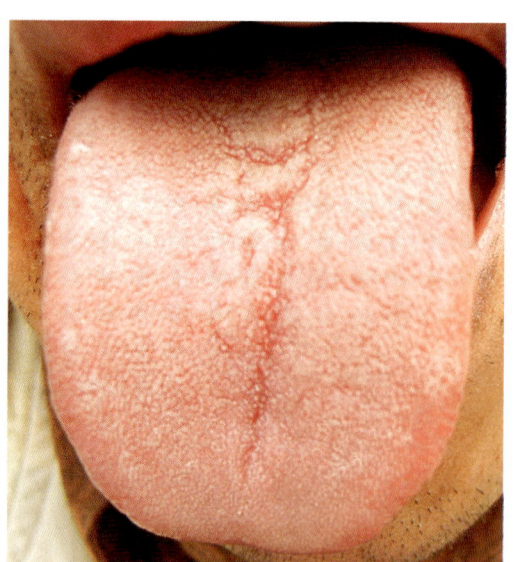

Fig 2.1-58

Patient, Male, 39years,

Case NO.: W345

Fig 2.1-59

Patient, Female, 33years,

Case NO.: W211

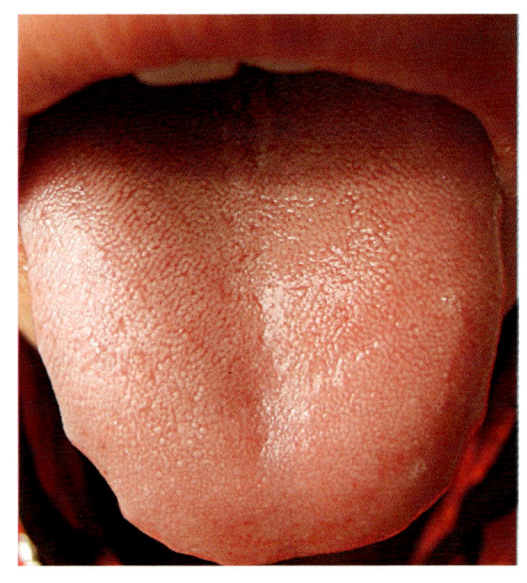

Fig 2.1-60

Patient, Female, 40years,

Case NO.: W210

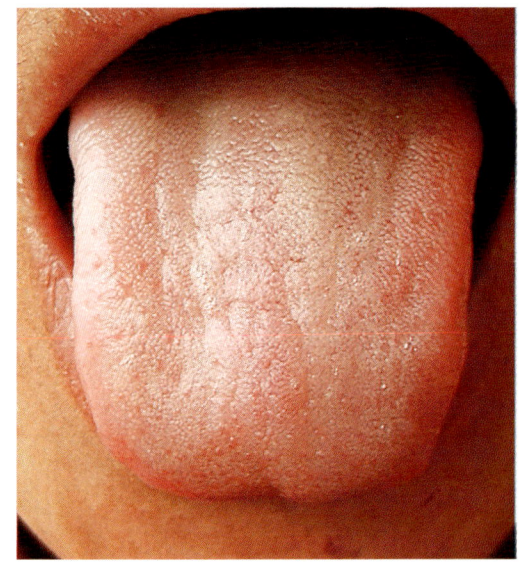

Light red tongue

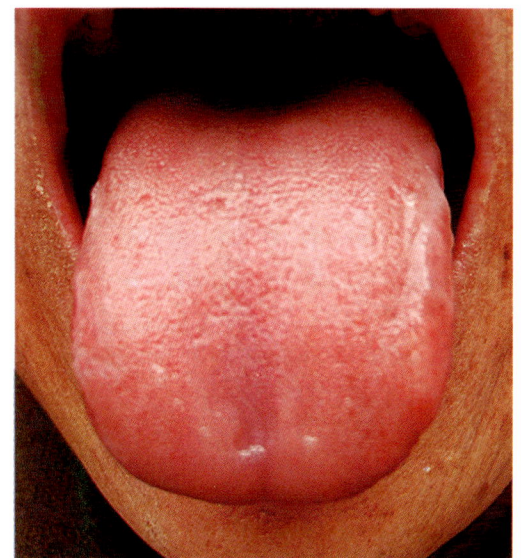

Fig 2.1-61

Patient, Female, 51years,

Case NO.: F171

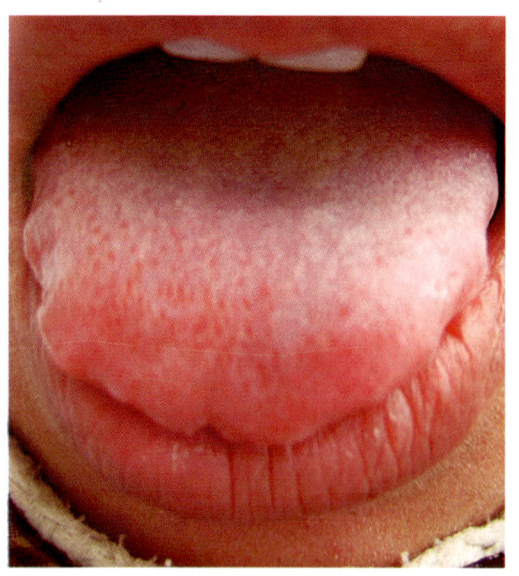

Fig 2.1-62

Patient, Female, 48years,

Case NO.: F282

Fig 2.1-63

Patient, Female, 35years,

Case NO.: F45

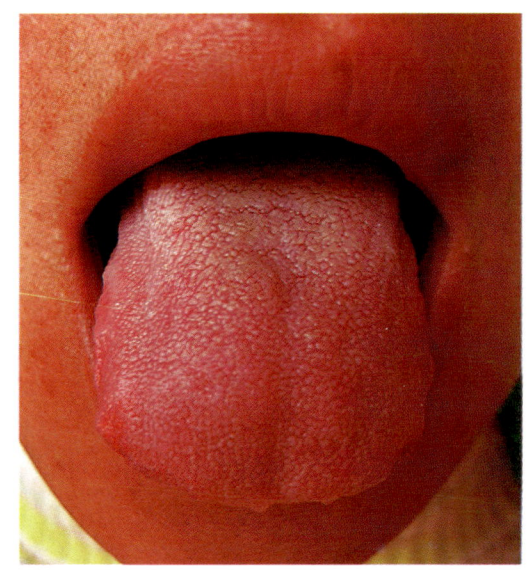

Fig 2.1-64

Patient, Female, 43years,

Case NO.: F38

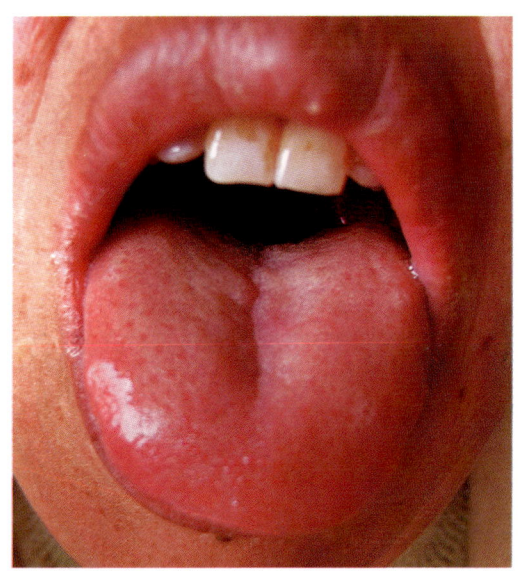

Light red tongue

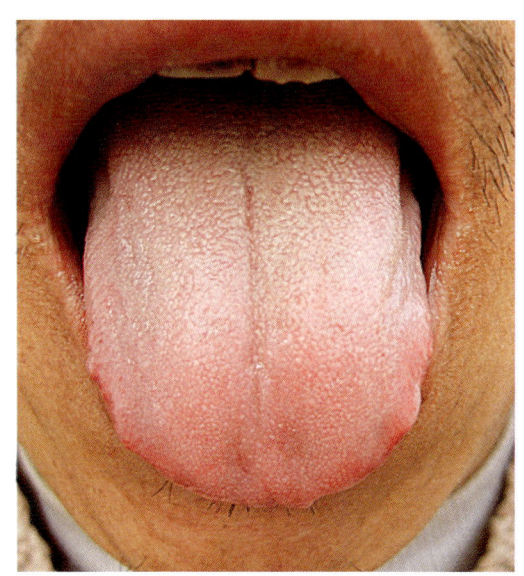

Fig 2.1-65

Patient, Male, 44years,

Case NO.: W577

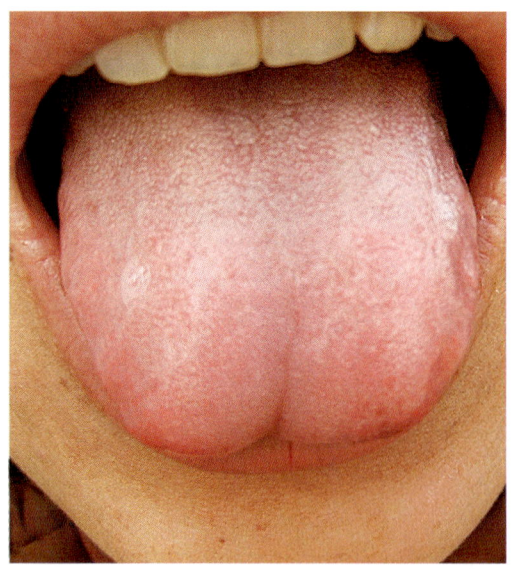

Fig 2.1-66

Patient, Female, 42years,

Case NO.: W572

Fig 2.1-67

Patient, Female, 38years,

Case NO.: W673

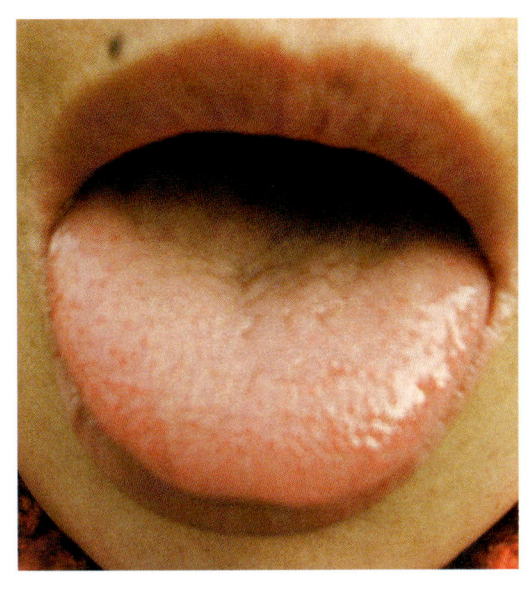

Fig 2.1-68

Patient, Female, 39years,

Case NO.: W643

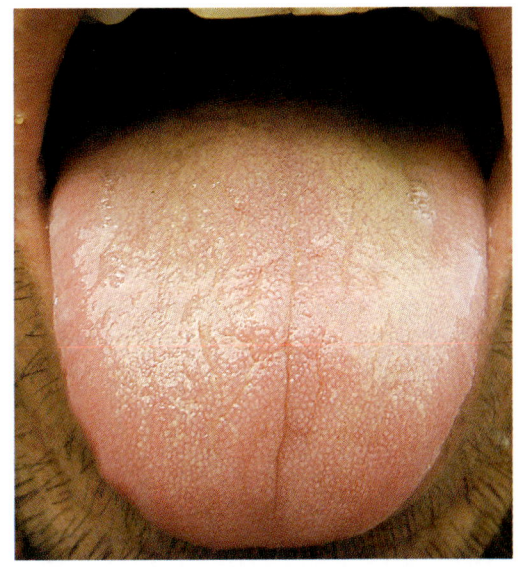

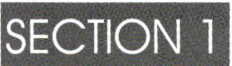

Light red tongue

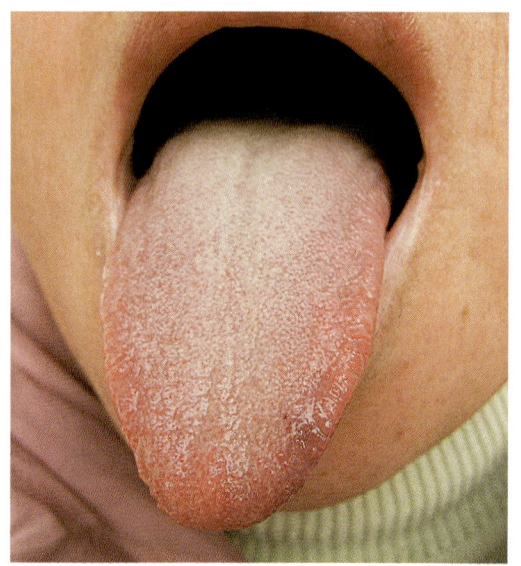

Fig 2.1-69

Patient, Female, 40years,

Case NO.: F225

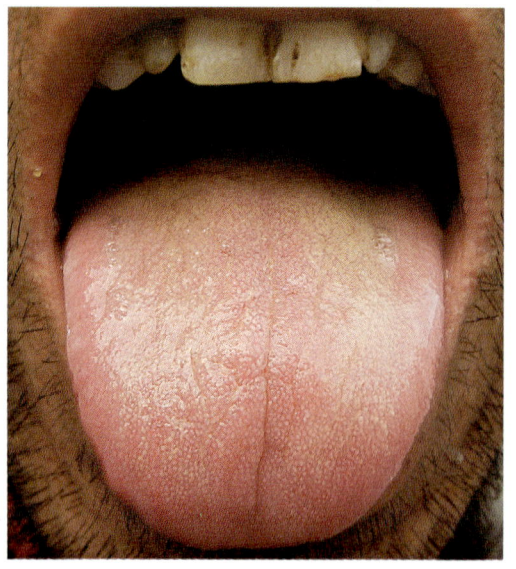

Fig 2.1-70

Patient, Male, 48years,

Case NO.: W632

Fig 2.1-71

Patient, Female, 46years,

Case NO.: W291

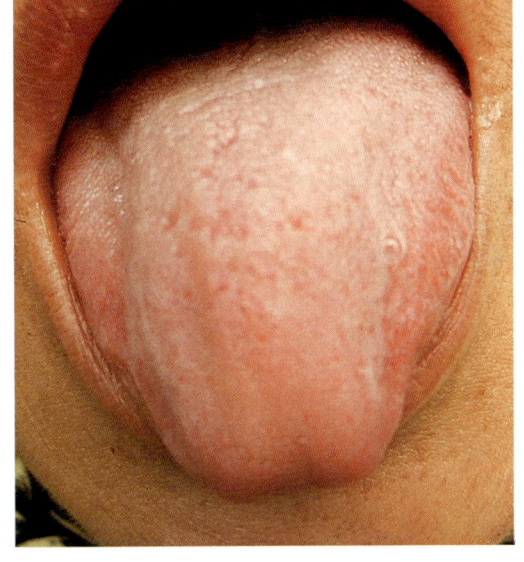

Fig 2.1-72

Patient, Male, 60years,

Case NO.: W605

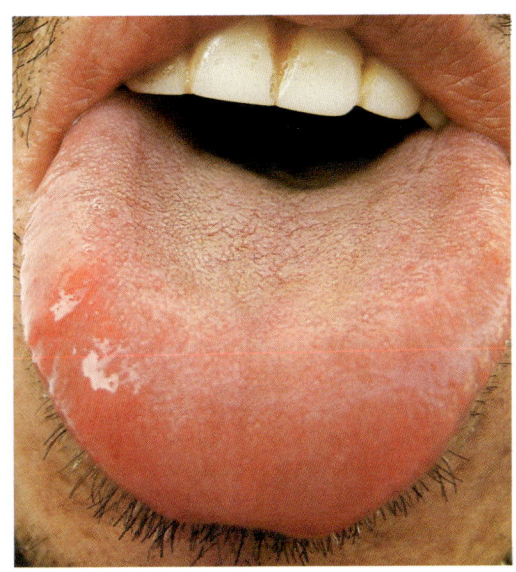

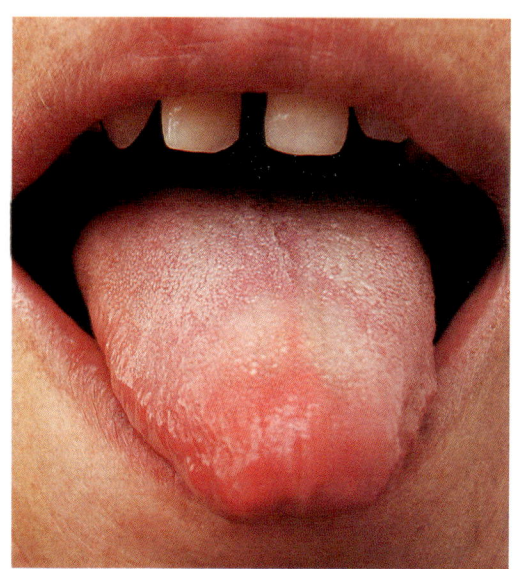

Fig 2.1-73

Patient, Female, 57years,

Case NO.: W579

Light red tongue

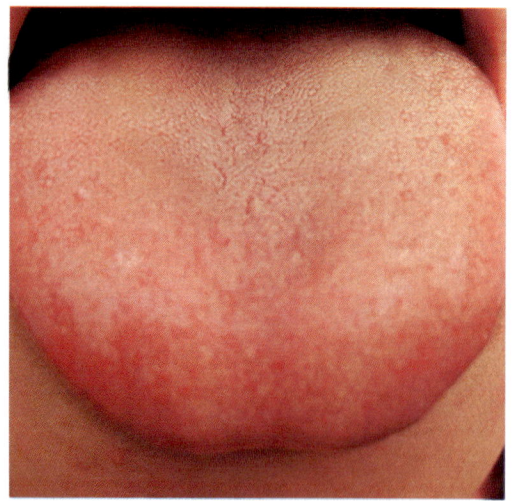

Fig 2.1-74

Patient, Female, 33years,

Case NO.: W265

Fig 2.1-75

Patient, Female, 49years,

Case NO.: F345

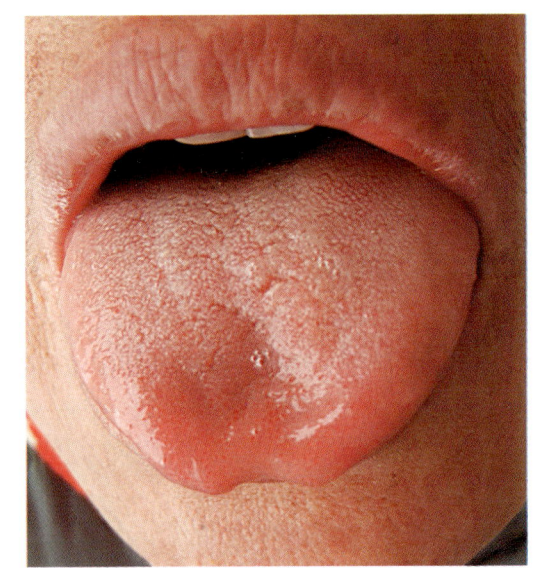

Fig 2.1-76

Patient, Female, 42years,

Case NO.: W388

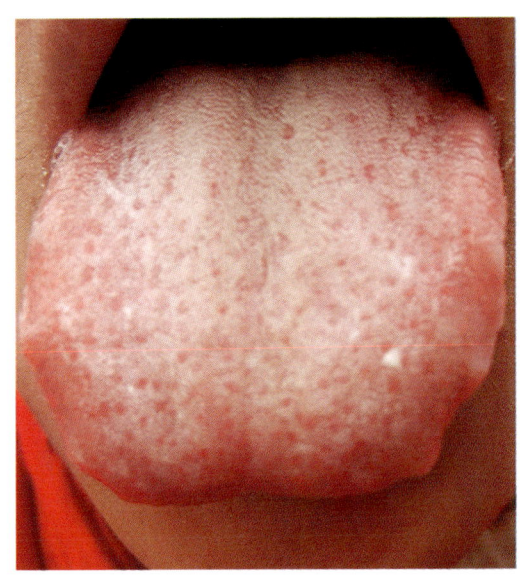

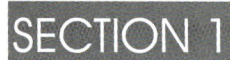

Light red tongue

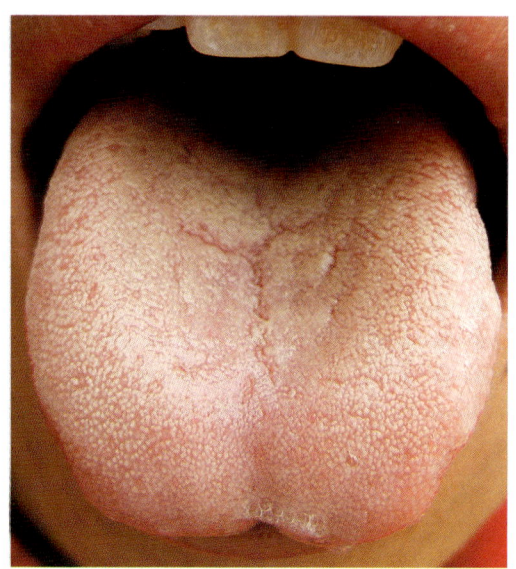

Fig 2.1-77

Patient, Female, 33years,

Case NO.: W163

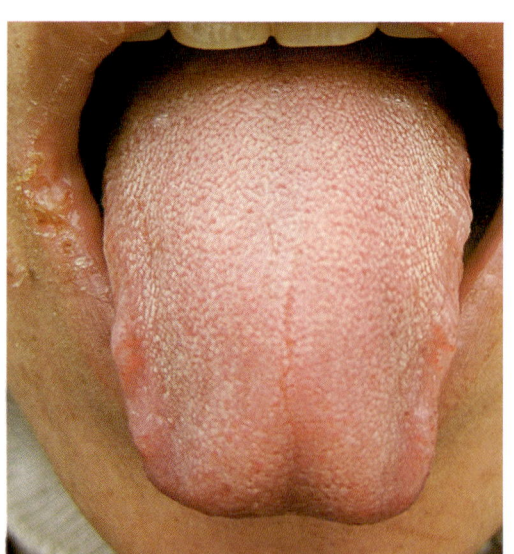

Fig 2.1-78

Patient, Female, 49years,

Case NO.: W571

Fig 2.1-79

Patient, Female, 41years,

Case NO.: W514

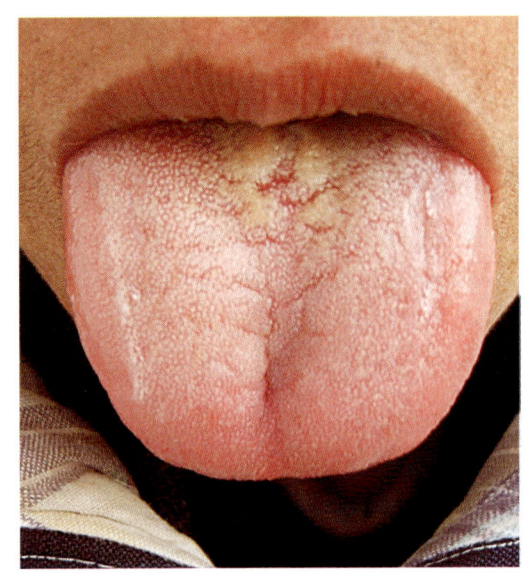

Fig 2.1-80

Patient, Male, 48years,

Case NO.: F169

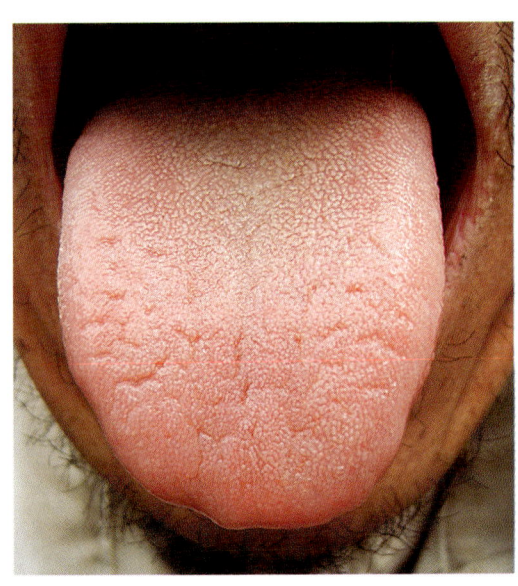

Light red tongue

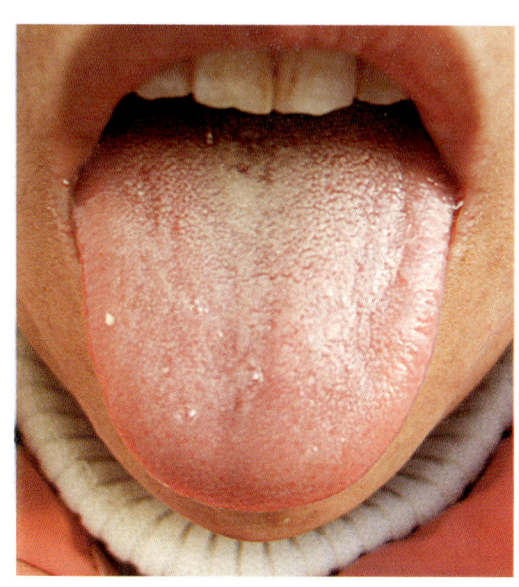

Fig 2.1-81

Patient, Female, 38years,

Case NO.: W504

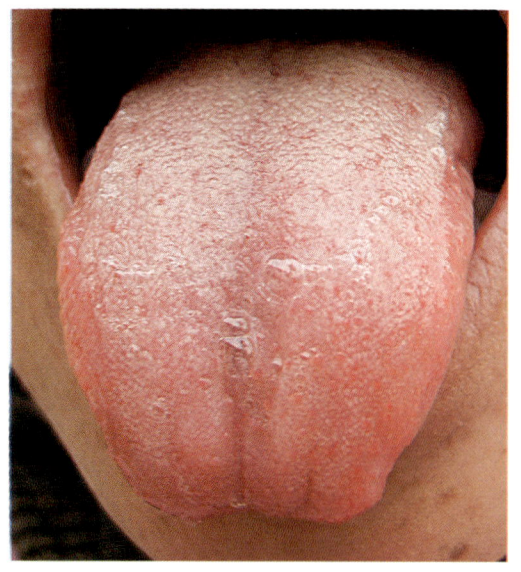

Fig 2.1-82

Patient, Female, 42years,

Case NO.: W561

Fig 2.1-83

Patient, Female, 33years,

Case NO.: F15

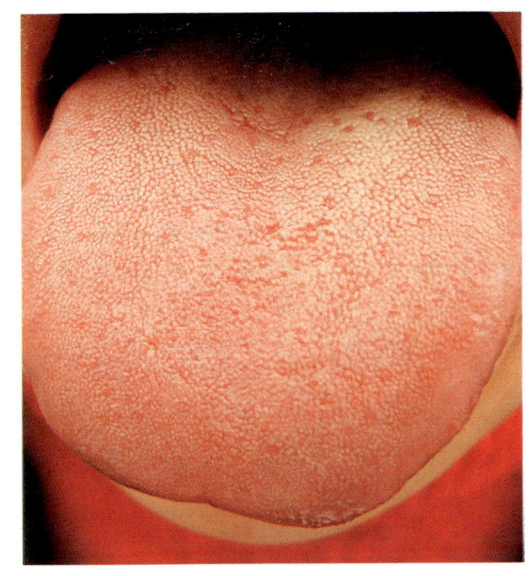

Fig 2.1-84

Patient, Male, 57years,

Case NO.: W676

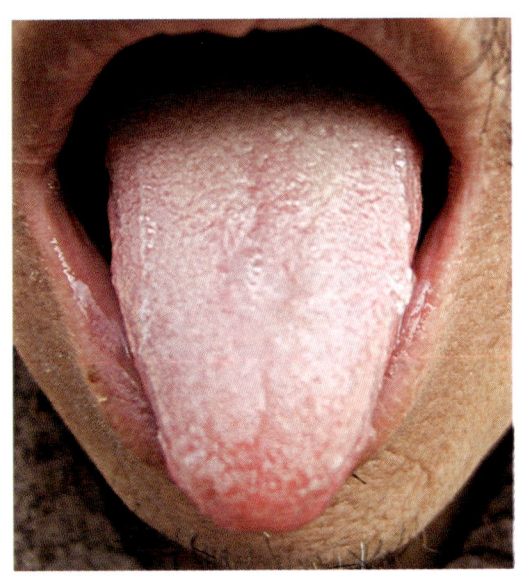

Light red tongue

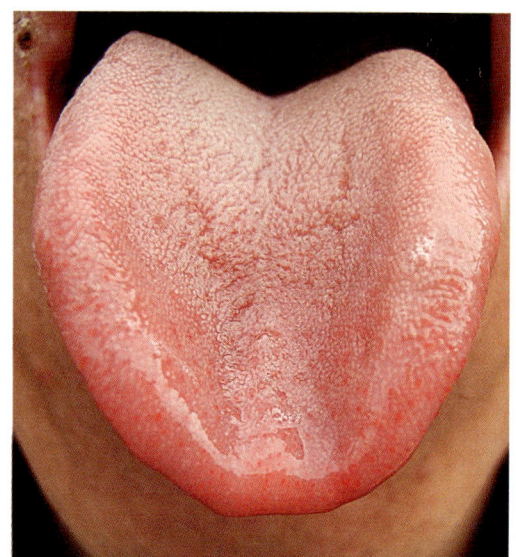

Fig 2.1-85

Patient, Male, 40years,

Case NO.: F161

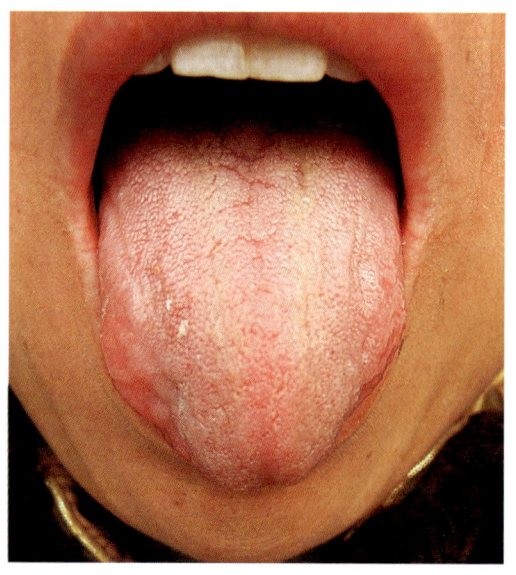

Fig 2.1-86

Patient, Female, 37years,

Case NO.: W274

Fig 2.1-87

Patient, Male, 40years,

Case NO.: F167

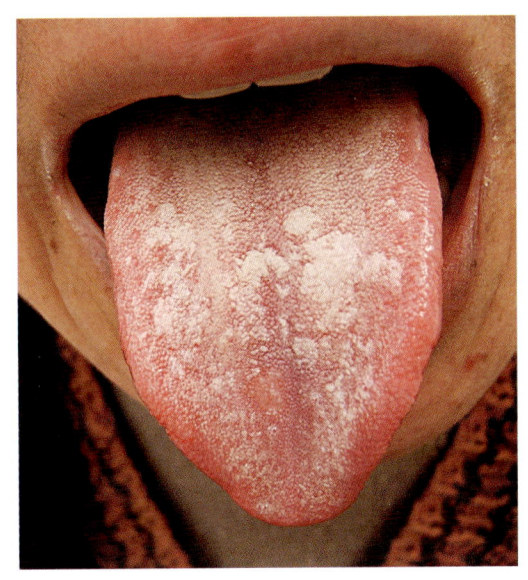

Fig 2.1-88

Patient, Male, 48years,

Case NO.: F230

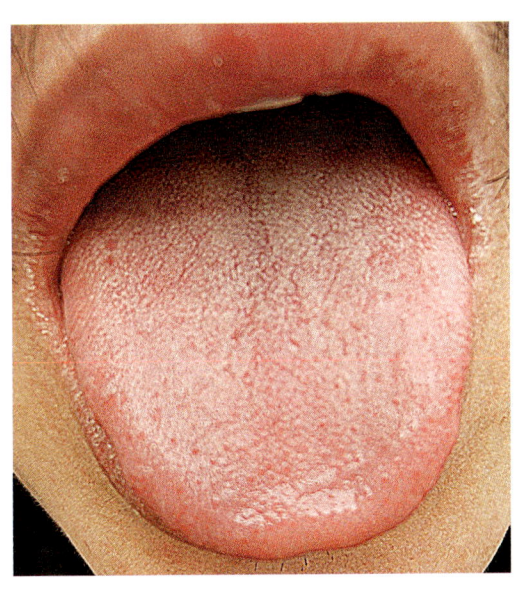

Light red tongue

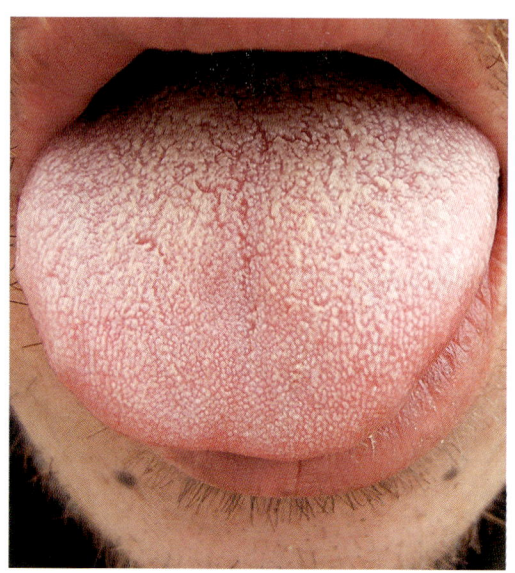

Fig 2.1-89

Patient, Male, 37years,

Case NO.: W556

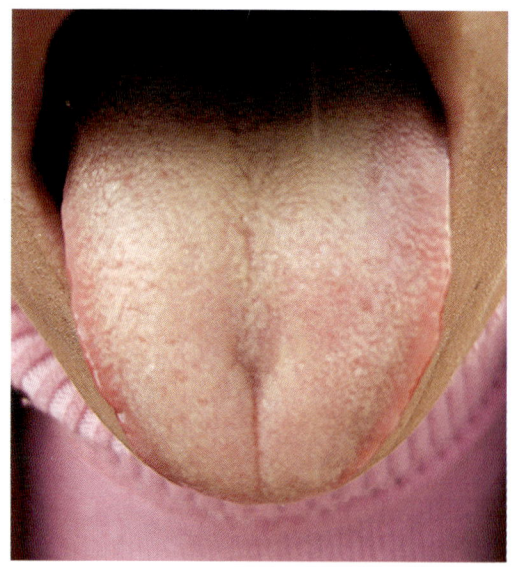

Fig 2.1-90

Patient, Female, 44years,

Case NO.: F58

Fig 2.1-91

Patient, Female, 29years,

Case NO.: W628

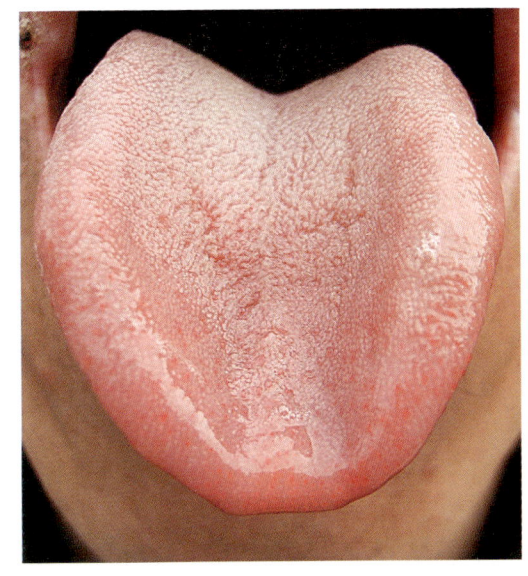

Fig 2.1-92

Patient, Female, 36years,

Case NO.: F74

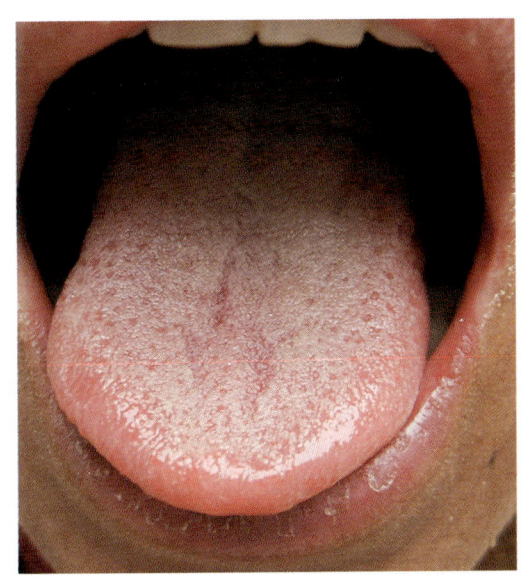

Light red tongue

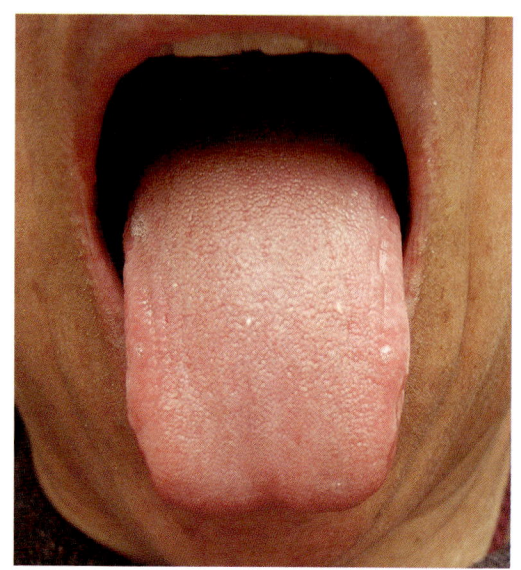

Fig 2.1-93

Patient, Female, 55years,

Case NO.: F84

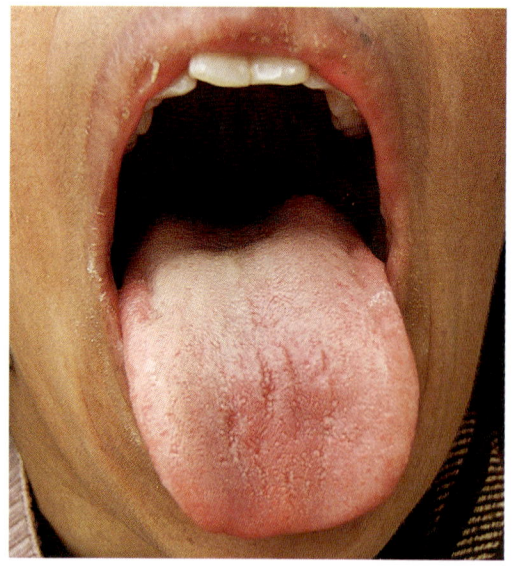

Fig 2.1-94

Patient, Female, 45years,

Case NO.: W67

Fig 2.1-95

Patient, Male, 35years,

Case NO.: W64

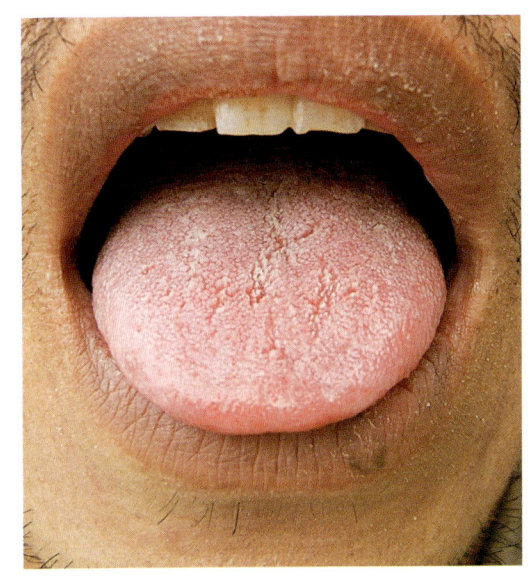

Fig 2.1-96

Patient, Female, 49years,

Case NO.: W102

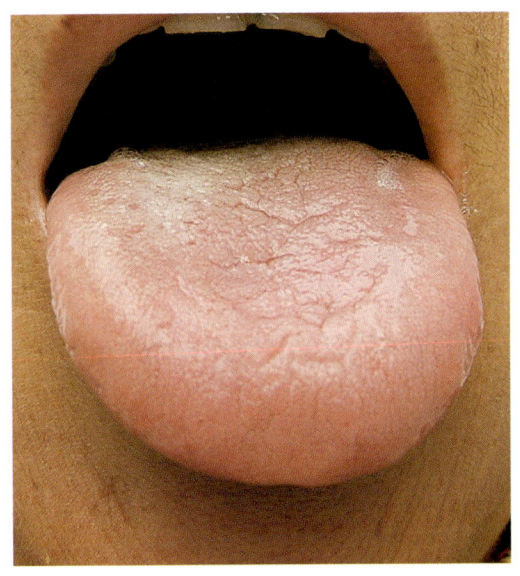

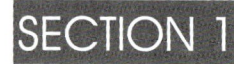
Light red tongue

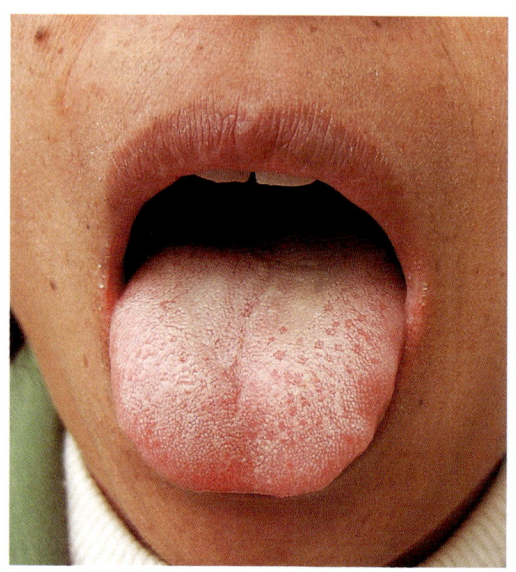

Fig 2.1-97

Patient, Female, 36years,

Case NO.: W54

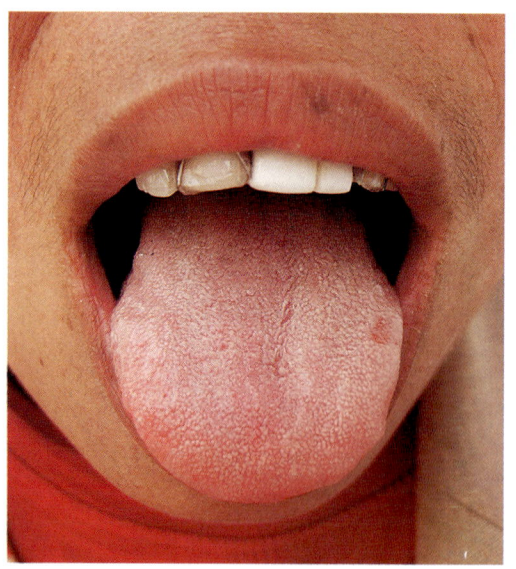

Fig 2.1-98

atient, Female, 37years,

Case NO.: W93

Fig 2.1-99

Patient, Female, 43years,

Case NO.: W86

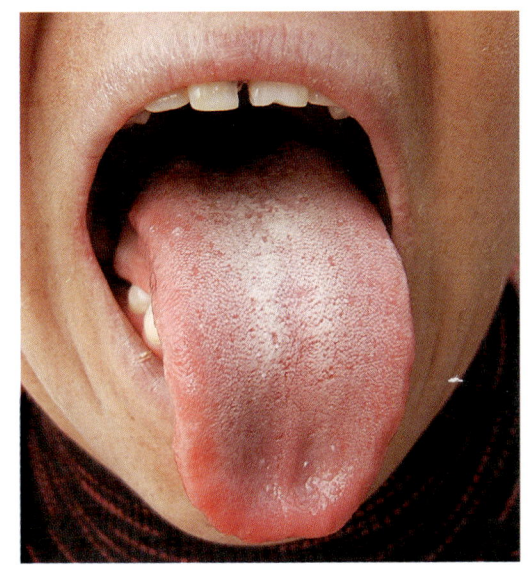

Fig 2.1-100

Patient, Female, 43years,

Case NO.: W241

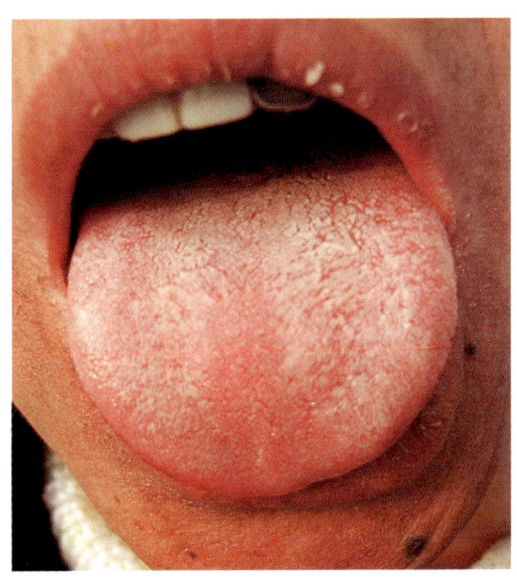

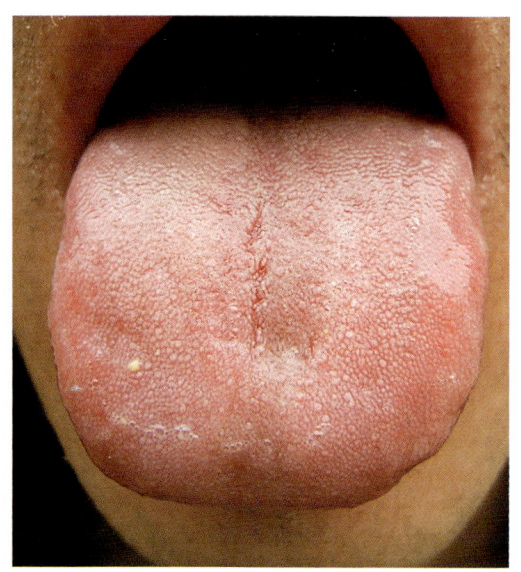

Fig 2.1-101

Patient, Male, 35years,

Case NO.: F73

Light red tongue

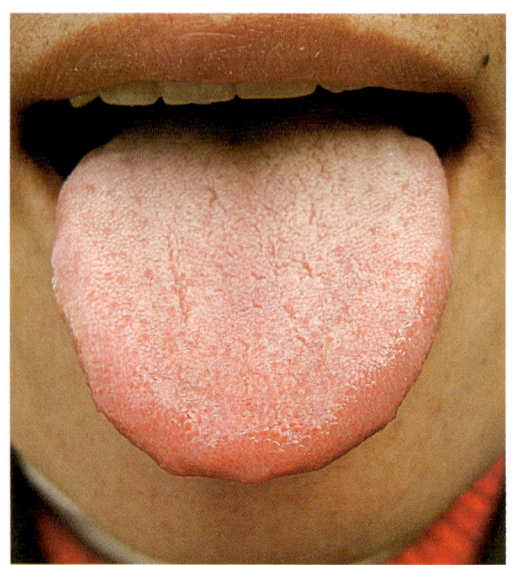

Fig 2.1-102

Patient, Female, 37years,

Case NO.: F120

Fig 2.1-103

Patient, Male, 51years,

Case NO.: W63

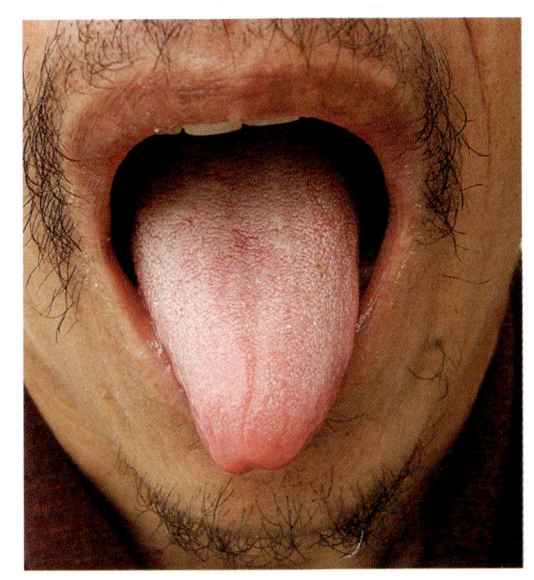

Fig 2.1-104

Patient, Female, 30years,

Case NO.: W87

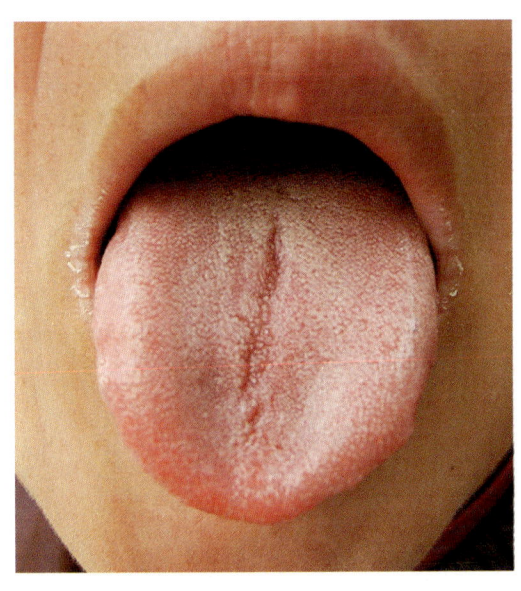

Light red tongue

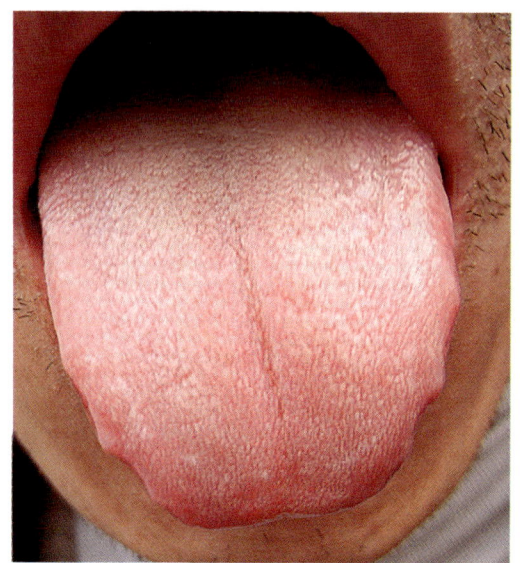

Fig 2.1-105

Patient, Male, 34years,

Case NO.: F133

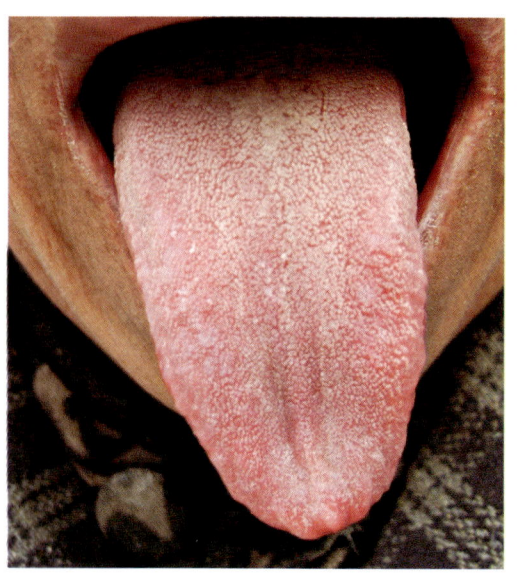

Fig 2.1-106

Patient, Female, 59years,

Case NO.: W338

Fig 2.1-107

Patient, Male, 47years,

Case NO.: W398

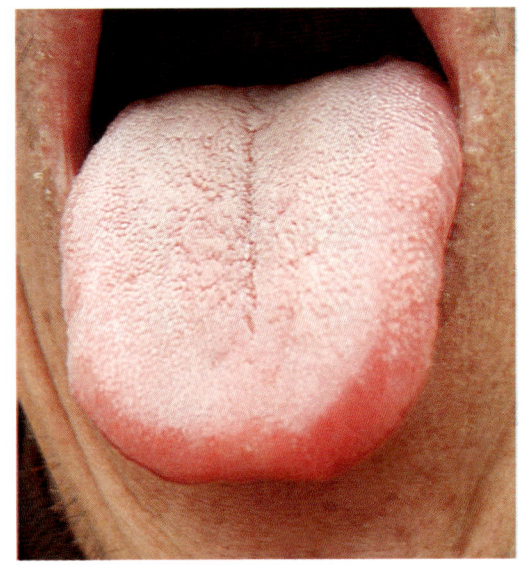

Fig 2.1-108

Patient, Female, 44years,

Case NO.: W408

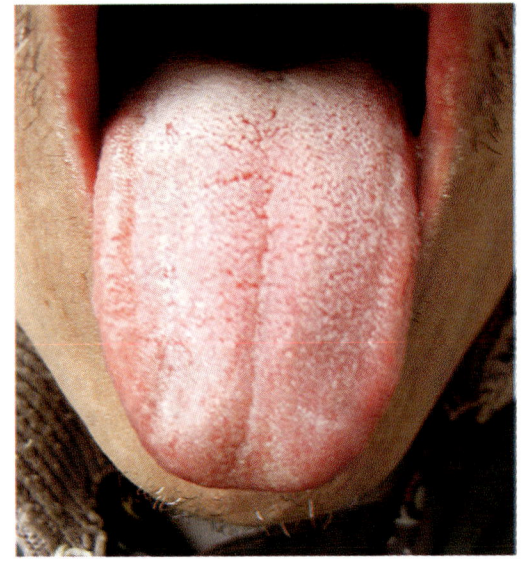

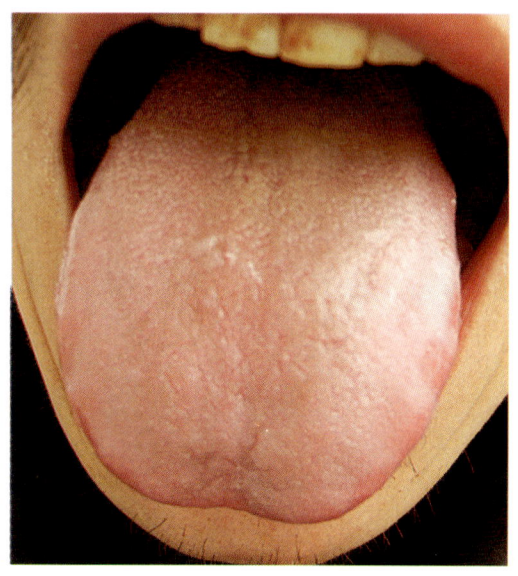

Fig 2.1-109

Patient, Male, 31years,

Case NO.: F293

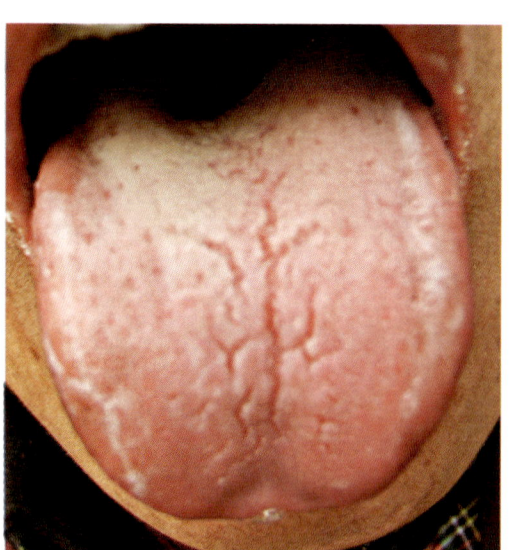

Fig 2.1-110

Patient, Female, 49years,

Case NO.: W689

Fig 2.1-111

Patient, Male, 43years,

Case NO.: W301

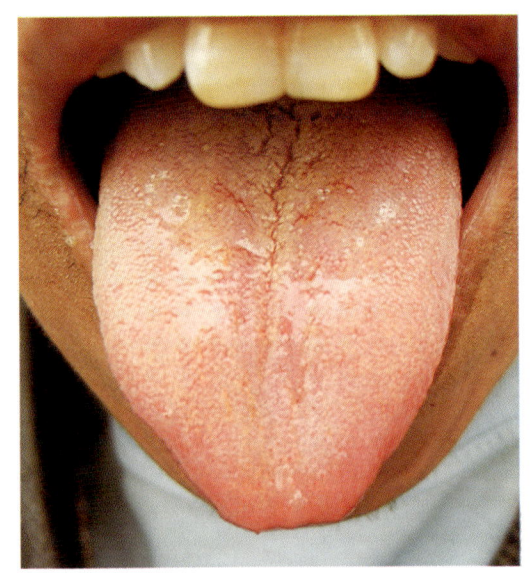

Fig 2.1-112

Patient, Female, 34years,

Case NO.: W61

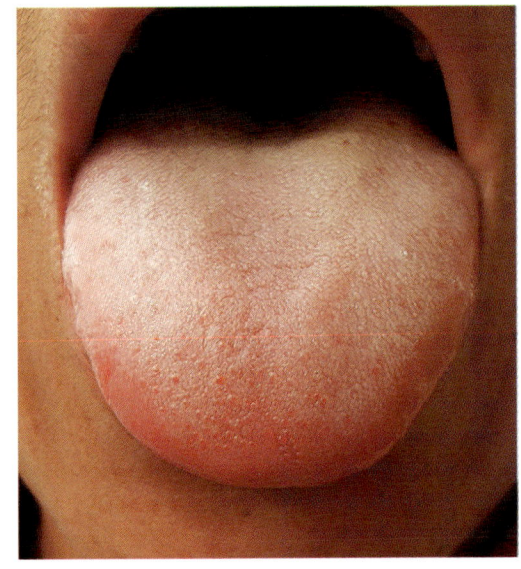

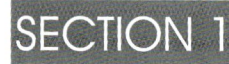

Light red tongue

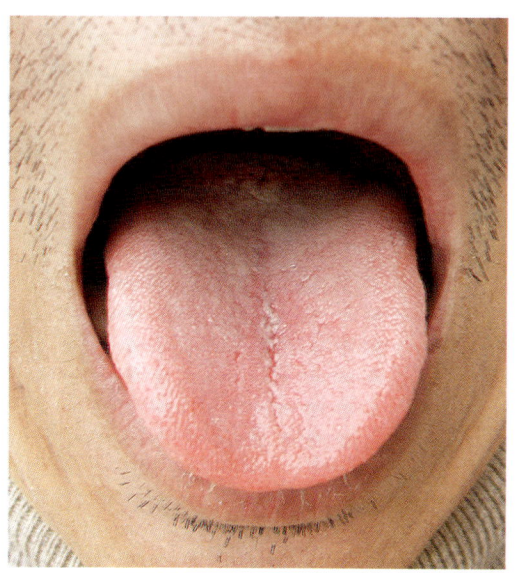

Fig 2.1-113

Patient, Male, 42years,

Case NO.: W72

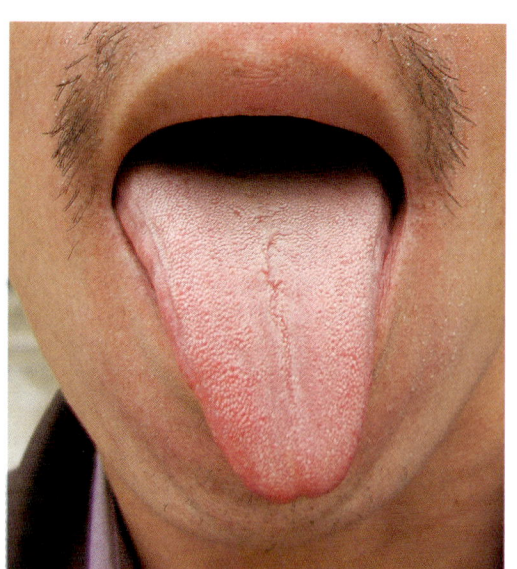

Fig 2.1-114

Patient, Female, 43years,

Case NO.: W43

Fig 2.1-115

Patient, Female, 37years,

Case NO.: W427

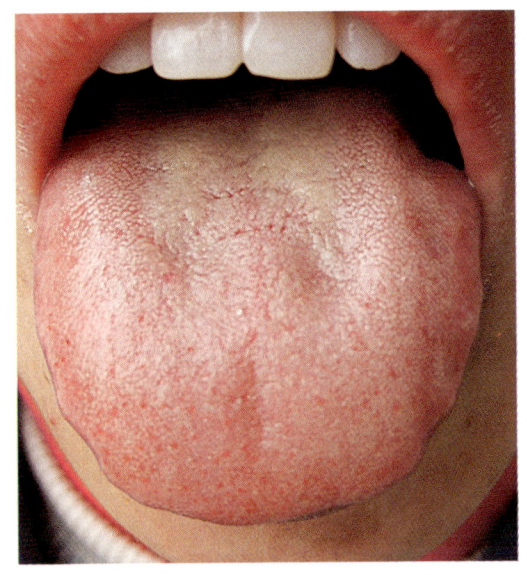

Fig 2.1-116

Patient, Female, 51years,

Case NO.: W92

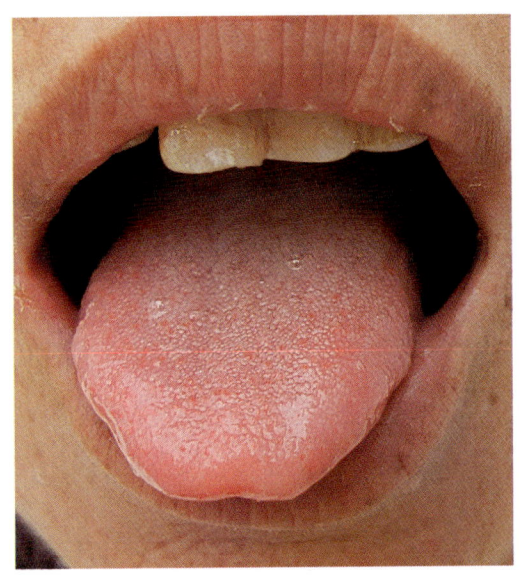

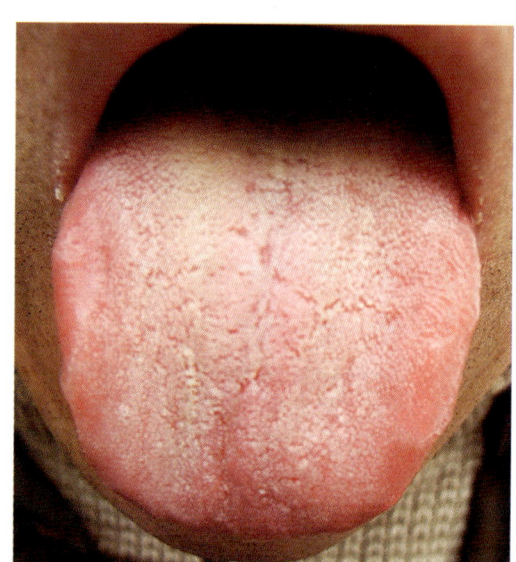

Fig 2.1-117

Patient, Male, 44years,

Case NO.: W253

Light red tongue

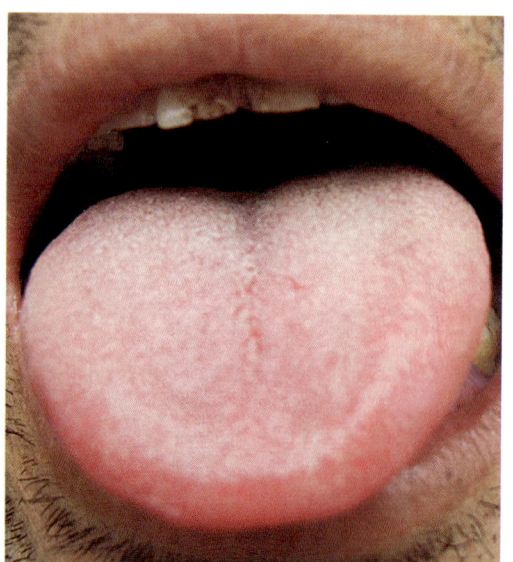

Fig 2.1-118

Patient, Male, 49years,

Case NO.: F23

Fig 2.1-119

Patient, Female, 37years,

Case NO.: W427

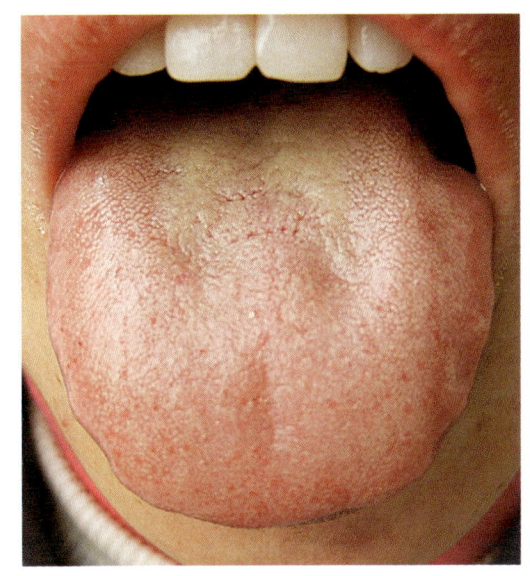

Fig 2.1-120

Patient, Male, 31years,

Case NO.: W386

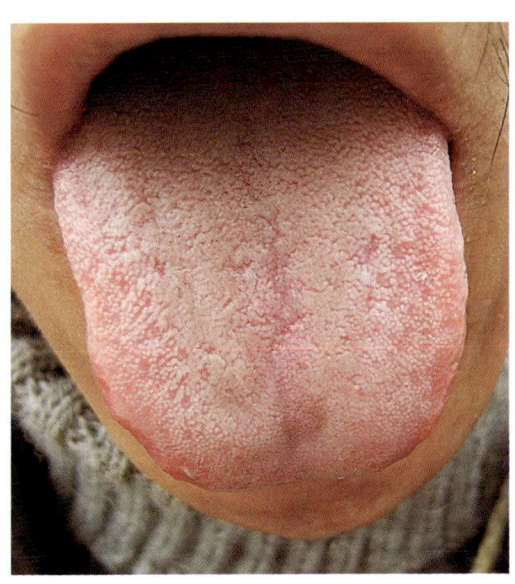

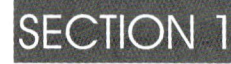
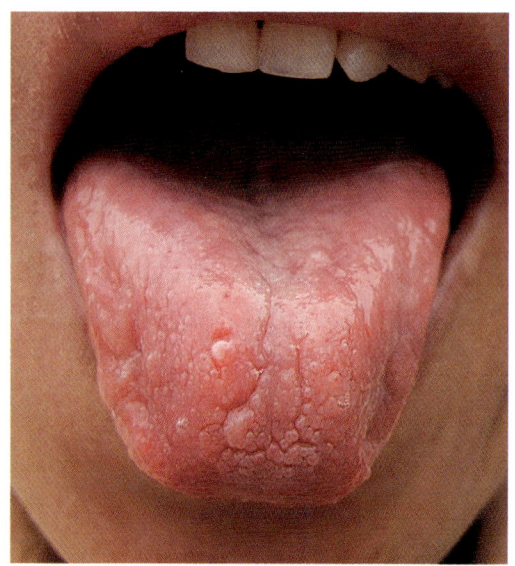

Fig 2.1-121

Patient, Male, 39years,

Case NO.: W404

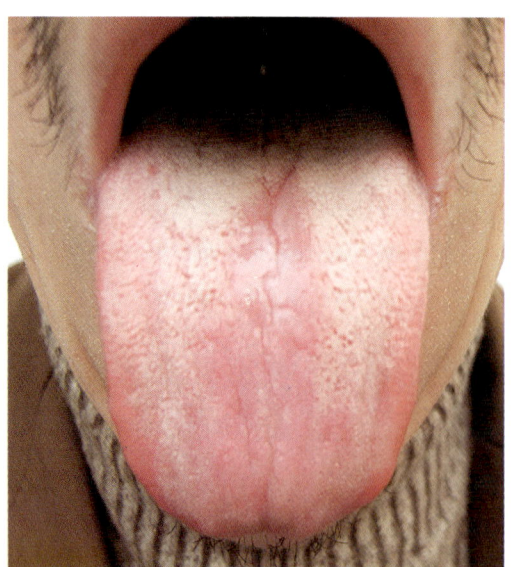

Fig 2.1-122

Patient, Male, 35years,

Case NO.: W270

Light red tongue

Fig 2.1-123

Patient, Male, 50years,

Case NO.: W212

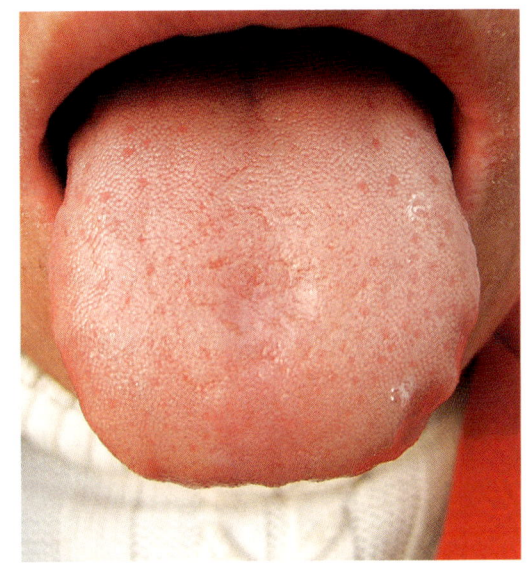

Fig 2.1-124

Patient, Male, 49years,

Case NO.: W65

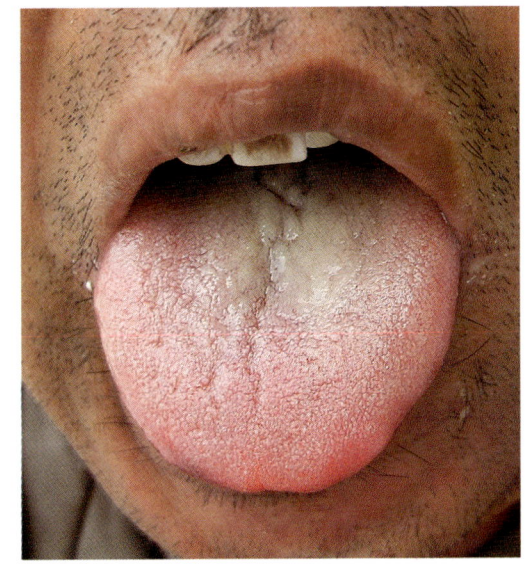

Light red tongue

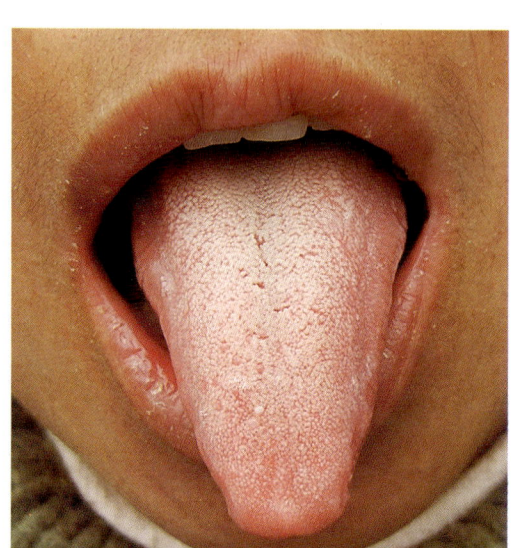

Fig 2.1-125

Patient, Female, 46years,

Case NO.: W35

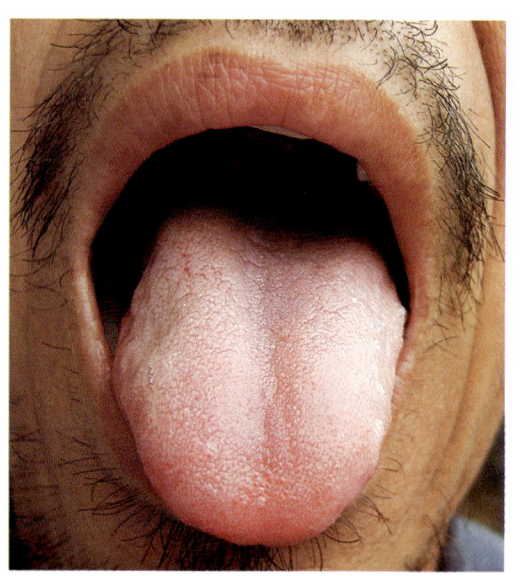

Fig 2.1-126

Patient, Male, 49years,

Case NO.: W157

Fig 2.1-127

Patient, Female, 48years,

Case NO.: F282

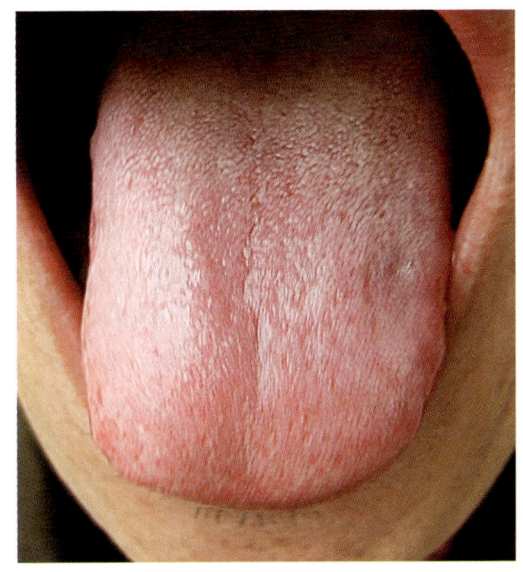

Fig 2.1-128

Patient, Female, 40years,

Case NO.: W678

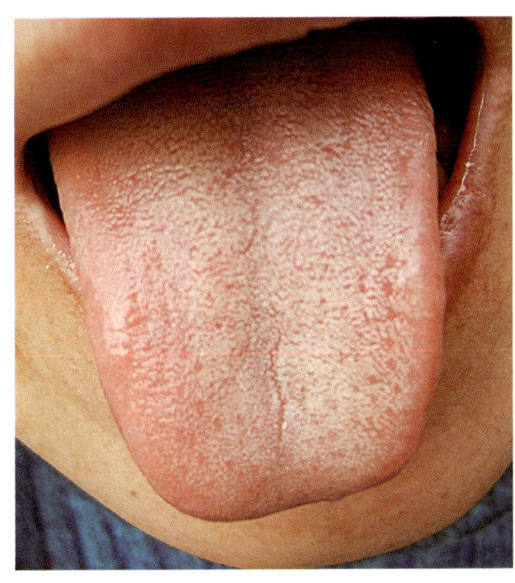

Light red tongue

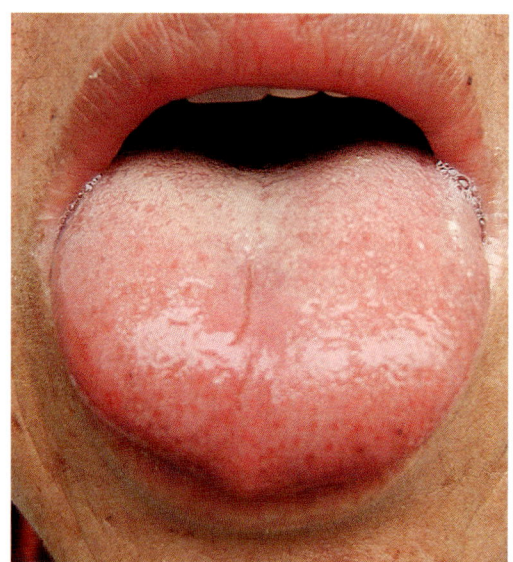

Fig 2.1-129

Patient, Female, 51years,

Case NO.: W110

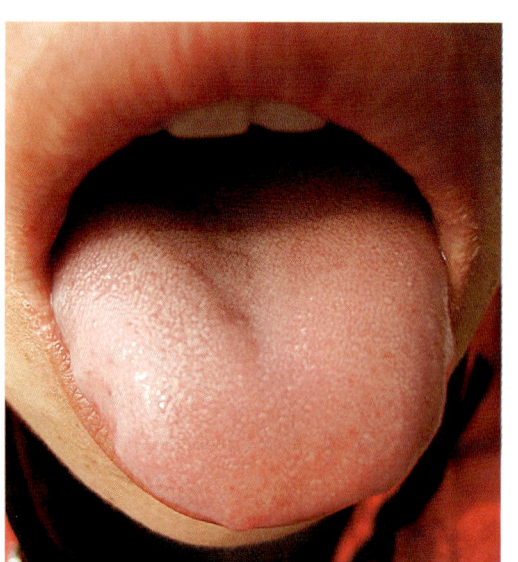

Fig 2.1-130

Patient, Female, 33years,

Case NO.: W211

Fig 2.1-131

Patient, Female, 46years,

Case NO.: W341

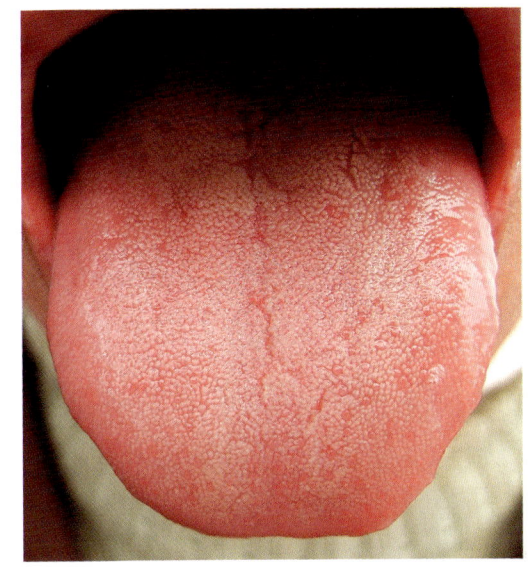

Fig 2.1-132

Patient, Male, 42years,

Case NO.: W39

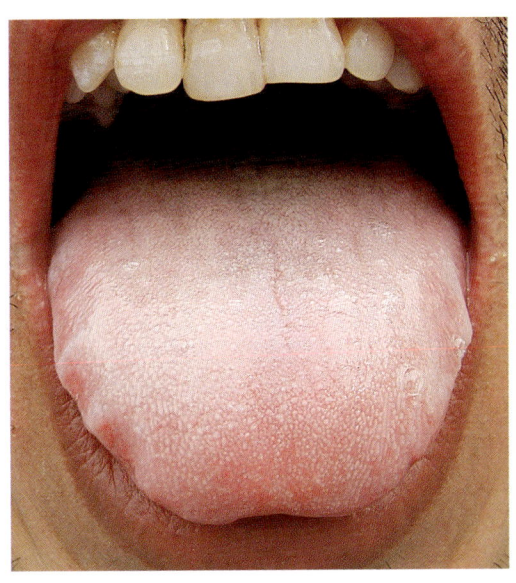

Light red tongue

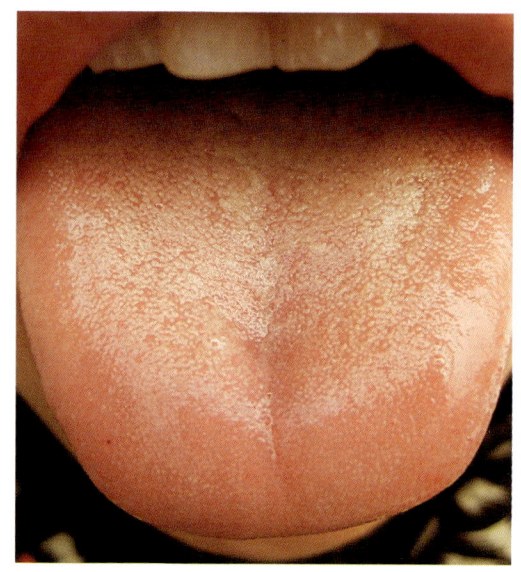

Fig 2.1-133

Patient, Female, 35years,

Case NO.: W363

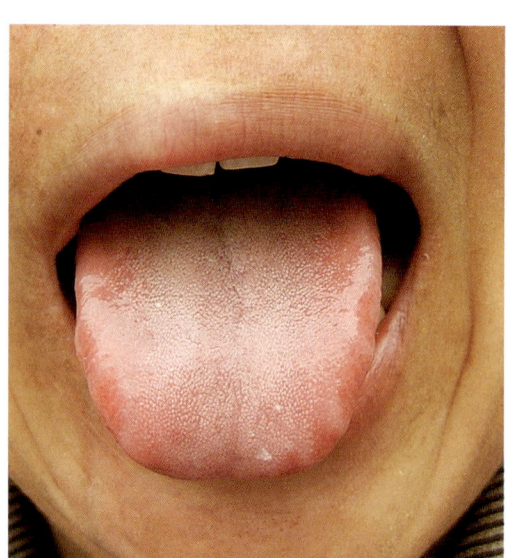

Fig 2.1-134

Patient, Female, 40years,

Case NO.: W37

Fig 2.1-135

Patient, Female, 54years,

Case NO.: W30

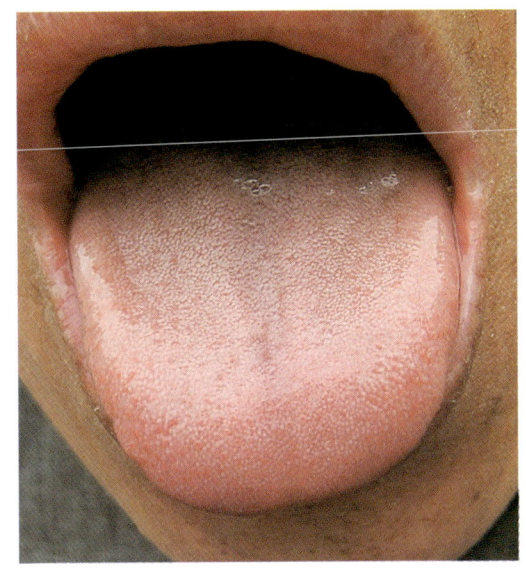

Fig 2.1-136

Patient, Female, 41years,

Case NO.: F174

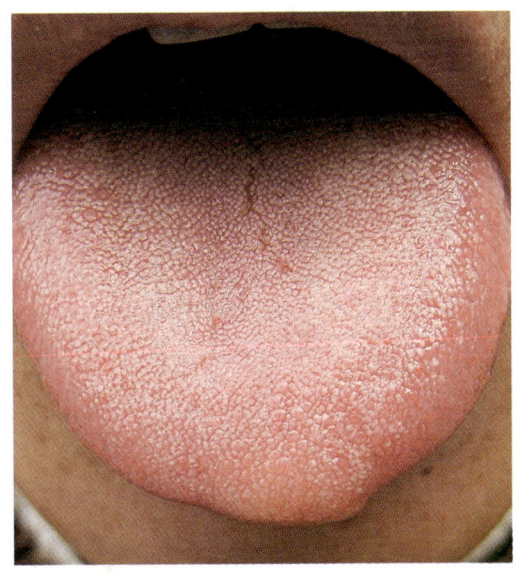

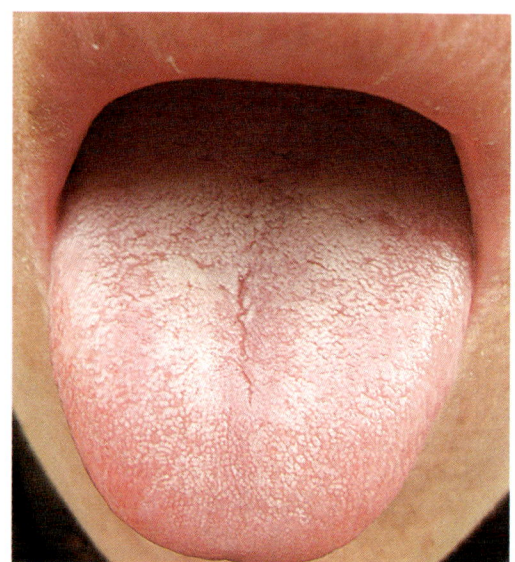

Fig 2.1-137

Patient, Female, 60years,

Case NO.: W667

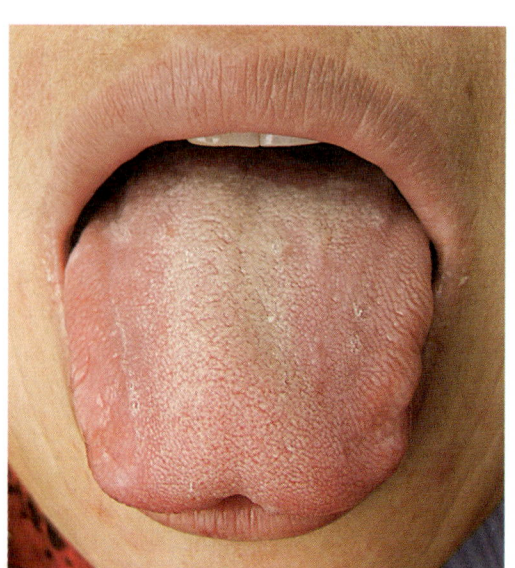

Fig 2.1-138

Patient, Female, 50years,

Case NO.: F335

Fig 2.1-139

Patient, Female, 48years,

Case NO.: W236

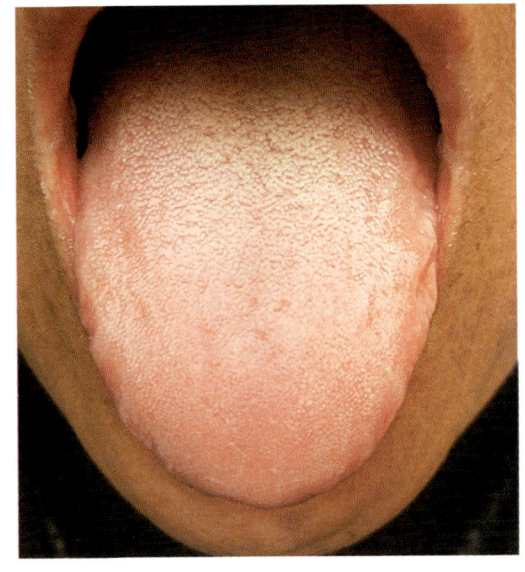

Fig 2.1-140

Patient, Female, 53years,

Case NO.: F332

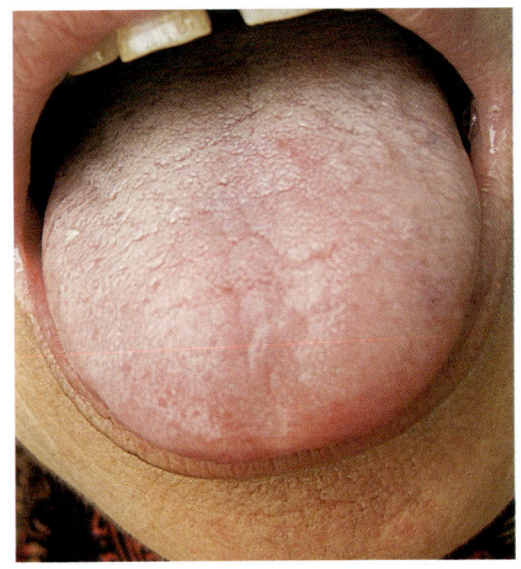

Light red tongue

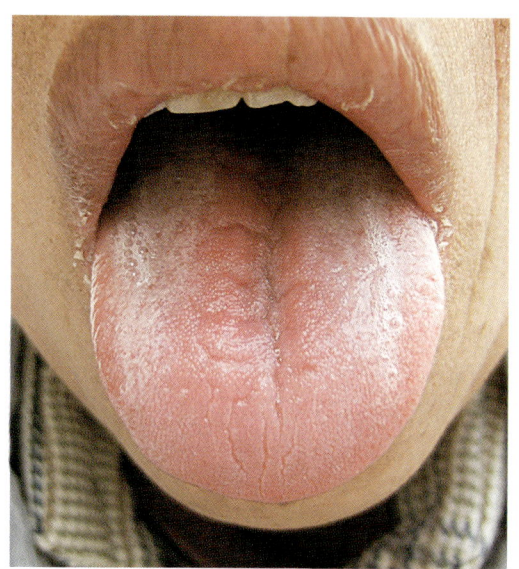

Fig 2.1-141

Patient, Female, 54years,

Case NO.: F53

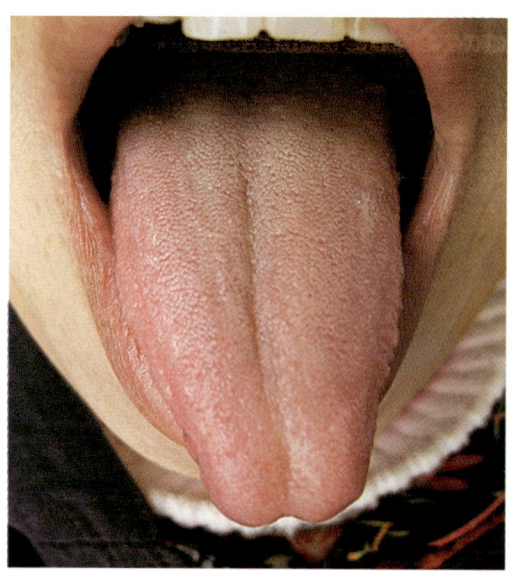

Fig 2.1-142

Patient, Female, 34years,

Case NO.: F328

Fig 2.1-143

Patient, Male, 47years,

Case NO.: F206

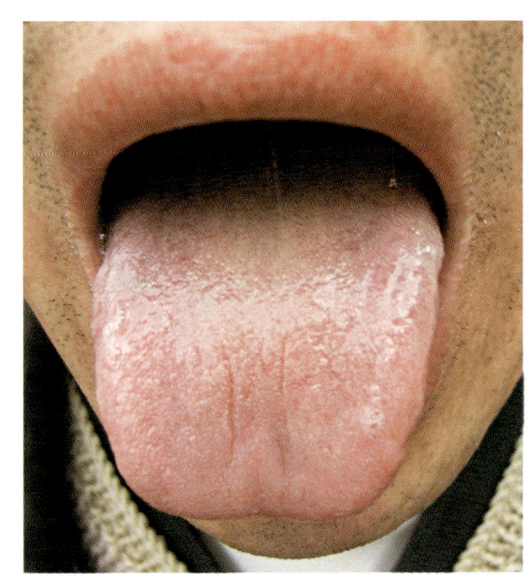

Fig 2.1-144

Patient, Female, 52years,

Case NO.: F56

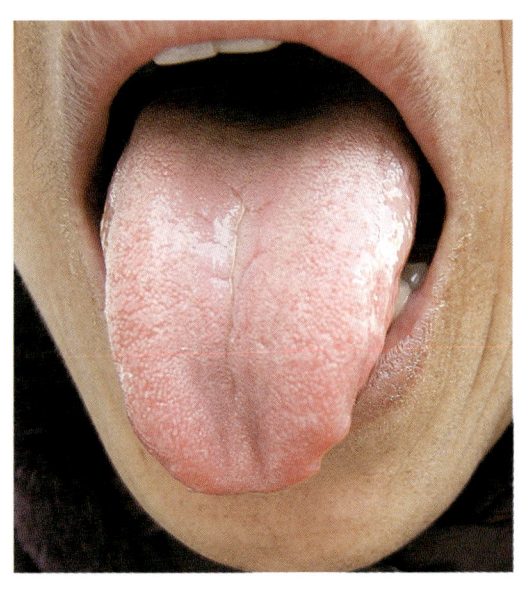

Light red tongue

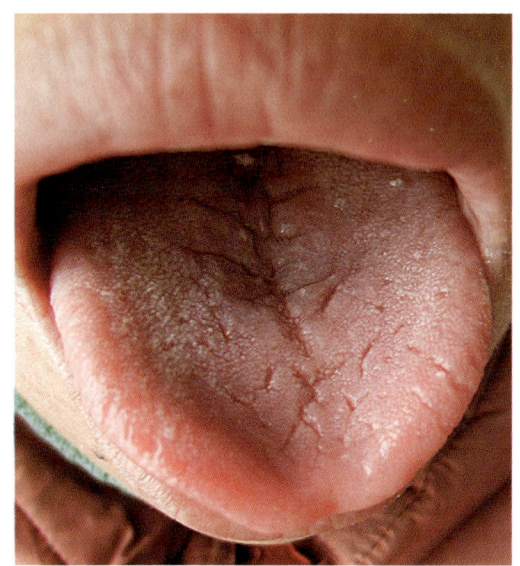

Fig 2.1-145

Patient, Female, 38years,

Case NO.: W736

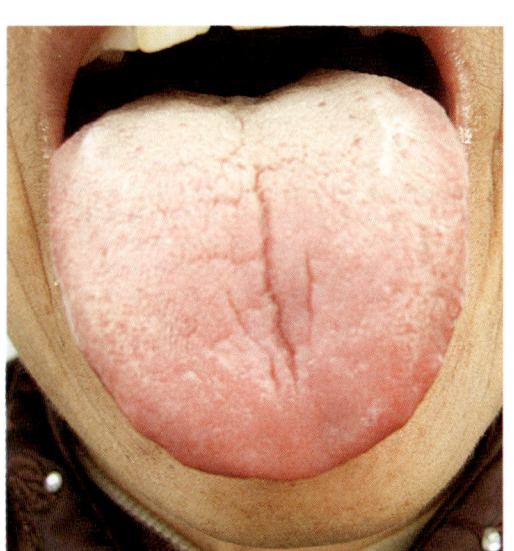

Fig 2.1-146

Patient, Female, 54years,

Case NO.: W237

Fig 2.1-147

Patient, Male, 40years,

Case NO.: F156

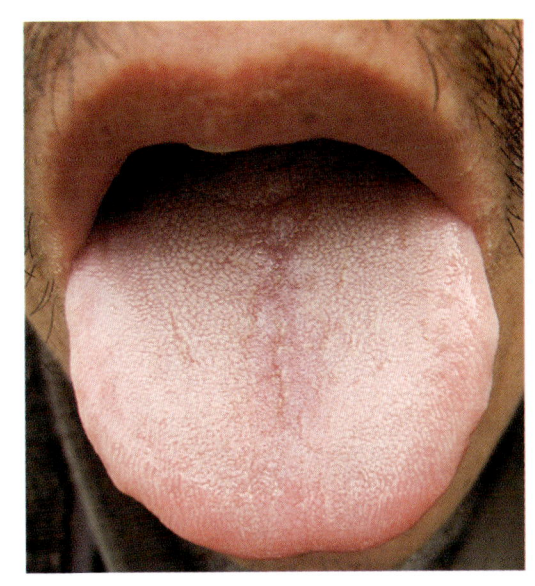

Fig 2.1-148

Patient, Male, 41years,

Case NO.: F353

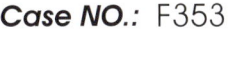

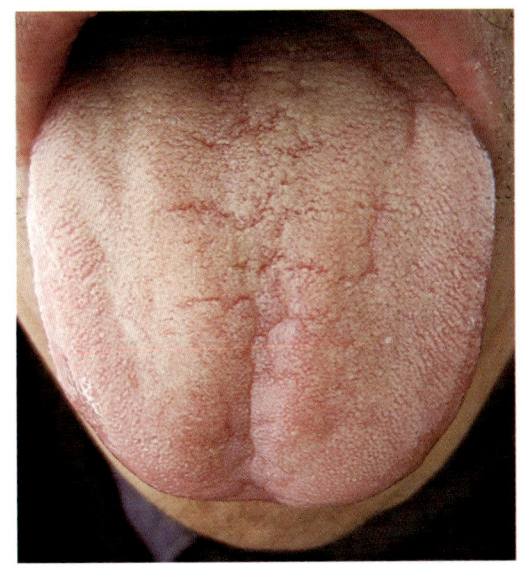

Light red tongue

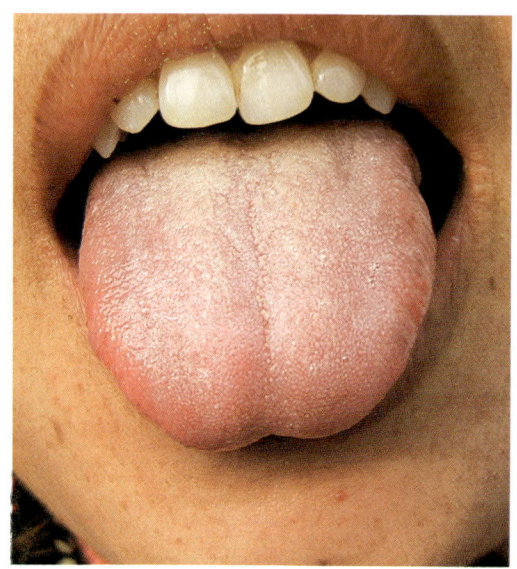

Fig 2.1-149

Patient, Female, 43years,

Case NO.: W216

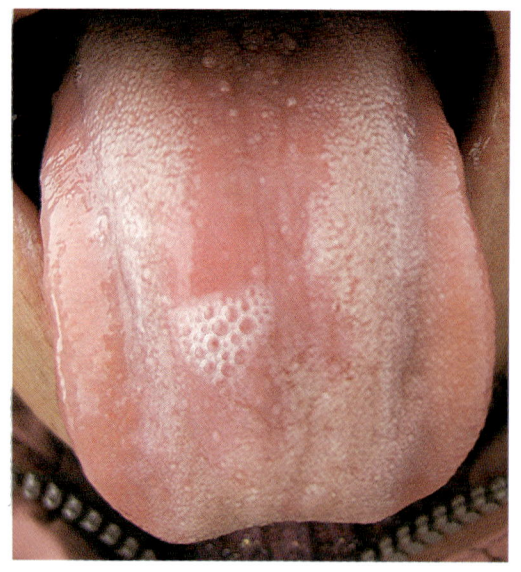

Fig 2.1-150

Patient, Female, 48years,

Case NO.: F361

Fig 2.1-151

Patient, Female, 34years,

Case NO.: W245

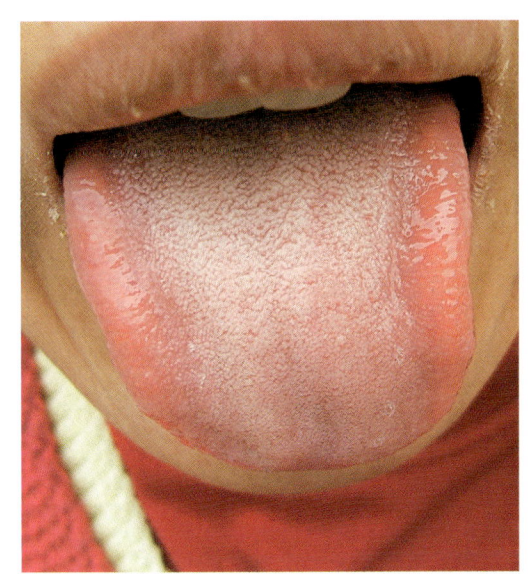

Fig 2.1-152

Patient, Male, 64years,

Case NO.: F276

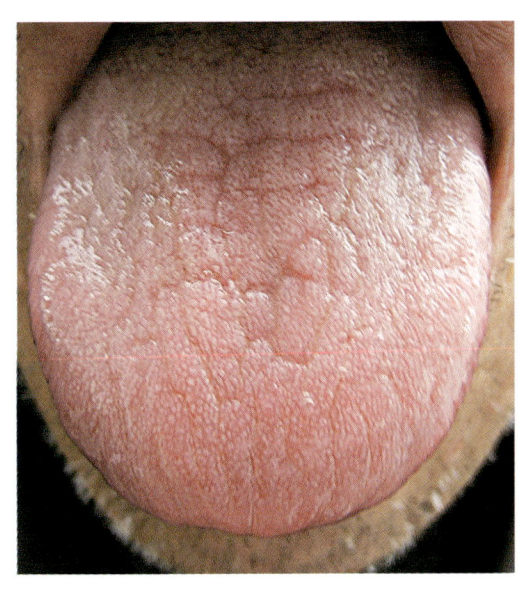

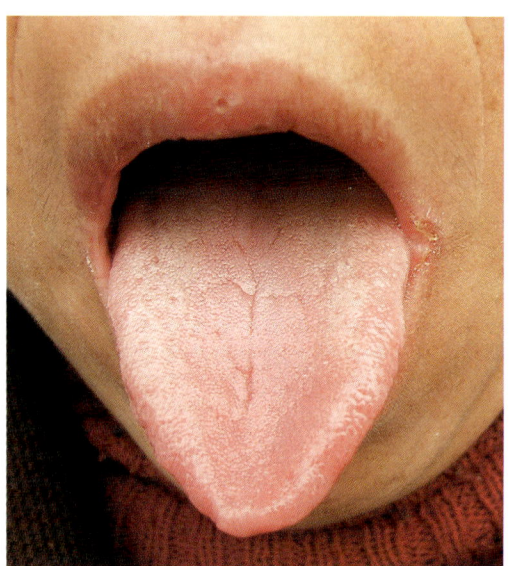

Fig 2.1-153

Patient, Female, 43years,

Case NO.: W290

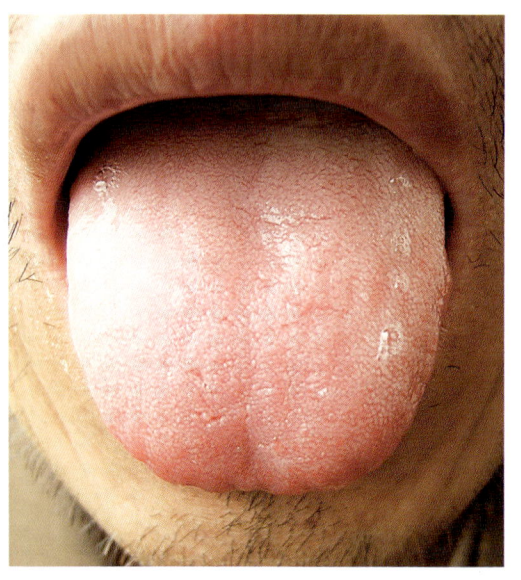

Fig 2.1-154

Patient, Male, 41years,

Case NO.: W214

Fig 2.1-155

Patient, Male, 51years,

Case NO.: W576

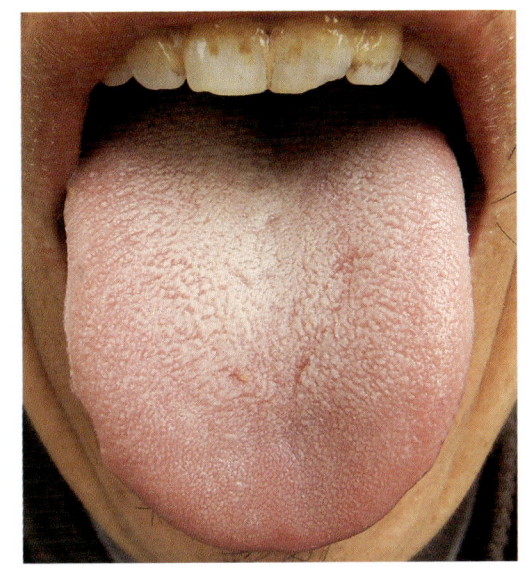

Fig 2.1-156

Patient, Male, 43years,

Case NO.: F347

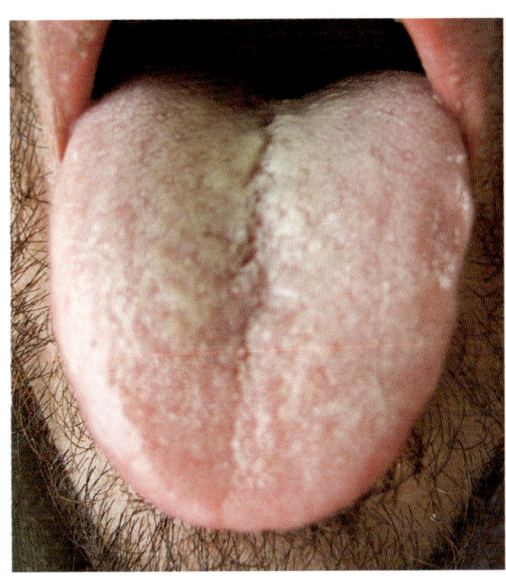

Light red tongue

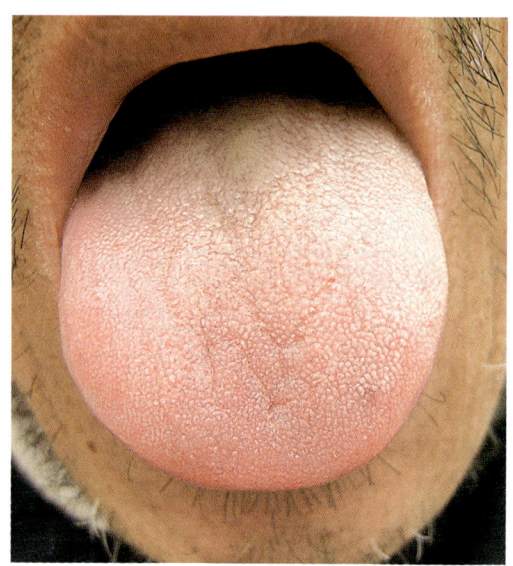

Fig 2.1-157

Patient, Male, 46years,

Case NO.: W586

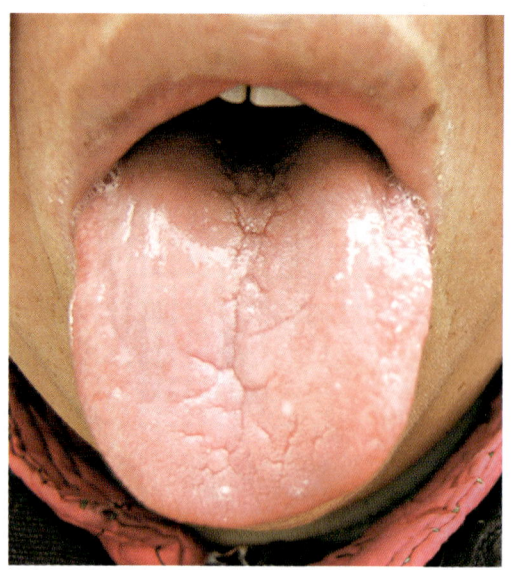

Fig 2.1-158

Patient, Female, 60years,

Case NO.: F54

Fig 2.1-159

Patient, Male, 38years,

Case NO.: F22

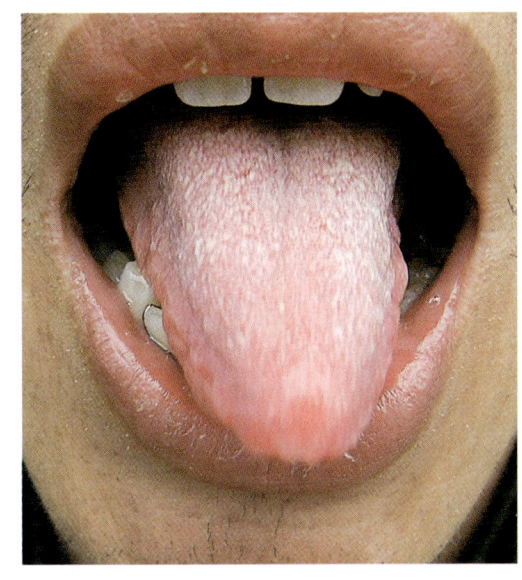

Fig 2.1-160

Patient, Female, 40years,

Case NO.: F222

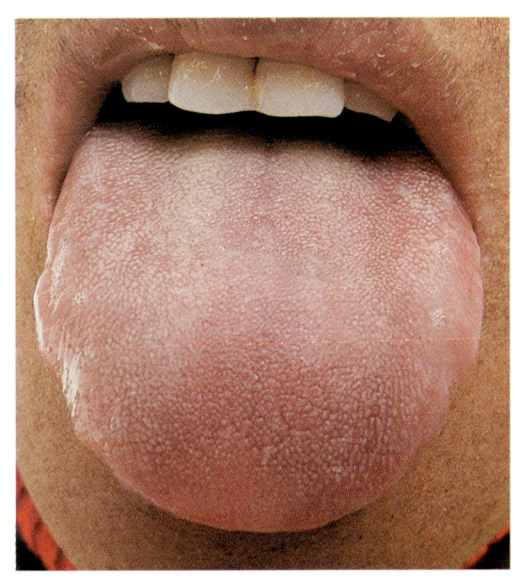

Light red tongue

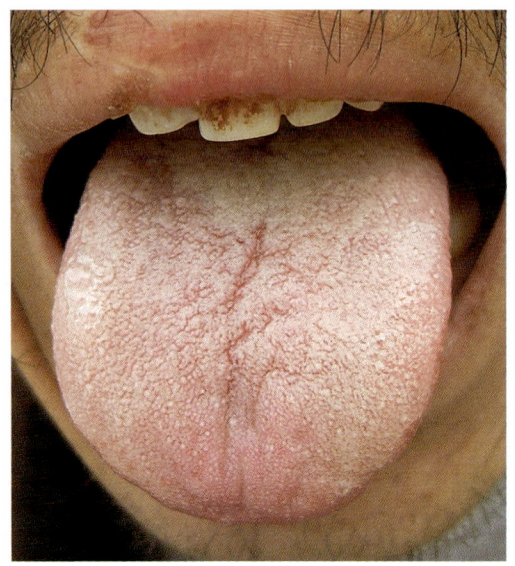

Fig 2.1-161

Patient, Male, 38years,

Case NO.: W46

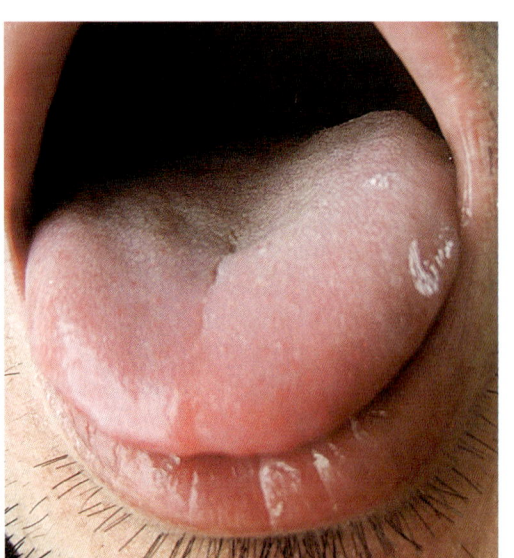

Fig 2.1-162

Patient, Male, 42years,

Case NO.: F307

Fig 2.1-163

Patient, Male, 42years,

Case NO.: F338

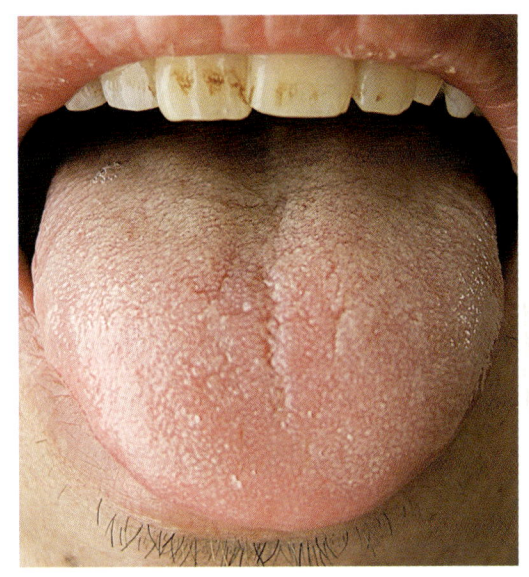

Fig 2.1-164

Patient, Male, 40years,

Case NO.: W315

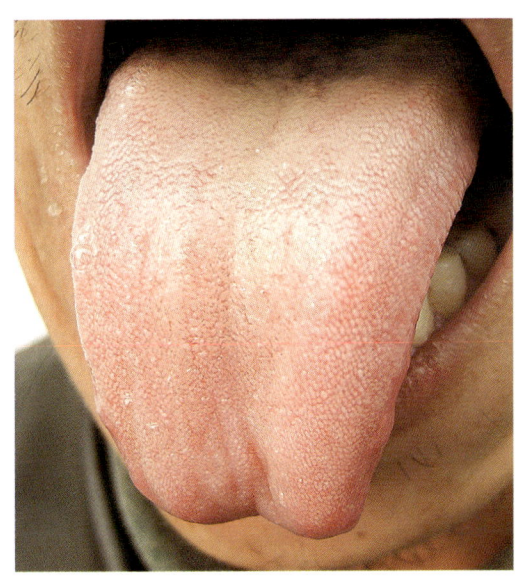

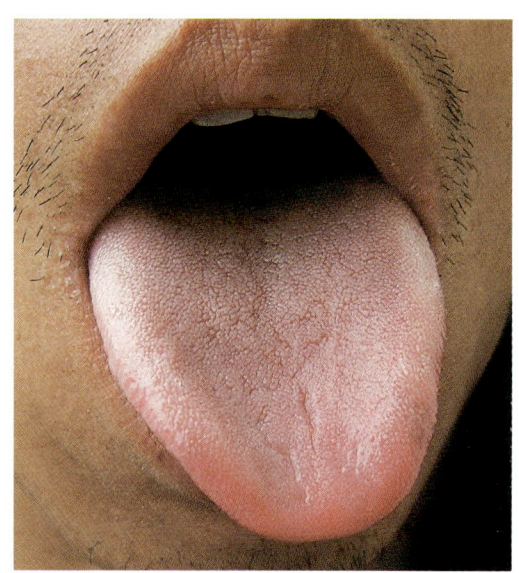

Fig 2.1-165

Patient, Male, 39years,

Case NO.: W4

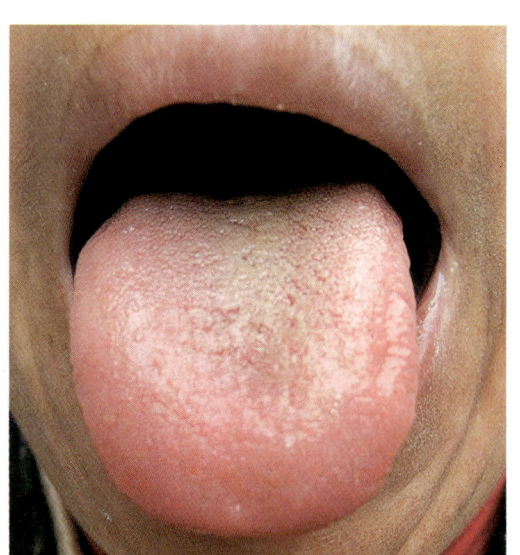

Fig 2.1-166

Patient, Female, 35years,

Case NO.: F83

Fig 2.1-167

Patient, Male, 43years,

Case NO.: W357

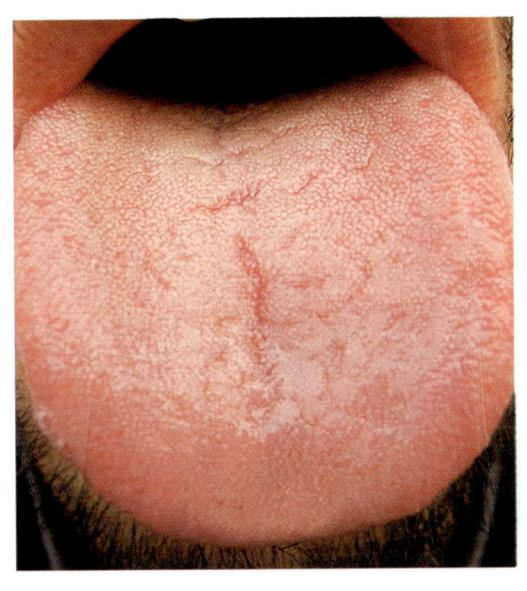

Fig 2.1-168

Patient, Male, 46years,

Case NO.: F277

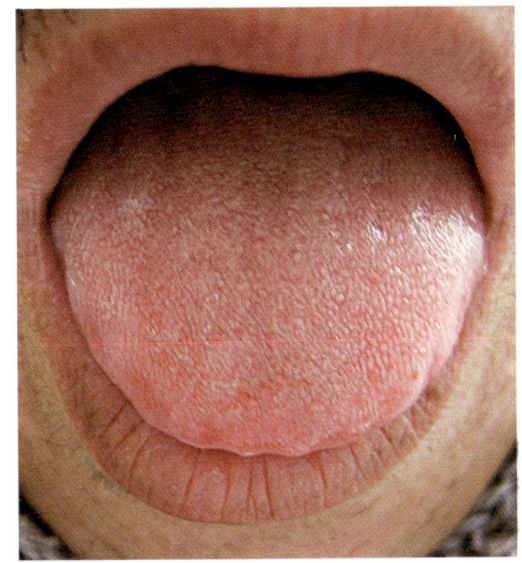

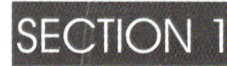

Light red tongue

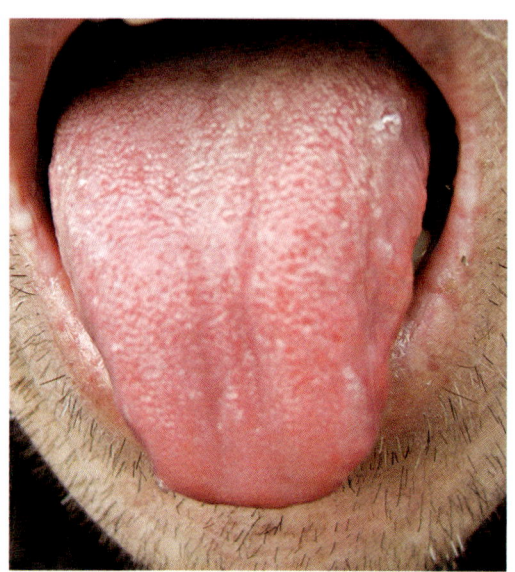

Fig 2.1-169

Patient, Male, 51years,

Case NO.: W690

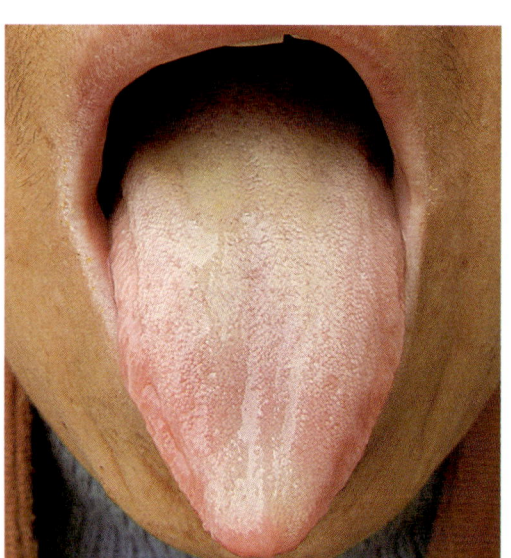

Fig 2.1-170

Patient, Female, 46years,

Case NO.: W70

Fig 2.1-171

Patient, Male, 49years,

Case NO.: W153

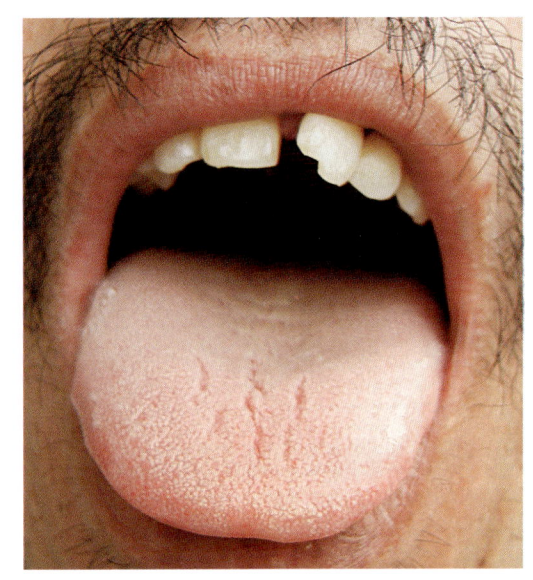

Fig 2.1-172

Patient, Female, 53years,

Case NO.: 111

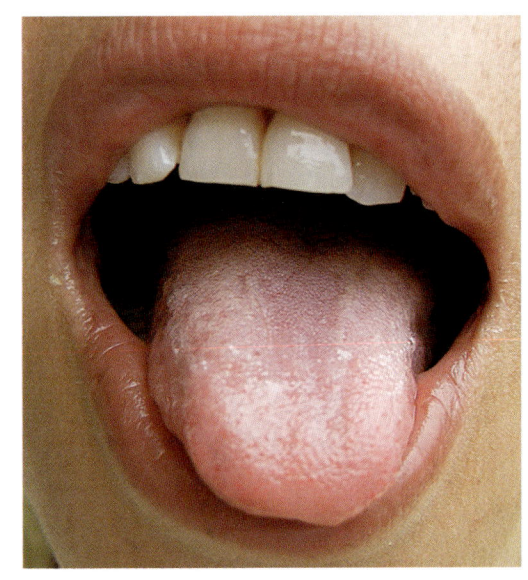

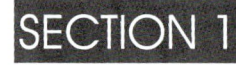

Light red tongue

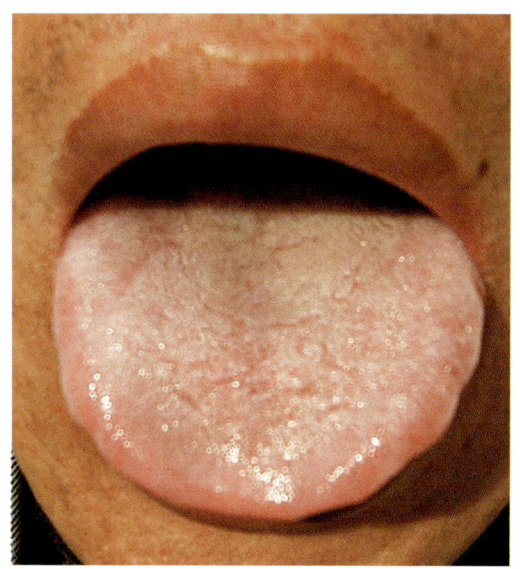

Fig 2.1-173

Patient, Male, 34years,

Case NO.: 306

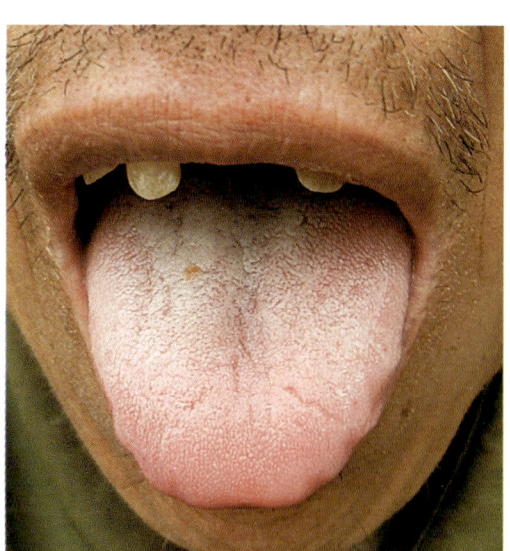

Fig 2.1-174

Patient, Male, 52years,

Case NO.: W36

Fig 2.1-175

Patient, Female, 33years,

Case NO.: F257

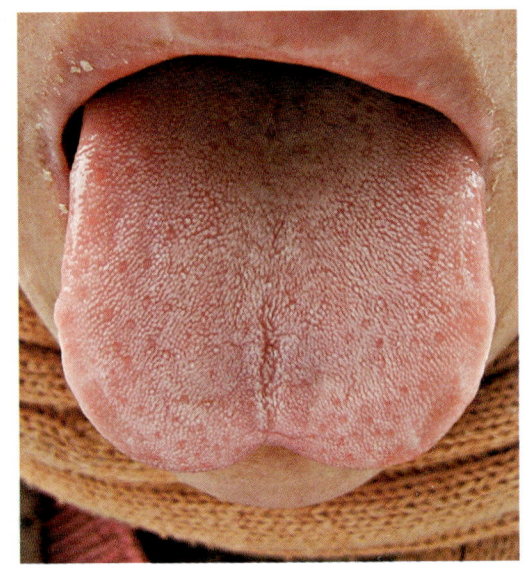

Fig 2.1-176

Patient, Male, 44years,

Case NO.: W574

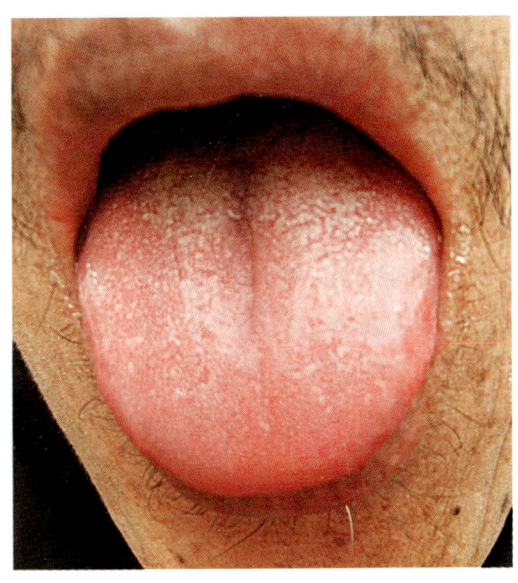

Light red tongue

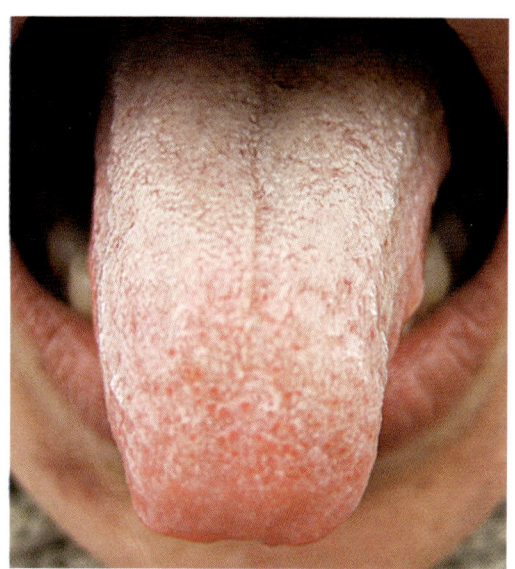

Fig 2.1-177

Patient, Male, 32years,

Case NO.: F248

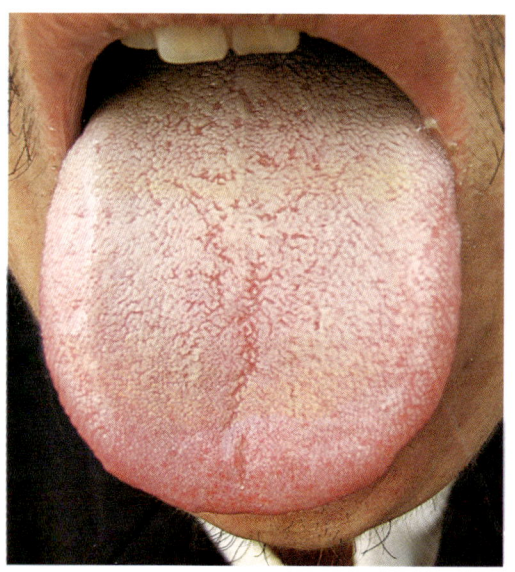

Fig 2.1-178

Patient, Male, 42years,

Case NO.: W679

Fig 2.1-179

Patient, Female, 47years,

Case NO.: W493

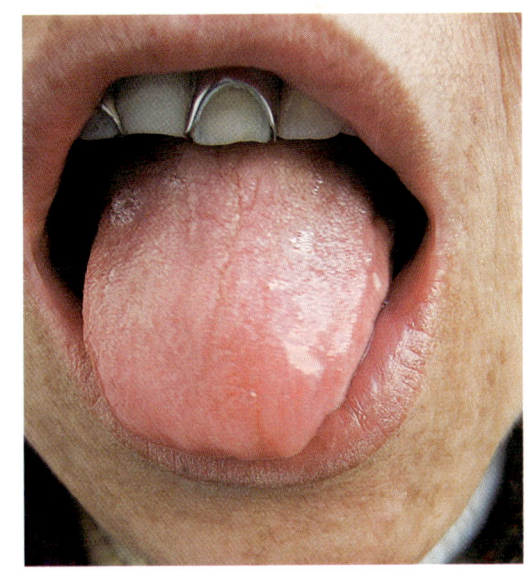

Fig 2.1-180

Patient, Male, 29years,

Case NO.: F275

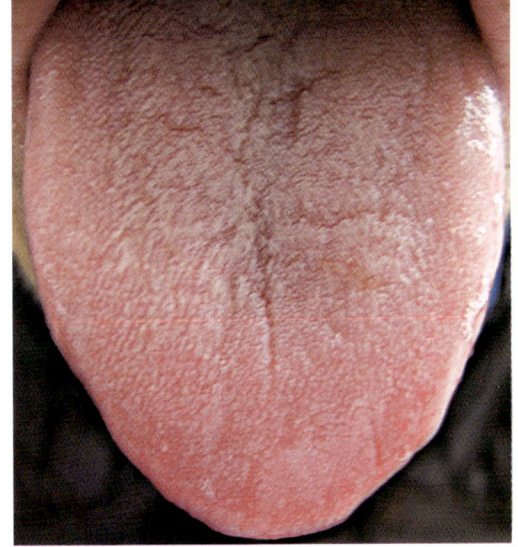

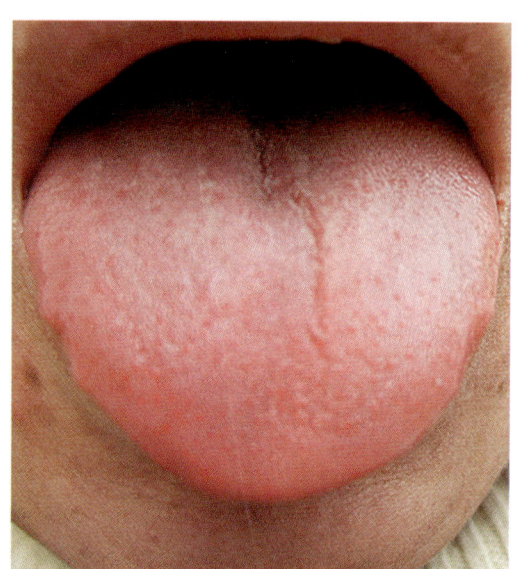

Fig 2.1-181

Patient, Female, 37years,

Case NO.: W581

Light red tongue

1.3 Red tongue

Infected with HIV yet clinically asymptomatic

Fig 2.1-182

Patient, Male, 59years,

Case NO.: W114

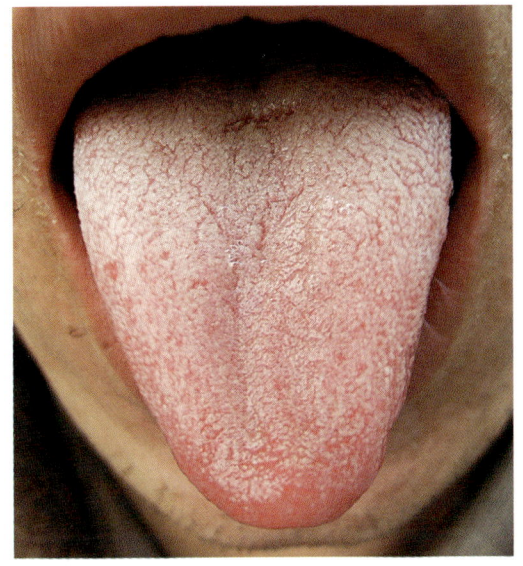

Fig 2.1-183

Patient, Male, 42years,

Case NO.: W557

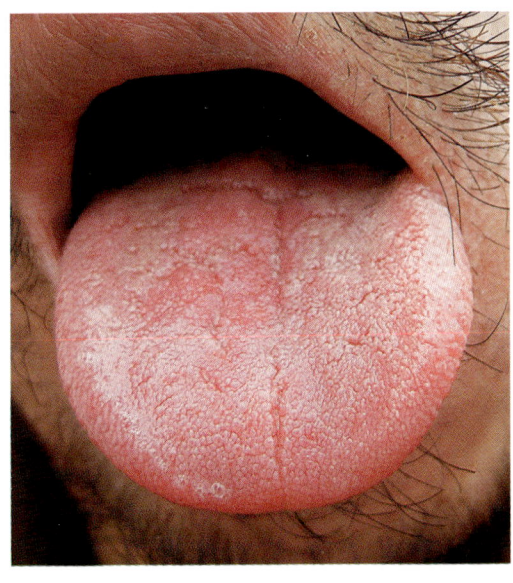

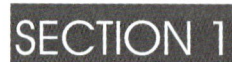

Red tongue

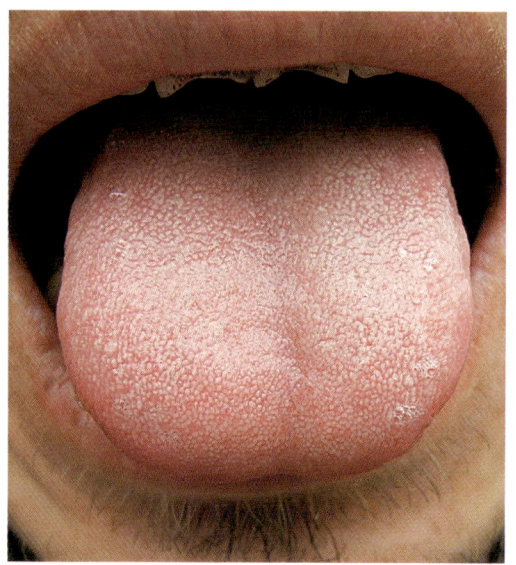

Fig 2.1-184

Patient, Male, 40years,

Case NO.: W558

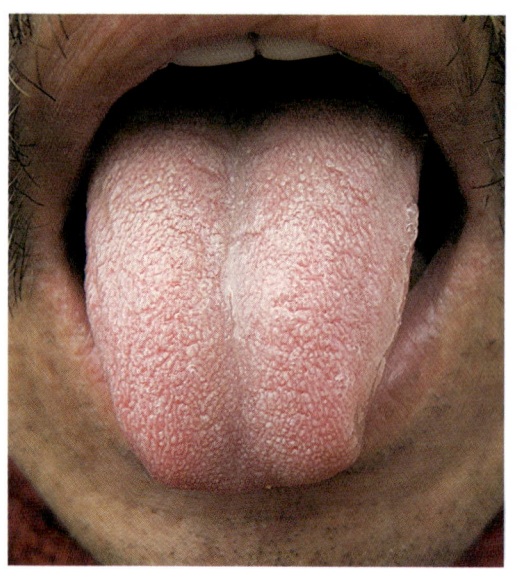

Fig 2.1-185

Patient, Male, 44years,

Case NO.: F158

Fig 2.1-186

Patient, Male, 40years,

Case NO.: W582

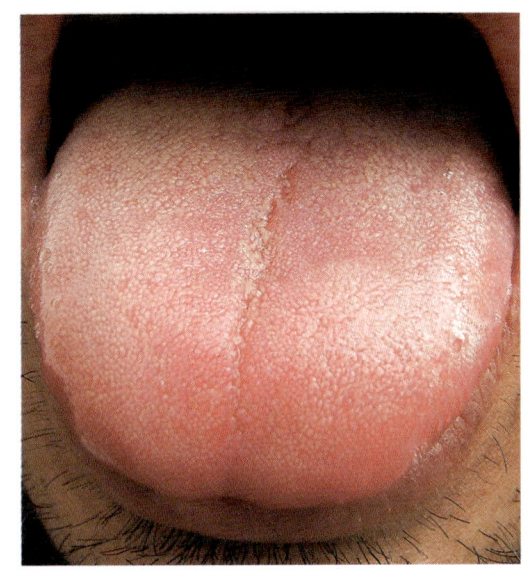

Fig 2.1-187

Patient, Female, 43years,

Case NO.: F221

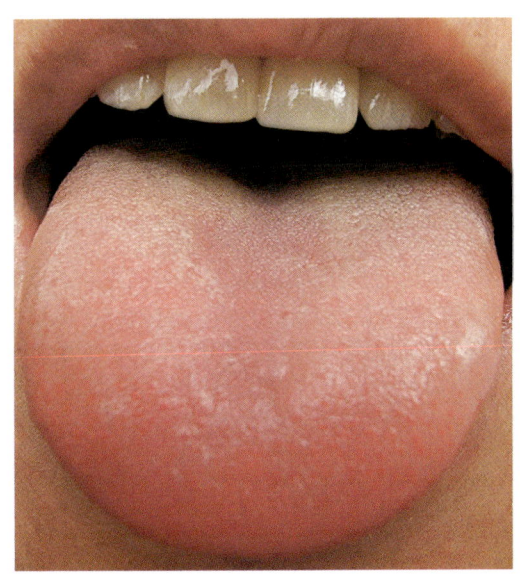

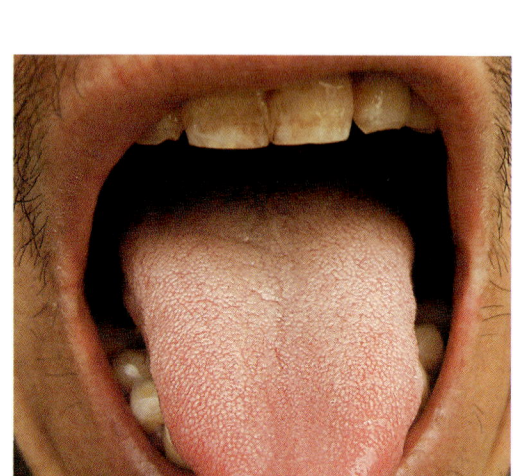

Fig 2.1-188

Patient, Male, 50years,

Case NO.: W258

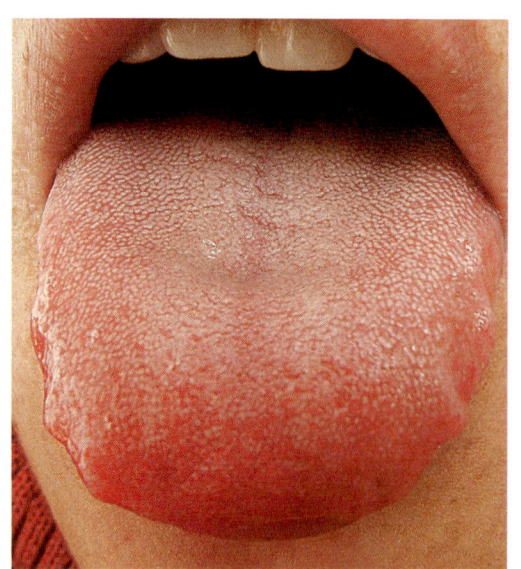

Fig 2.1-189

Patient, Female, 38years,

Case NO.: W545

Fig 2.1-190

Patient, Male, 34years,

Case NO.: W666

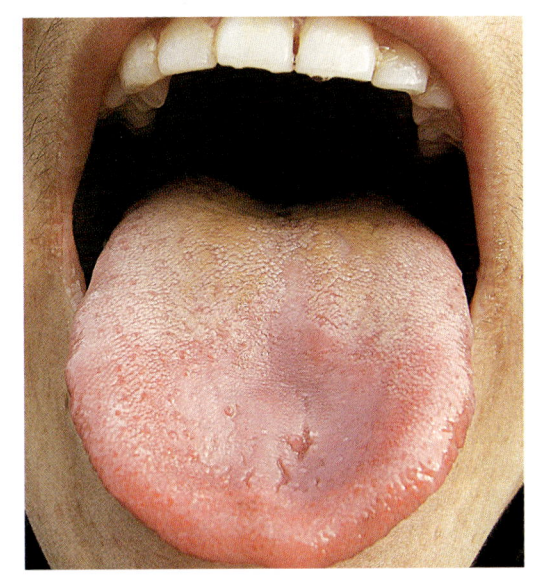

Fig 2.1-191

Patient, Male, 40years,

Case NO.: F30

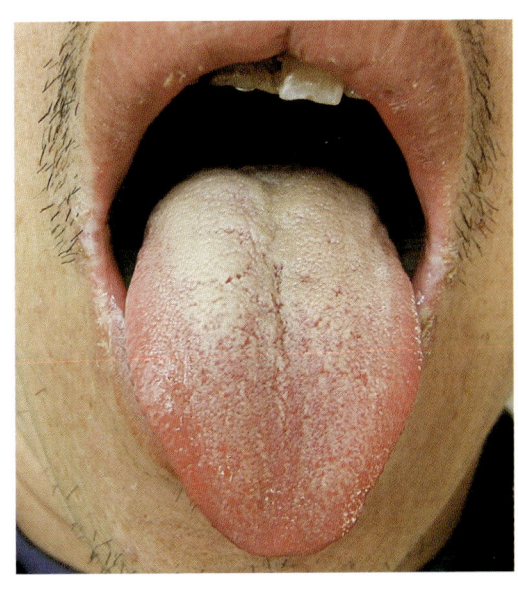

Red tongue

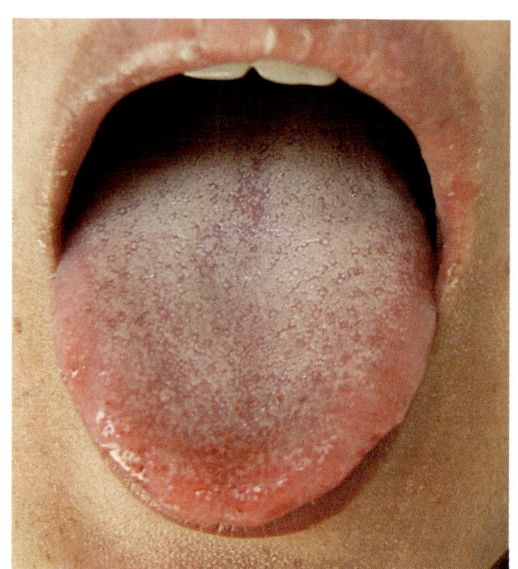

Fig 2.1-192

Patient, Male, 38years,

Case NO.: F44

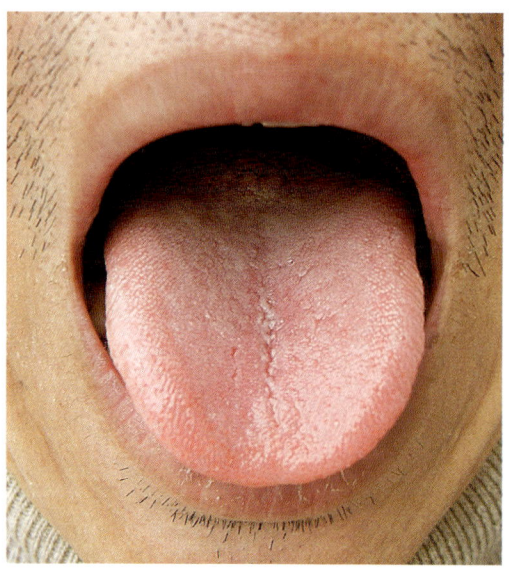

Fig 2.1-193

Patient, Male, 42years,

Case NO.: W72

Fig 2.1-194

Patient, Male, 36years,

Case NO.: W23

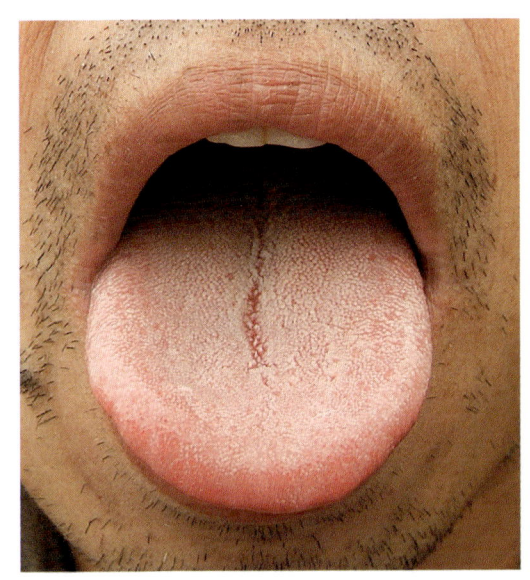

Fig 2.1-195

Patient, Female, 43years,

Case NO.: W86

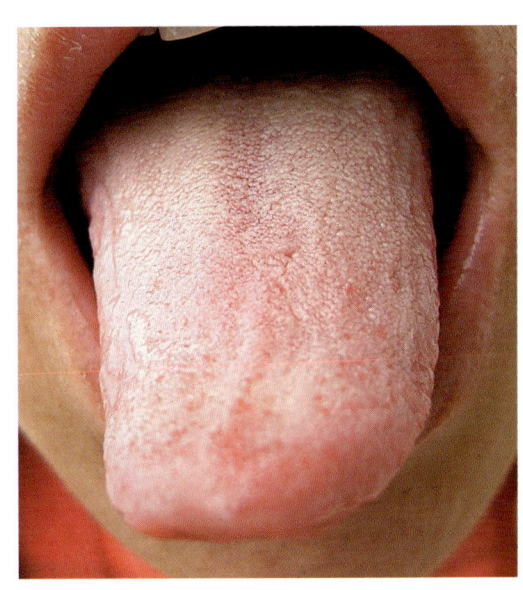

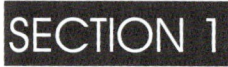

Red tongue

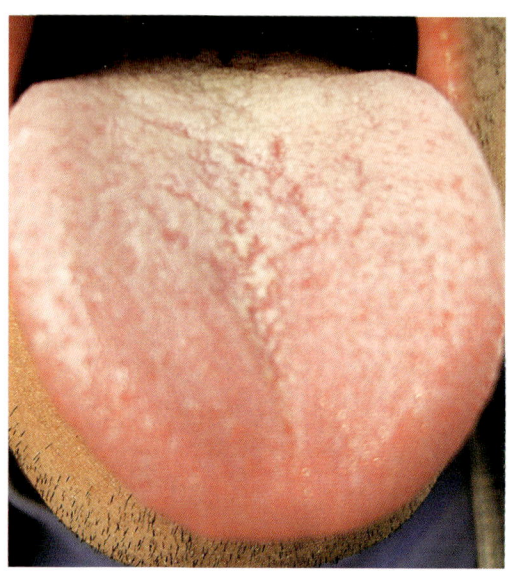

Fig 2.1-196

Patient, Male, 42years,

Case NO.: W233

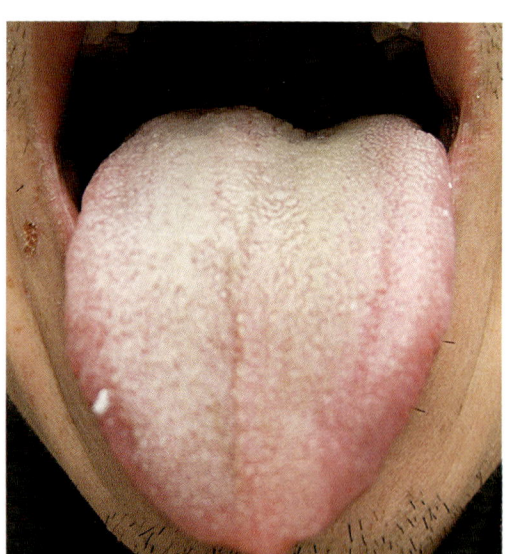

Fig 2.1-197

Patient, Male, 33years,

Case NO.: F81

Fig 2.1-198

Patient, Male, 34years,

Case NO.: F20

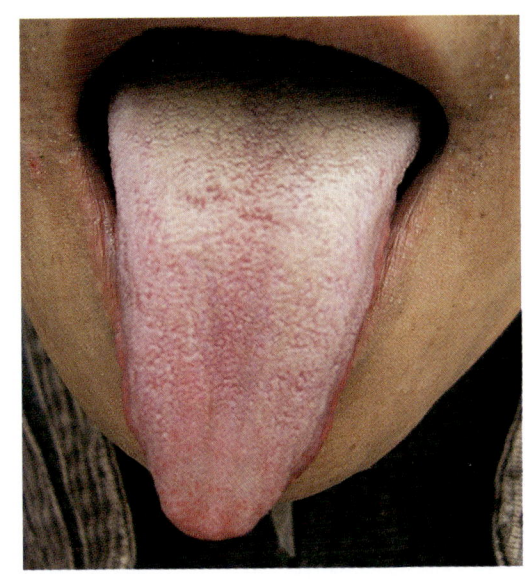

Fig 2.1-199

Patient, Male, 58years,

Case NO.: F229

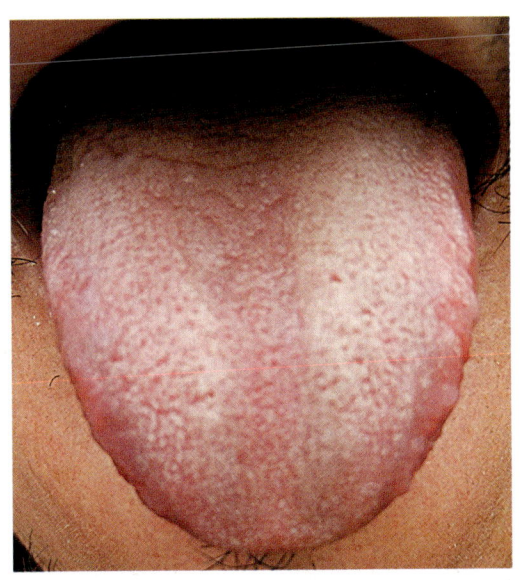

Red tongue

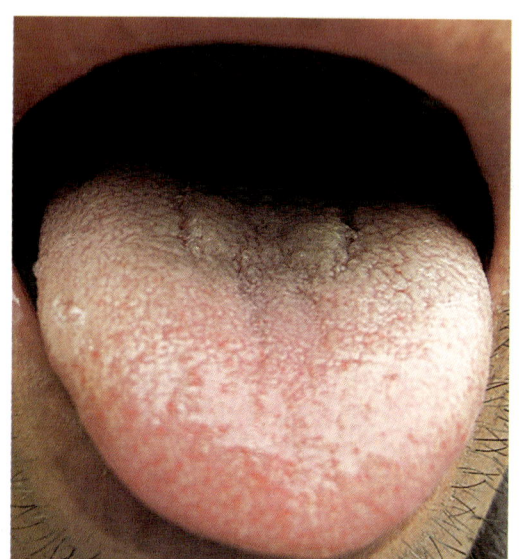

Fig 2.1-200

Patient, Male, 51years,

Case NO.: F64

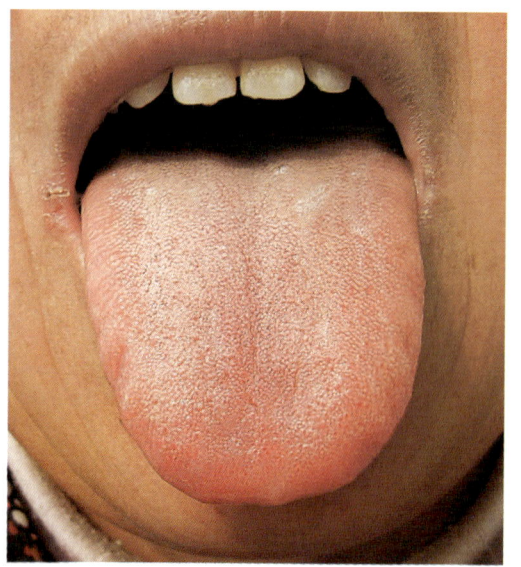

Fig 2.1-201

Patient, Female, 48years,

Case NO.: W202

Fig 2.1-202

Patient, Male, 35years,

Case NO.: W352

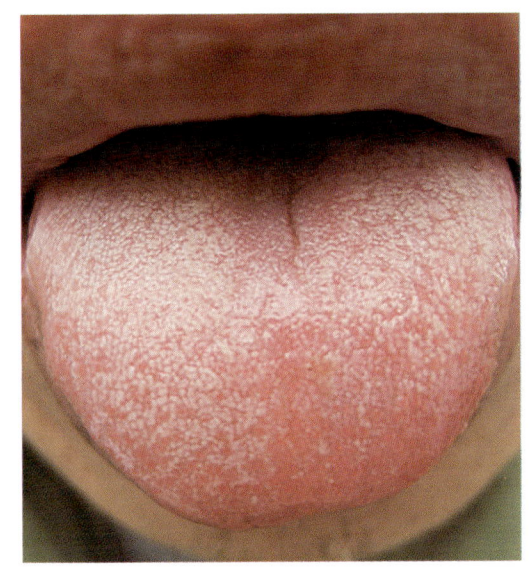

Fig 2.1-203

Patient, Male, 46years,

Case NO.: W283

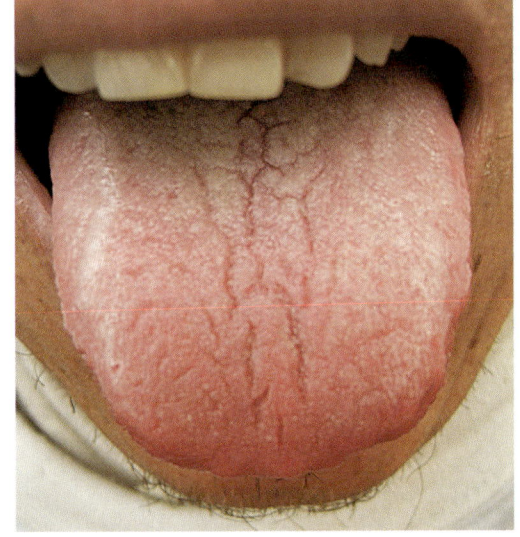

Red tongue

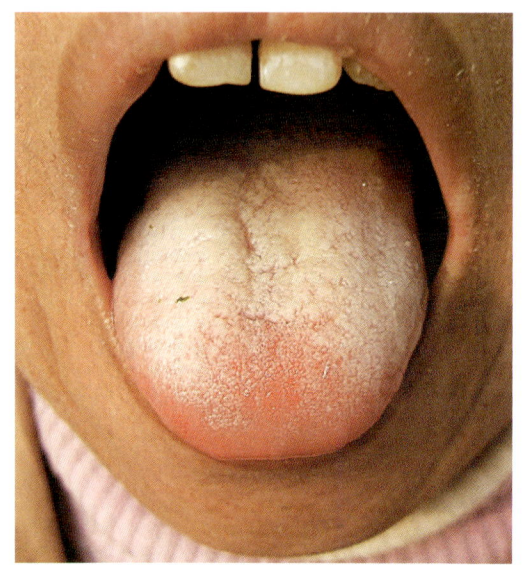

Fig 2.1-204

Patient, Female, 43years,

Case NO.: W232

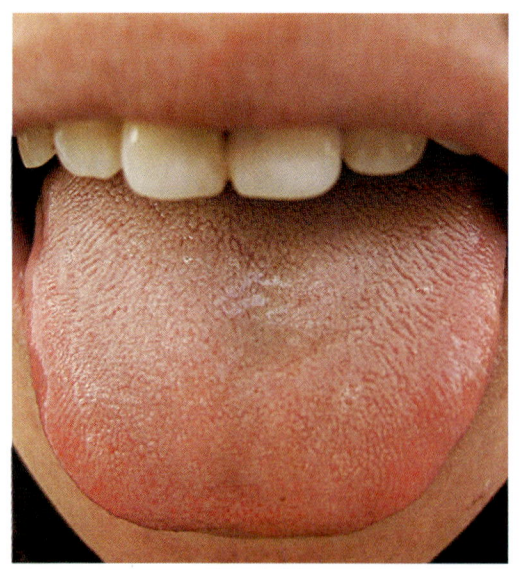

Fig 2.1-205

Patient, Female, 37years,

Case NO.: W597

Fig 2.1-206

Patient, Male, 52years,

Case NO.: W224

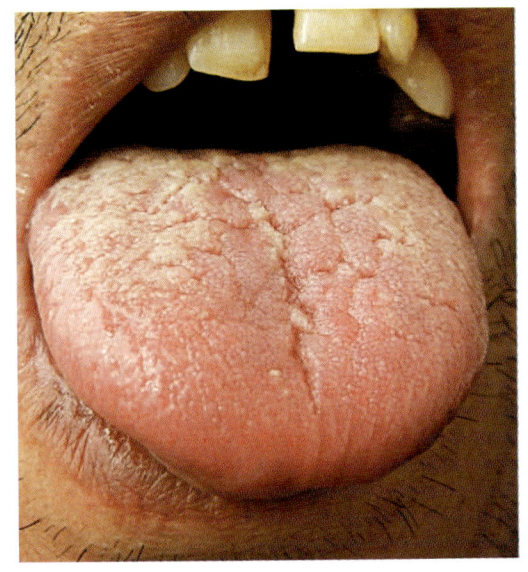

Fig 2.1-207

Patient, Female, 39years,

Case NO.: W127

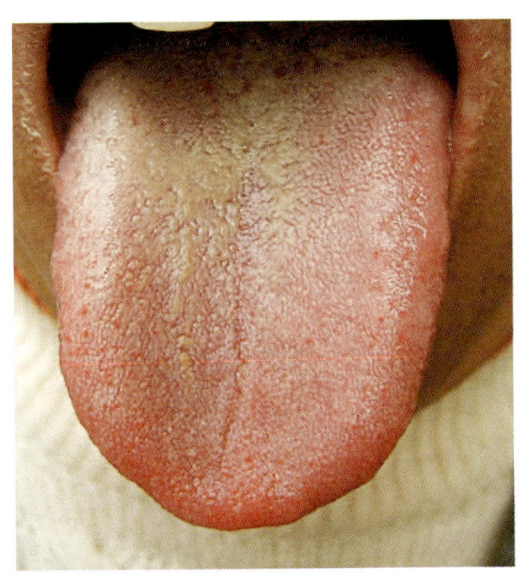

Red tongue

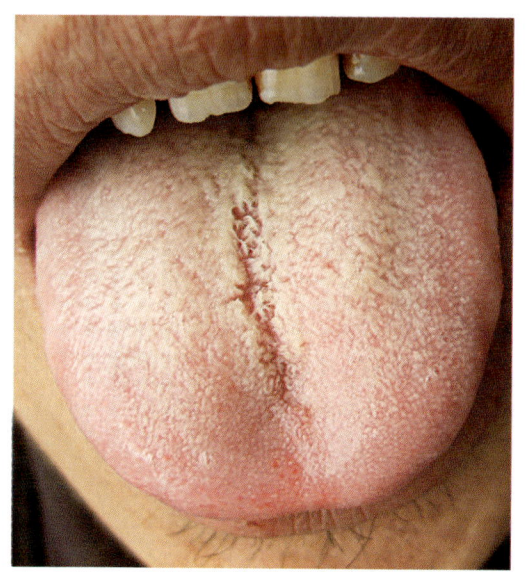

Fig 2.1-208

Patient, Male, 55years,

Case NO.: F334

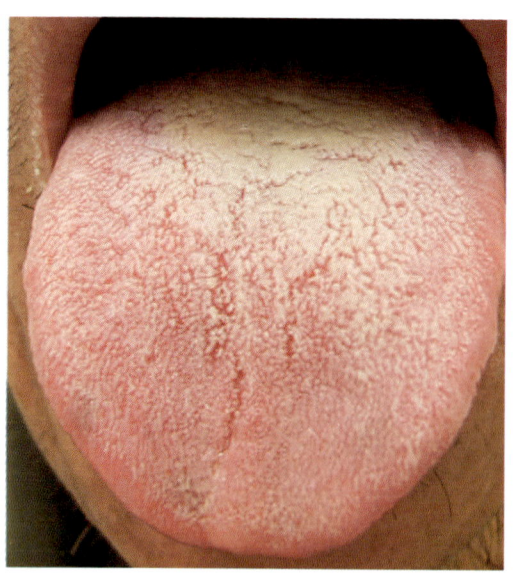

Fig 2.1-209

Patient, Male, 48years,

Case NO.: W133

Fig 2.1-210

Patient, Female, 38years,

Case NO.: W205

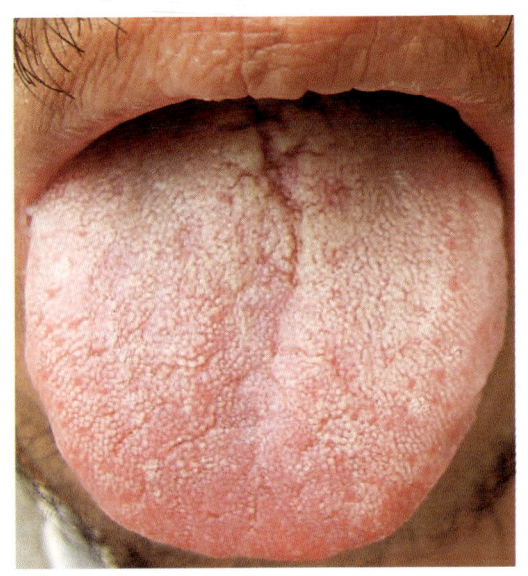

Fig 2.1-211

Patient, Male, 35years,

Case NO.: W731

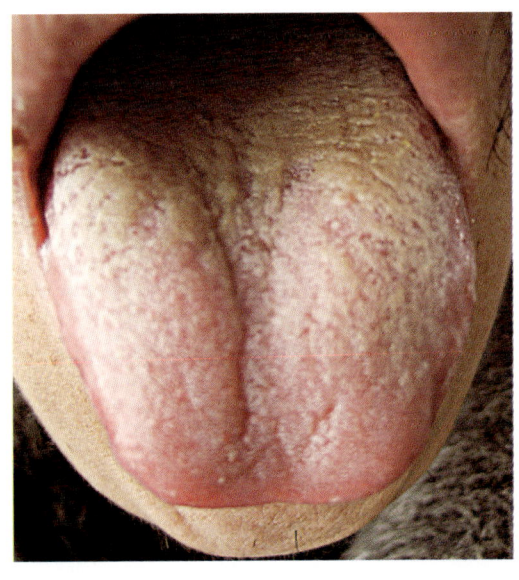

Red tongue

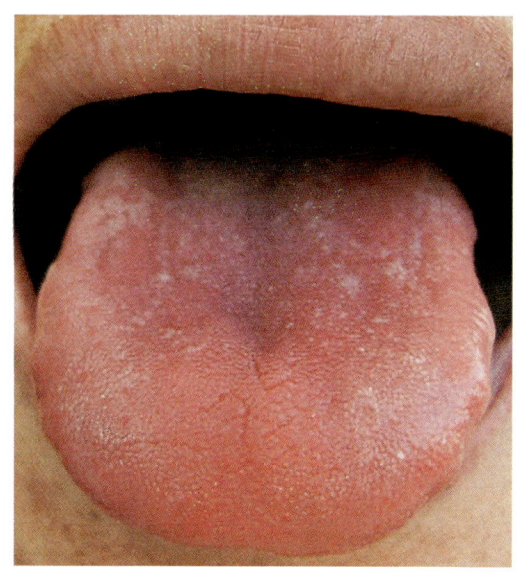

Fig 2.1-212

Patient, Female, 30years,

Case NO.: W464

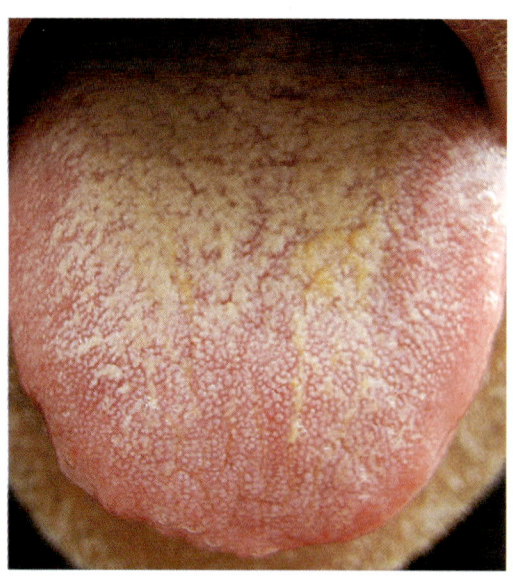

Fig 2.1-213

Patient, Male, 59years,

Case NO.: F101

Fig 2.1-214

Patient, Female, 38years,

Case NO.: W490

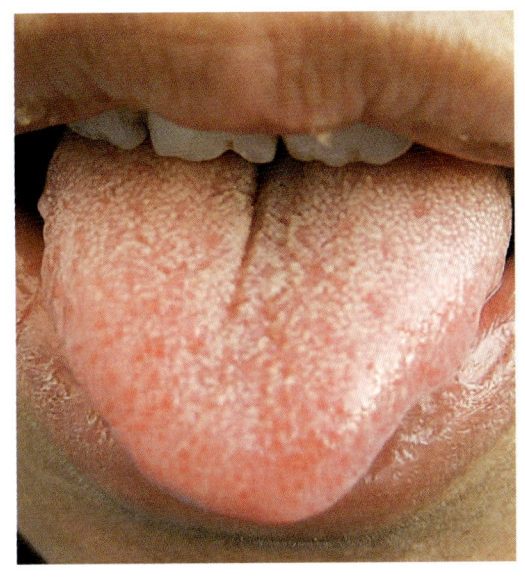

Fig 2.1-215

Patient, Male, 52years,

Case NO.: F114

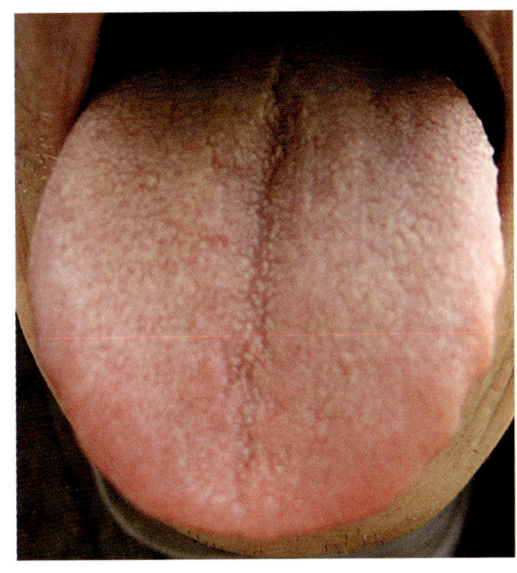

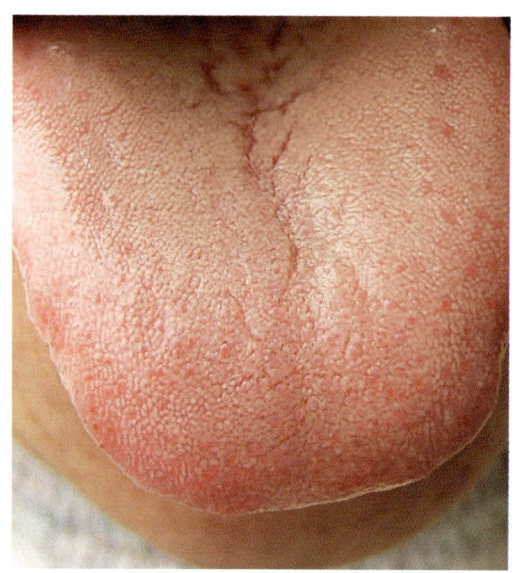

Fig 2.1-216

Patient, Female, 40years,

Case NO.: W193

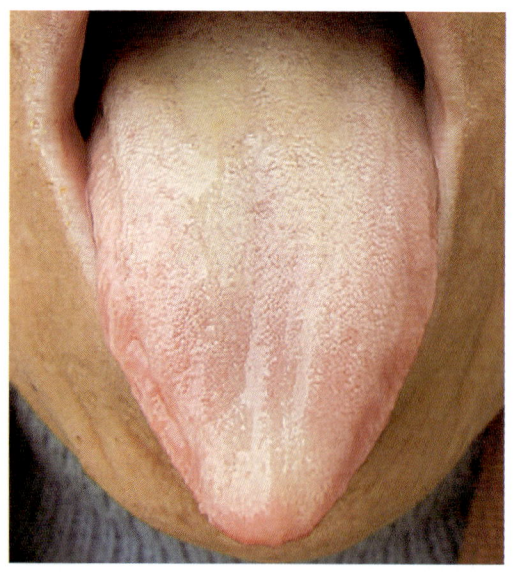

Fig 2.1-217

Patient, Female, 46years,

Case NO.: W70

Red tongue

Fig 2.1-218

Patient, Male, 55years,

Case NO.: W637

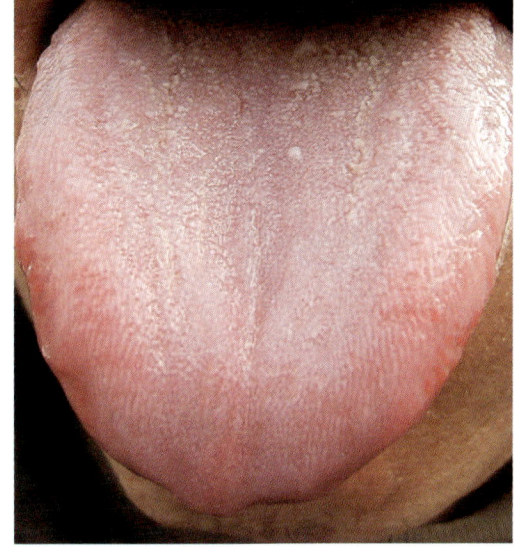

Fig 2.1-219

Patient, Female, 36years,

Case NO.: F68

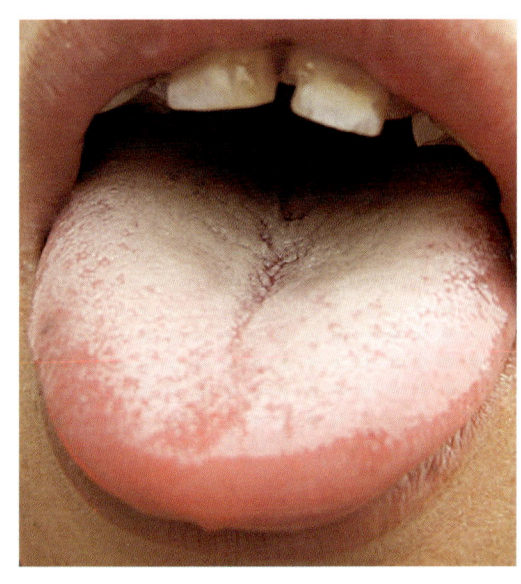

Red tongue

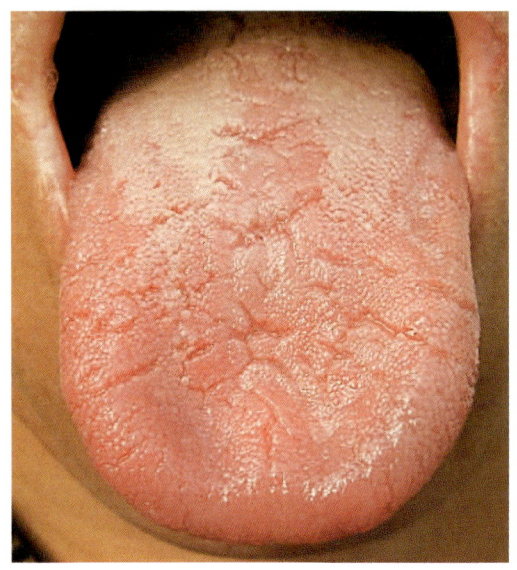

Fig 2.1-220

Patient, Female, 42years,

Case NO.: W225

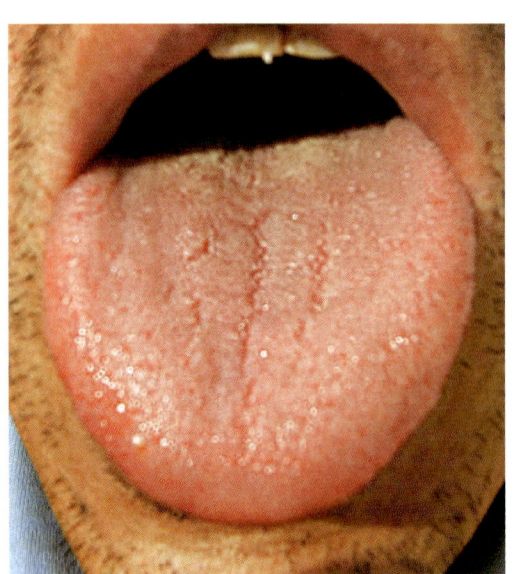

Fig 2.1-221

Patient, Male, 36years,

Case NO.: 234

Fig 2.1-222

Patient, Female, 50years,

Case NO.: 311

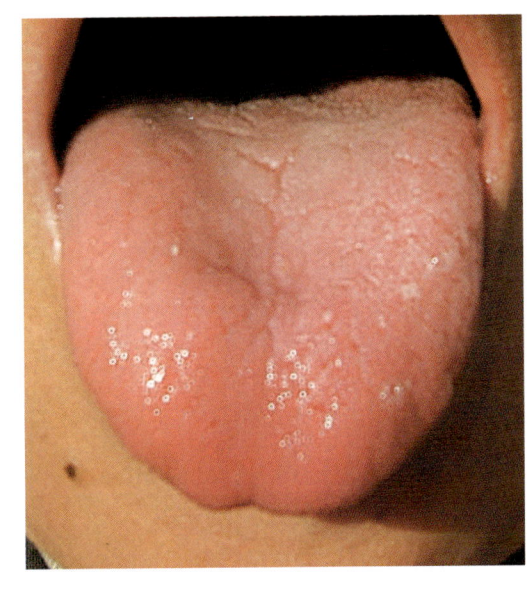

Fig 2.1-223

Patient, Female, 36years,

Case NO.: W164

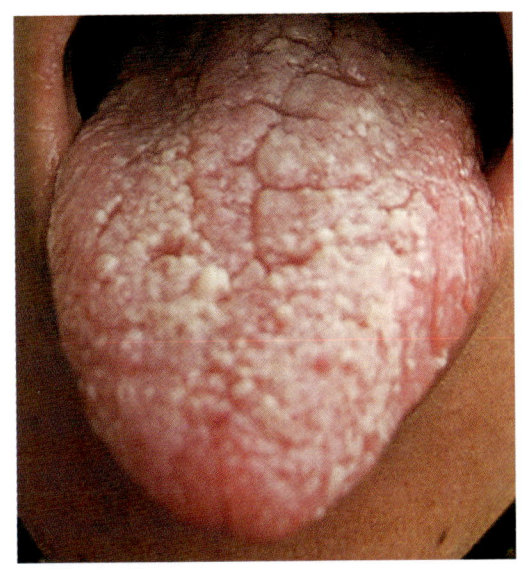

Red tongue

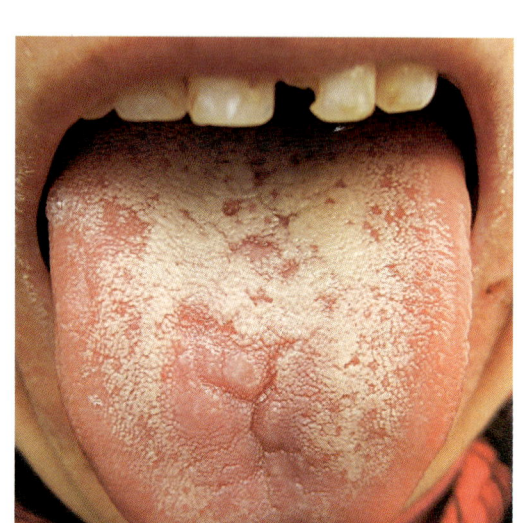

Fig 2.1-224

Patient, Female, 41years,

Case NO.: W355

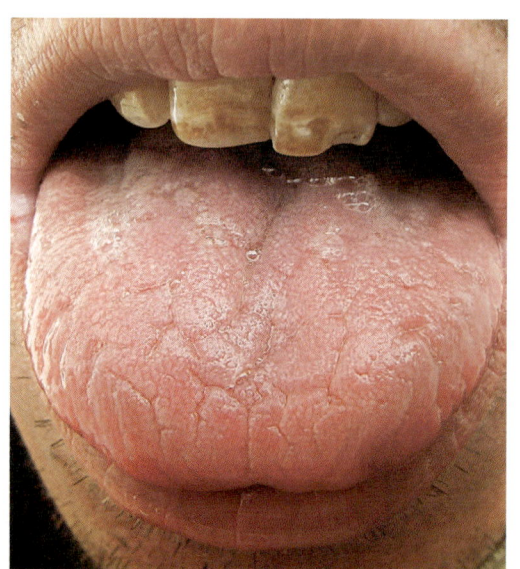

Fig 2.1-225

Patient, Male, 49years,

Case NO.: F227

Fig 2.1-226

Patient, Male, 37years,

Case NO.: W27

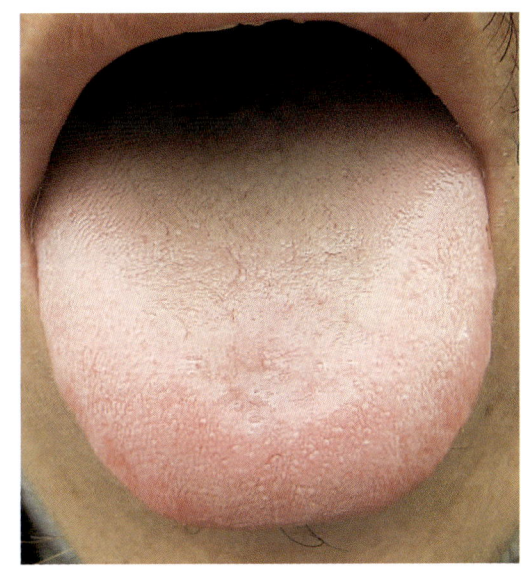

Fig 2.1-227

Patient, Male, 34years,

Case NO.: W307

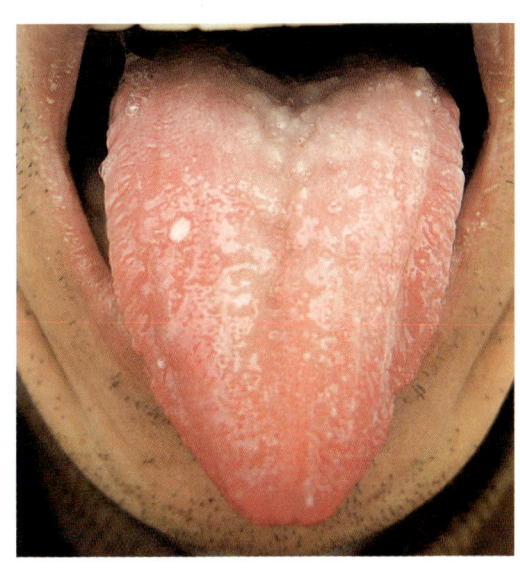

Red tongue

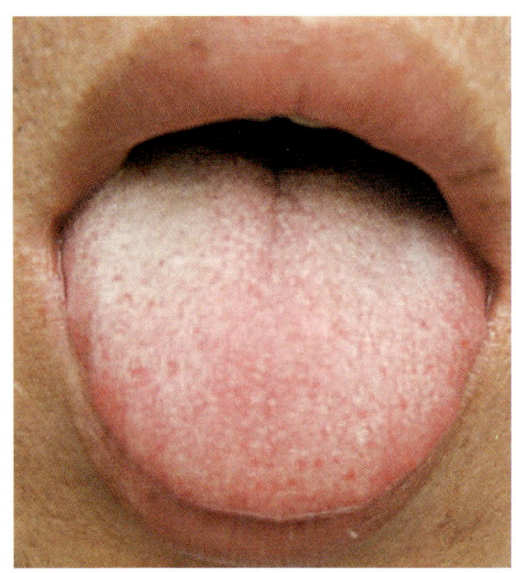

Fig 2.1-228

Patient, Male, 36years,

Case NO.: W117

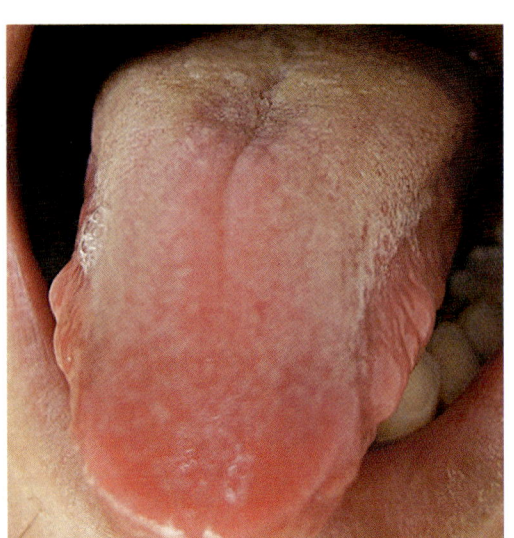

Fig 2.1-229

Patient, Male, 35years,

Case NO.: F21

Fig 2.1-230

Patient, Female, 39years,

Case NO.: W228

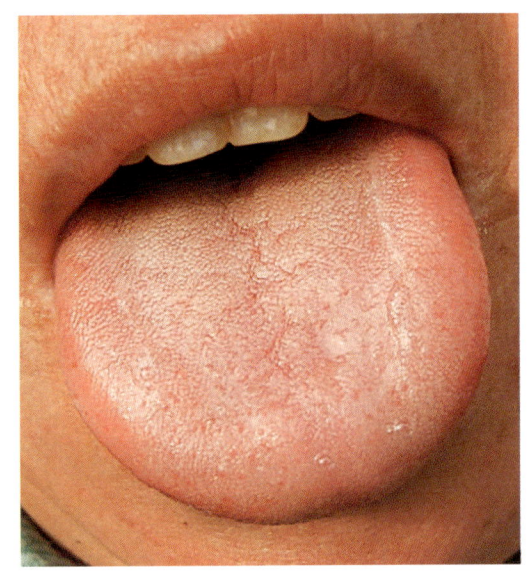

Fig 2.1-231

Patient, Male, 34years,

Case NO.: W590

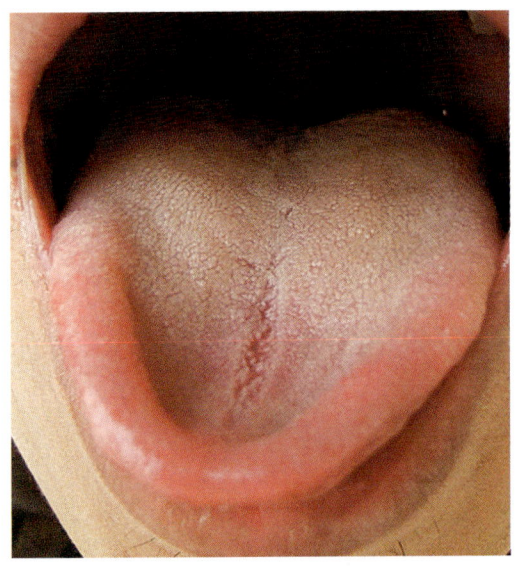

Red tongue

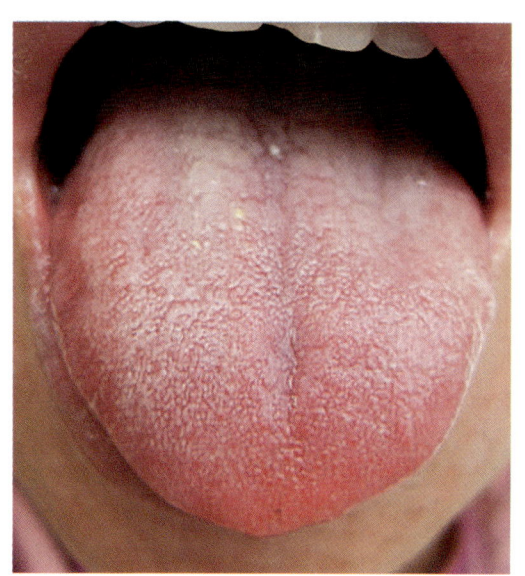

Fig 2.1-232

Patient, Male, 34years,

Case NO.: 308

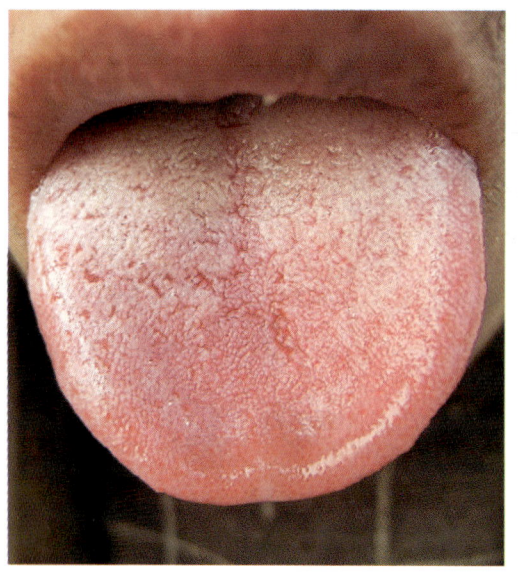

Fig 2.1-233

Patient, Male, 35years,

Case NO.: W360

CHAPTER ONE

Fig 2.1-234

Patient, Female, 40years,

Case NO.: W565

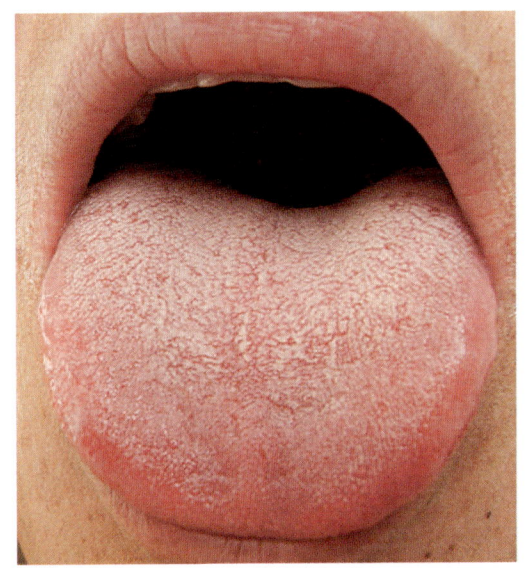

Fig 2.1-235

Patient, Female, 44years,

Case NO.: F236

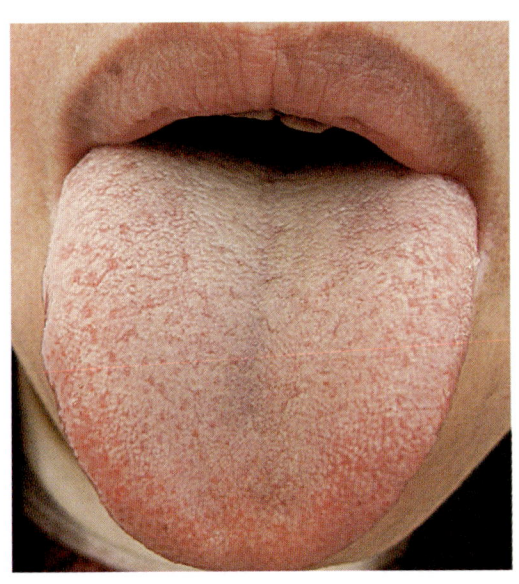

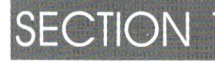

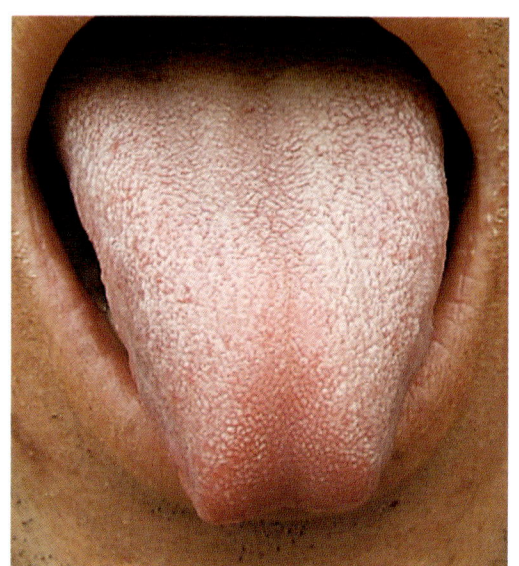

Fig 2.1-236

Patient, Male, 34years,

Case NO.: W38

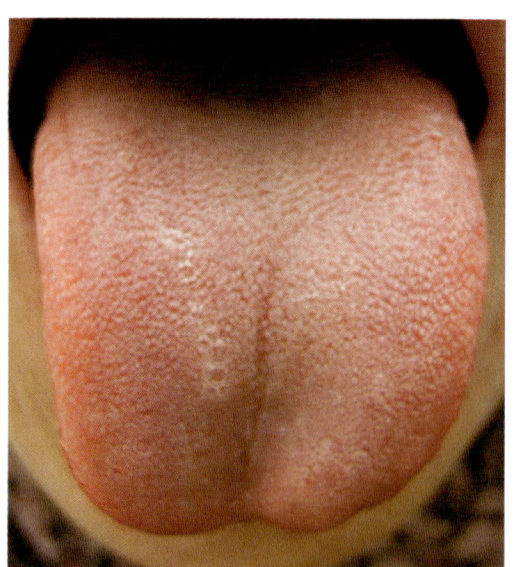

Fig 2.1-237

Patient, Female, 49years,

Case NO.: F145

Fig 2.1-238

Patient, Female, 48years,

Case NO.: F267

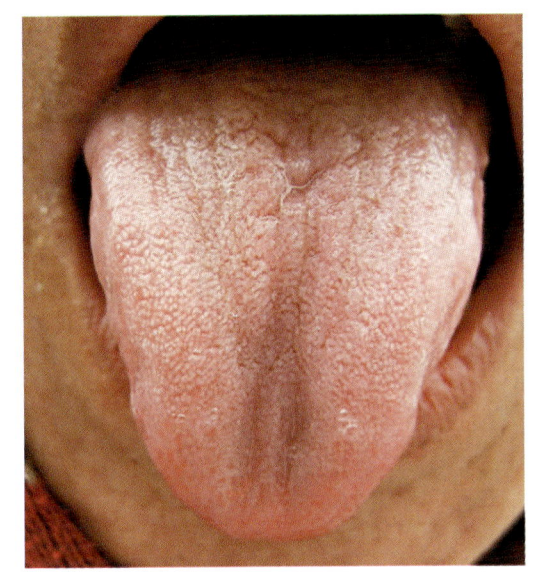

Fig 2.1-239

Patient, Male, 45years,

Case NO.: W660

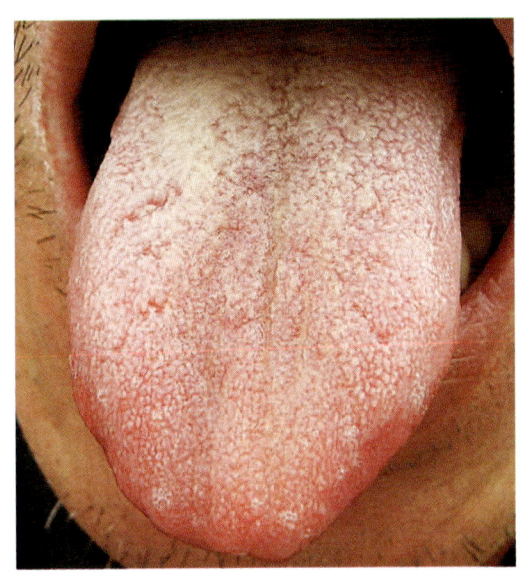

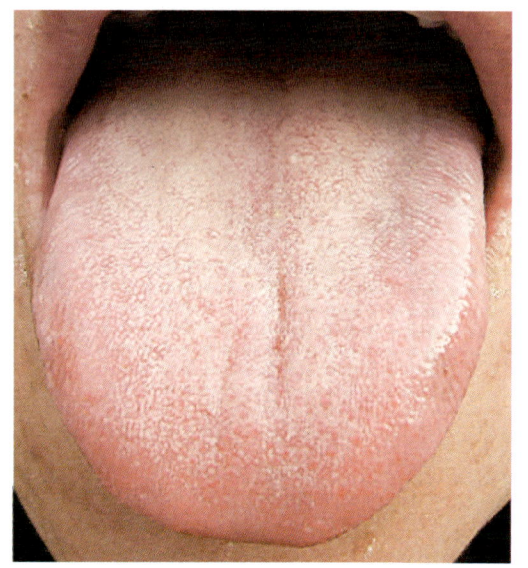

Fig 2.1-240

Patient, Female, 58years,

Case NO.: W641

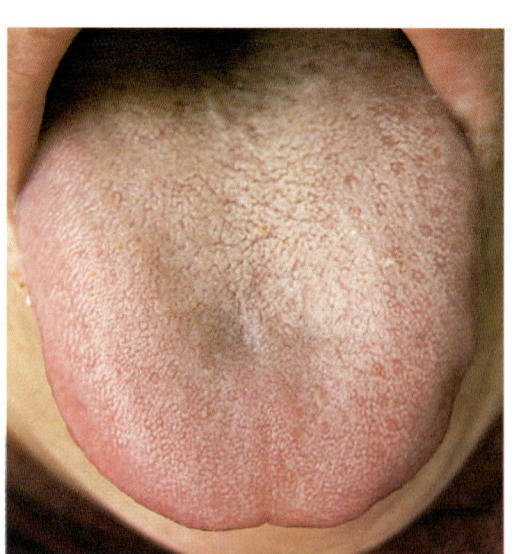

Fig 2.1-241

Patient, Female, 52years,

Case NO.: F336

Fig 2.1-242

Patient, Male, 41years,

Case NO.: W630

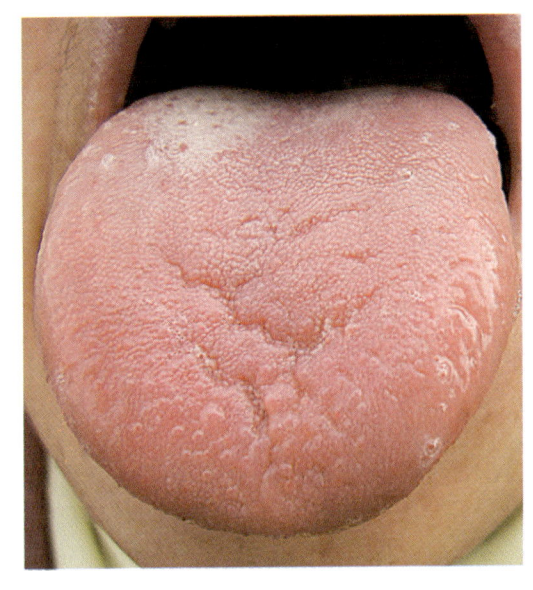

Fig 2.1-243

Patient, Male, 42years,

Case NO.: W698

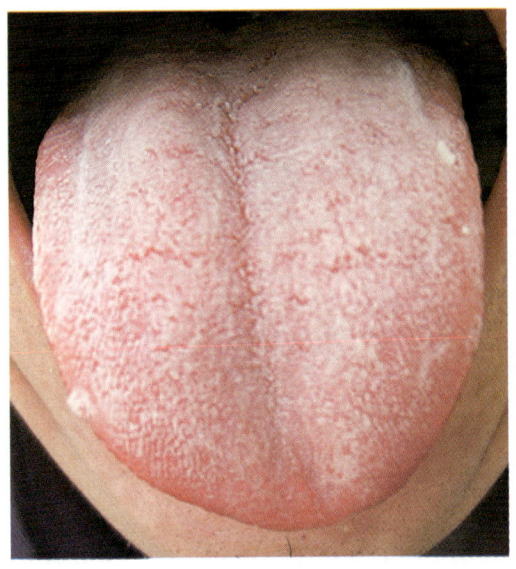

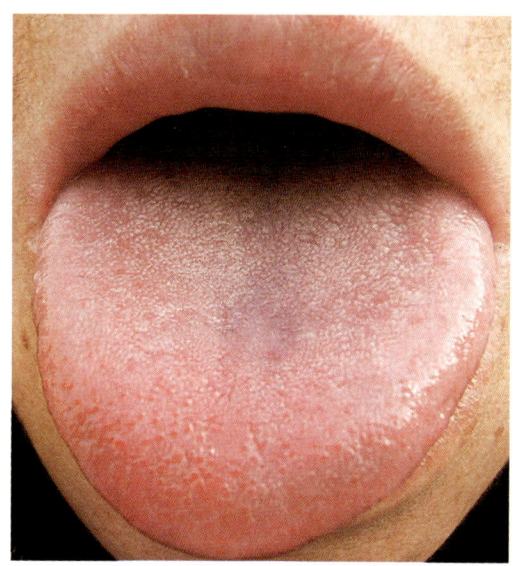

Fig 2.1-244

Patient, Female, 48years,

Case NO.: W636

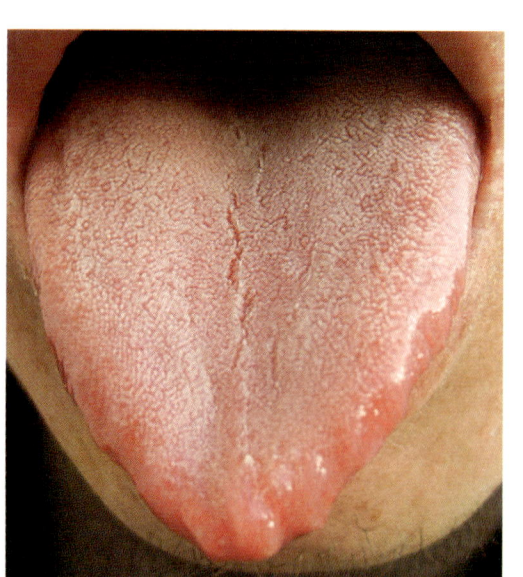

Fig 2.1-245

Patient, Male, 43years,

Case NO.: F207

Fig 2.1-246

Patient, Male, 48years,

Case NO.: W588

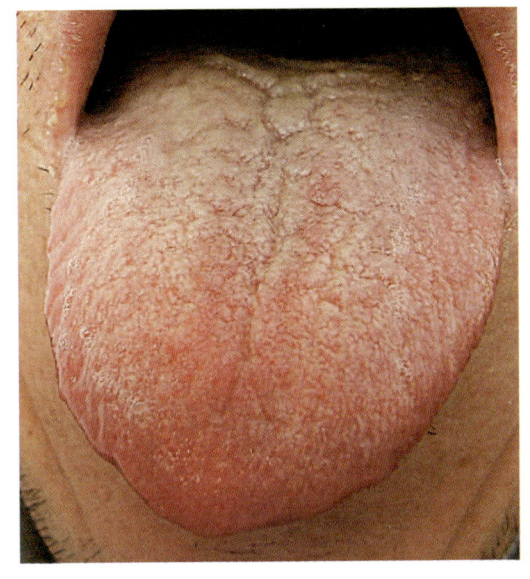

Fig 2.1-247

Patient, Male, 38years,

Case NO.: W115

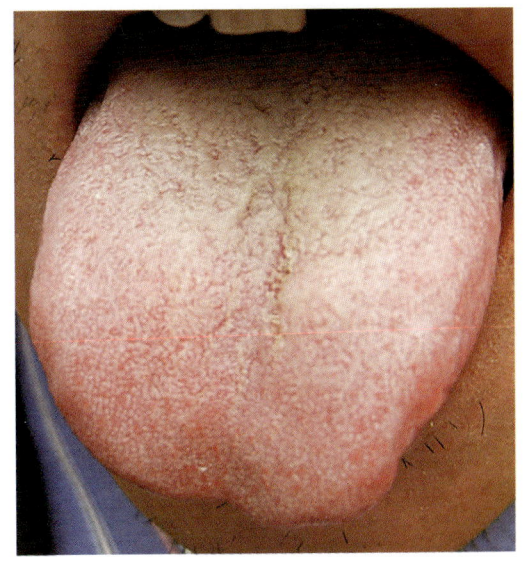

Red tongue

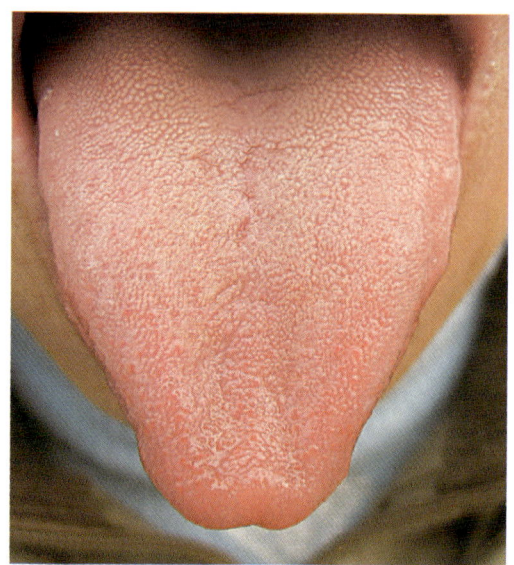

Fig 2.1-248

Patient, Female, 41years,

Case NO.: W350

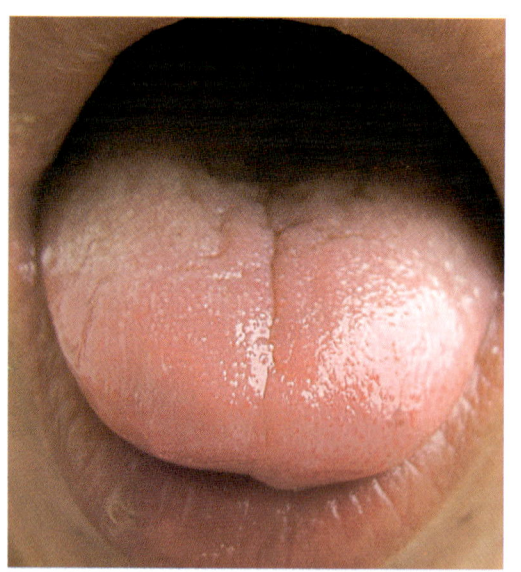

Fig 2.1-249

Patient, Female, 32years,

Case NO.: 133

Fig 2.1-250

Patient, Male, 45years,

Case NO.: F266

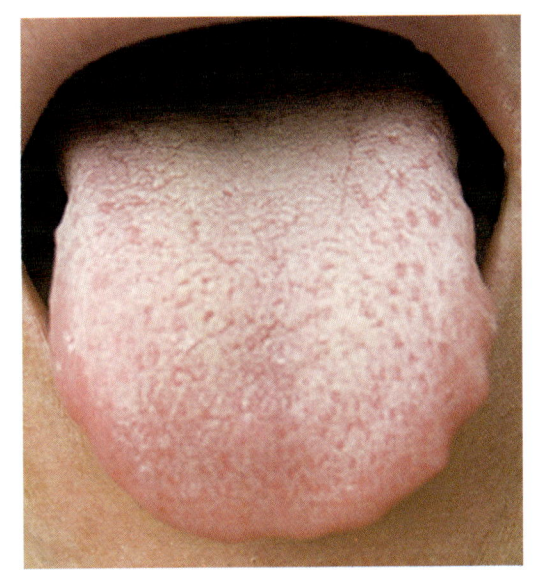

Fig 2.1-251

Patient, Female, 36years,

Case NO.: F351

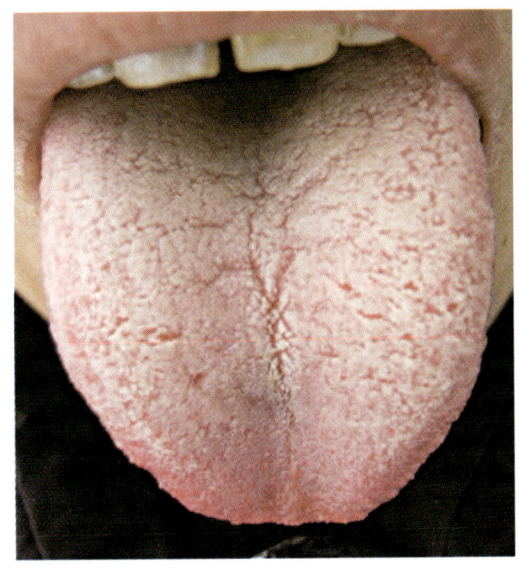

Red tongue

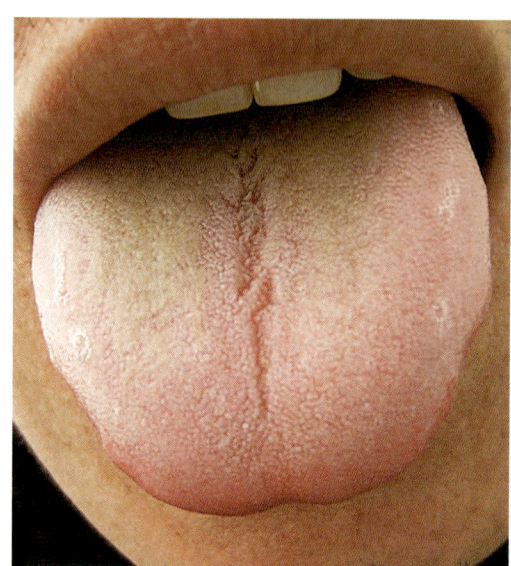

Fig 2.1-252

Patient, Male, 37years,

Case NO.: W752

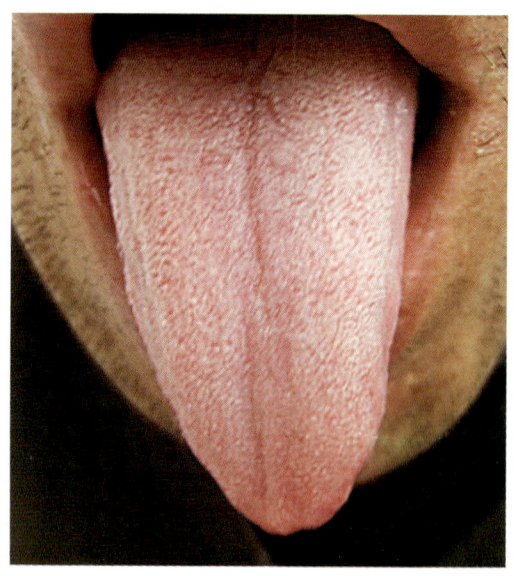

Fig 2.1-253

Patient, Male, 40years,

Case NO.: F295

Fig 2.1-254

Patient, Male, 37years,

Case NO.: W154

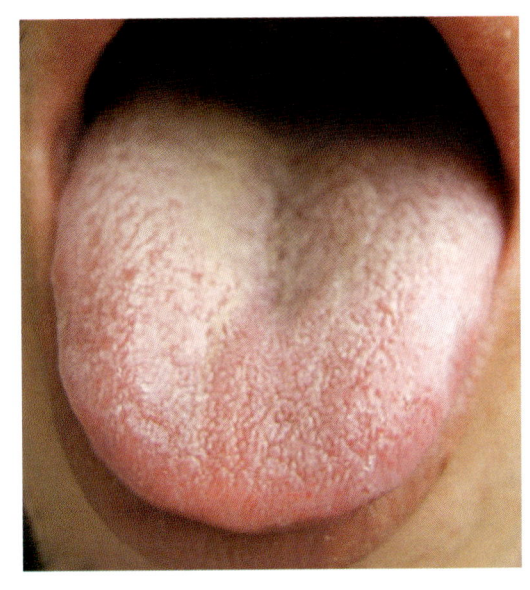

Fig 2.1-255

Patient, Male, 34years,

Case NO.: W284

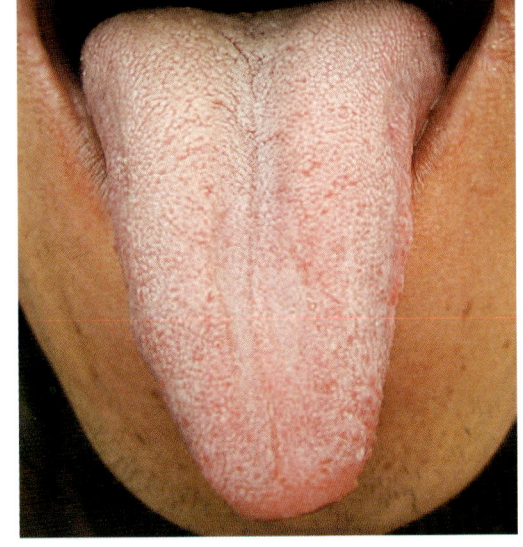

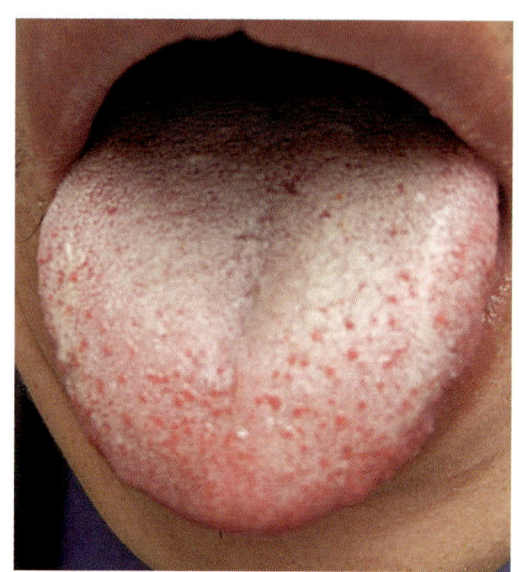

Fig 2.1-256

Patient, Male, 32years,

Case NO.: W166\171

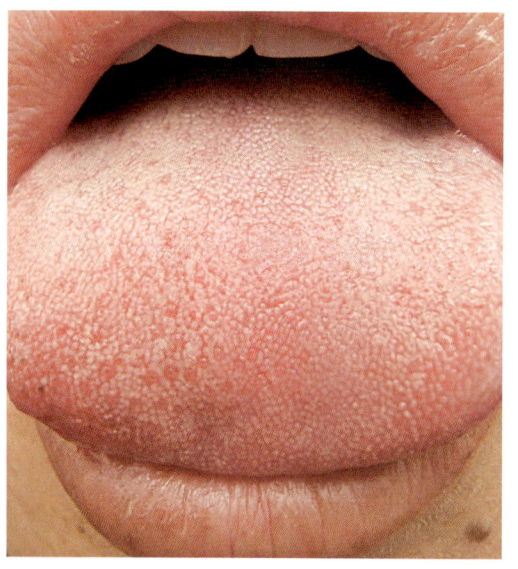

Fig 2.1-257

Patient, Female, 44years,

Case NO.: F219

Fig 2.1-258

Patient, Female, 46years,

Case NO.: W538

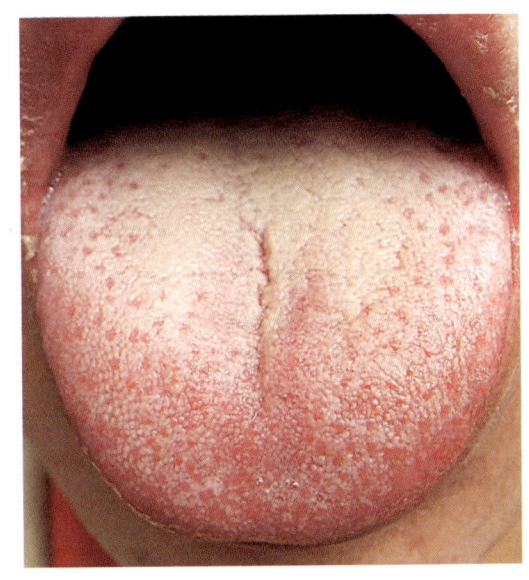

Fig 2.1-259

Patient, Female, 46years,

Case NO.: W347

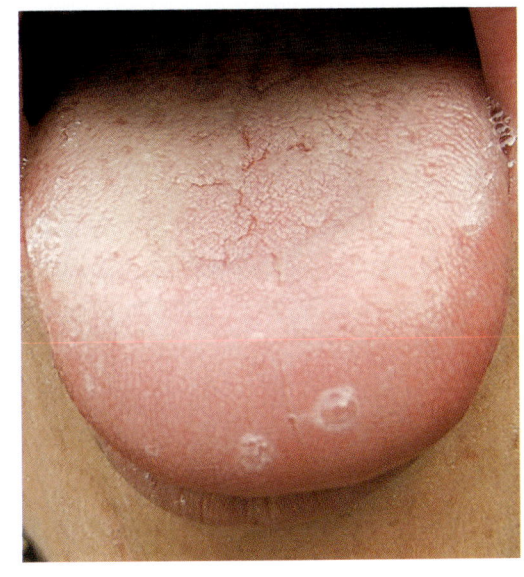

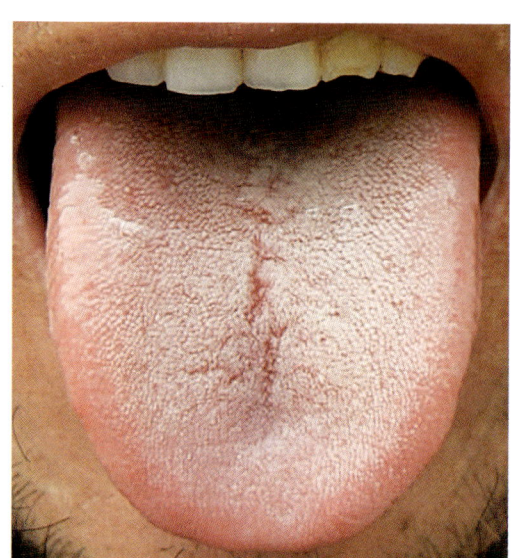

Fig 2.1-260

Patient, Male, 39years,

Case NO.: W42

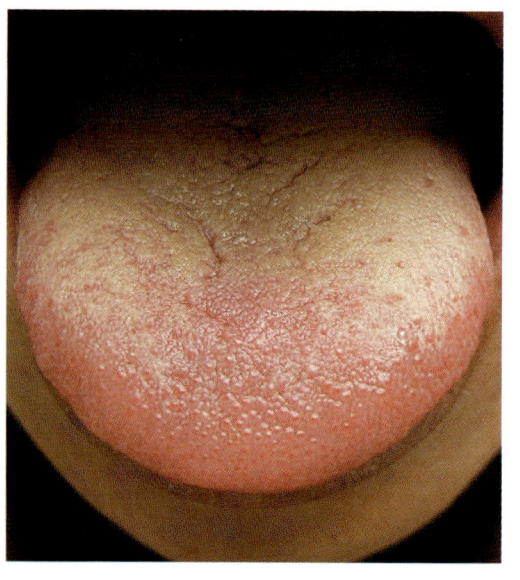

Fig 2.1-261

Patient, Female, 39years,

Case NO.: F87

Fig 2.1-262

Patient, Male, 44years,

Case NO.: W136

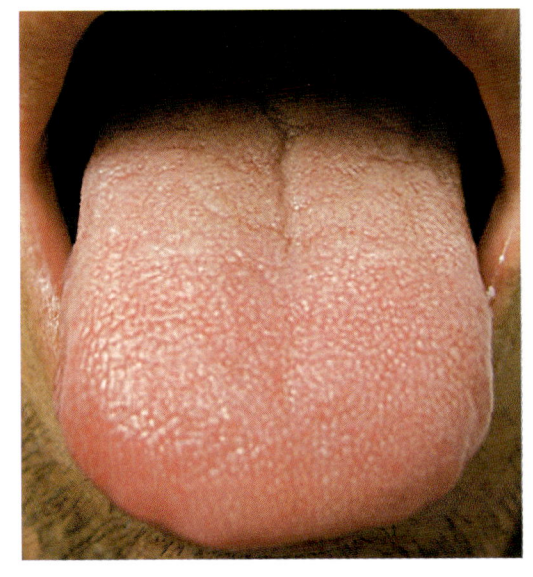

Fig 2.1-263

Patient, Male, 35years,

Case NO.: W98

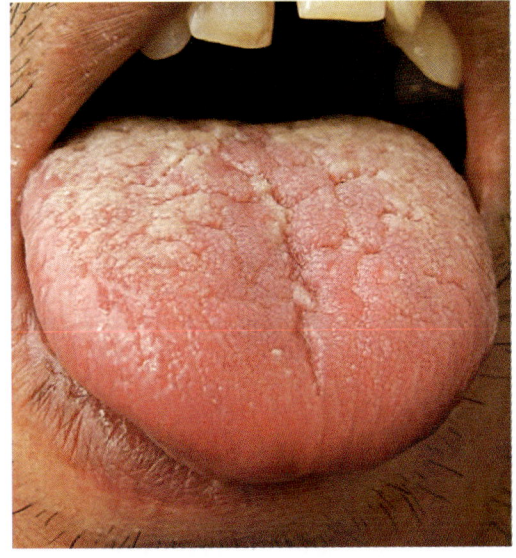

Red tongue

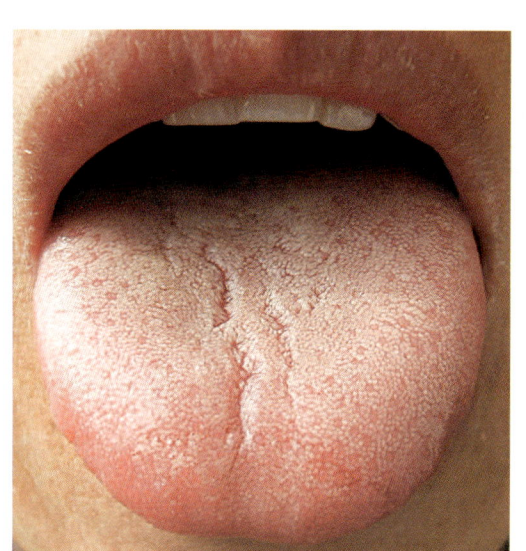

Fig 2.1-264

Patient, Female, 43years,

Case NO.: W175

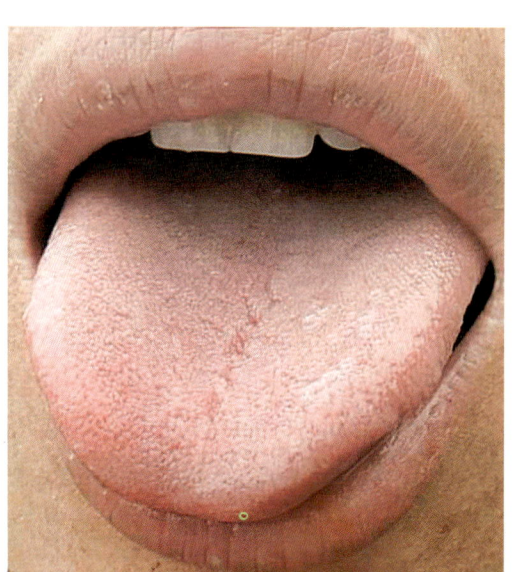

Fig 2.1-265

Patient, Female, 32years,

Case NO.: W25

Fig 2.1-266

Patient, Male, 53years,

Case NO.: W208

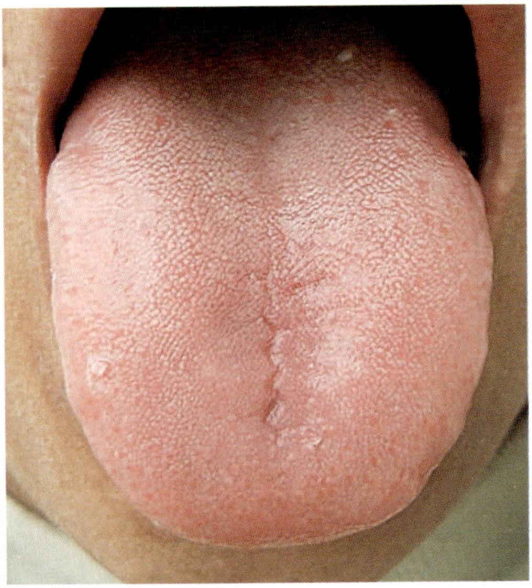

Fig 2.1-267

Patient, Male, 54years,

Case NO.: W604

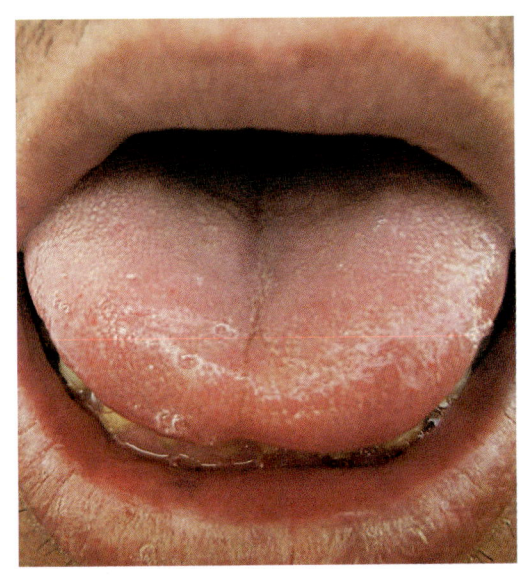

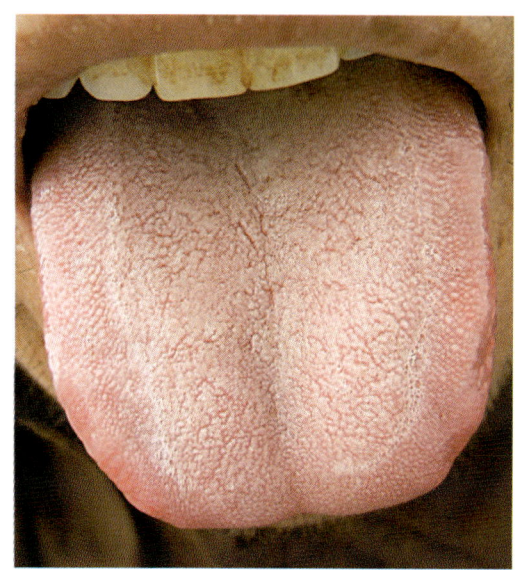

Fig 2.1-268

Patient, Male, 39years,

Case NO.: F366

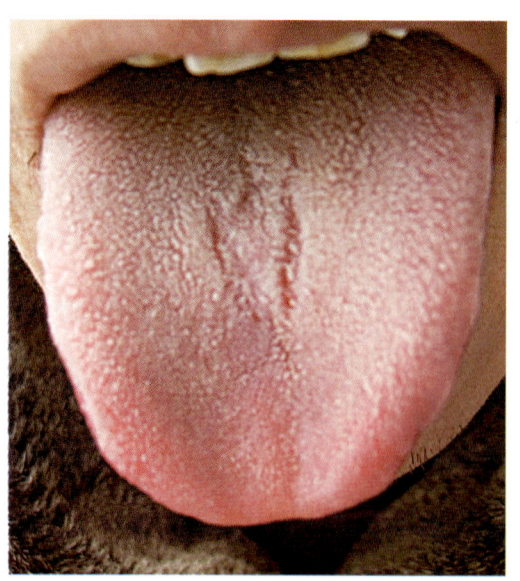

Fig 2.1-269

Patient, Male, 41years,

Case NO.: F353

Fig 2.1-270

Patient, Female, 32years,

Case NO.: W616

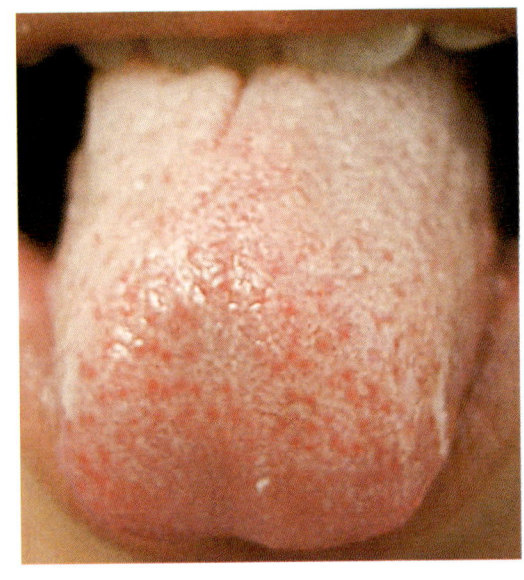

Fig 2.1-271

Patient, Female, 30years,

Case NO.: W568

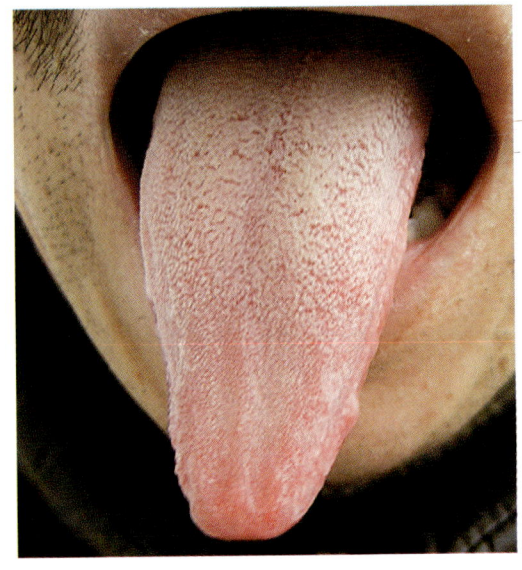

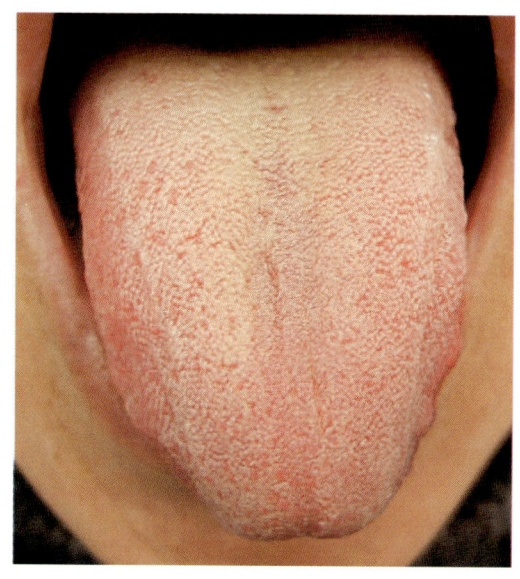

Fig 2.1-272

Patient, Female, 46years,

Case NO.: W235

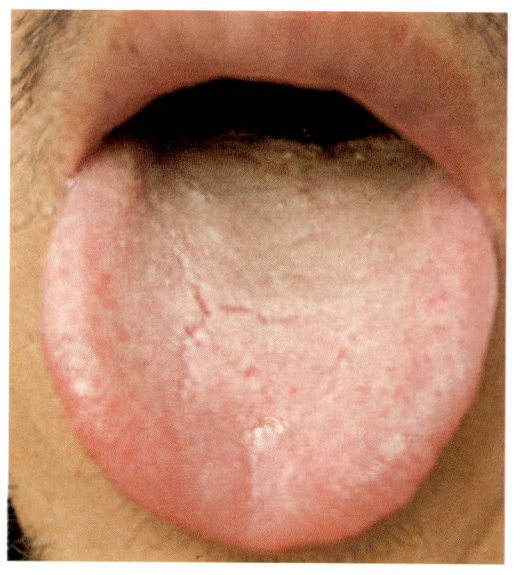

Fig 2.1-273

Patient, Male, 34years,

Case NO.: 291

Fig 2.1-274

Patient, Female, 40years,

Case NO.: W327

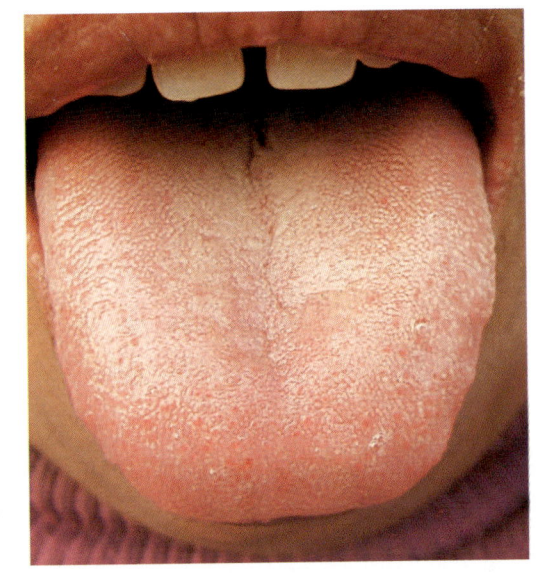

Fig 2.1-275

Patient, Female, 43years,

Case NO.: F103

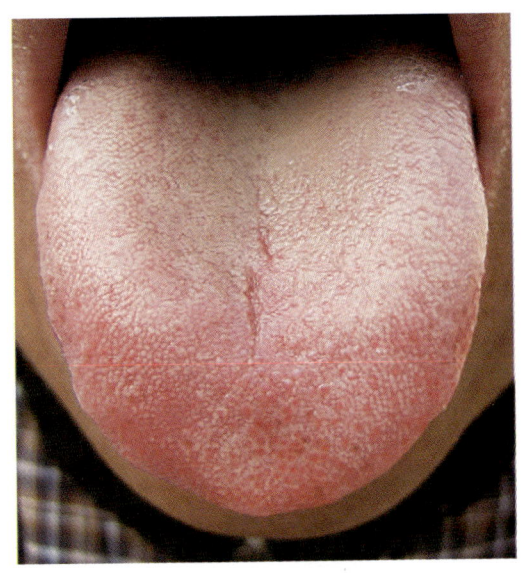

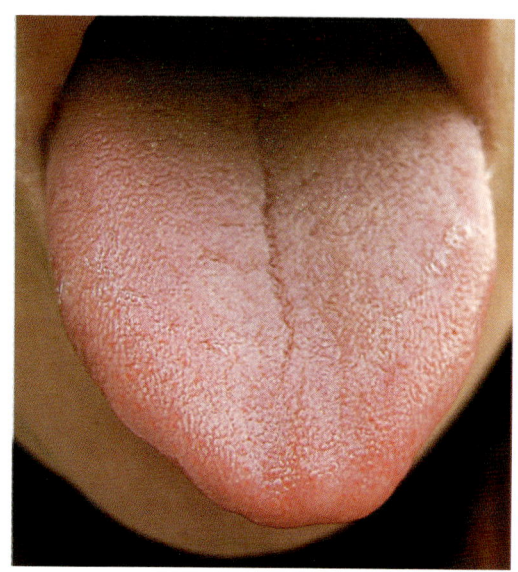

Fig 2.1-276

Patient, Female, 44years,

Case NO.: F49

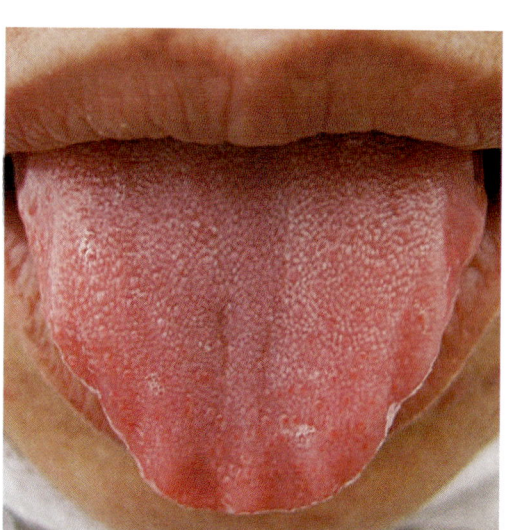

Fig 2.1-277

Patient, Female, 46years,

Case NO.: F242

Fig 2.1-278

Patient, Male, 36years,

Case NO.: F124

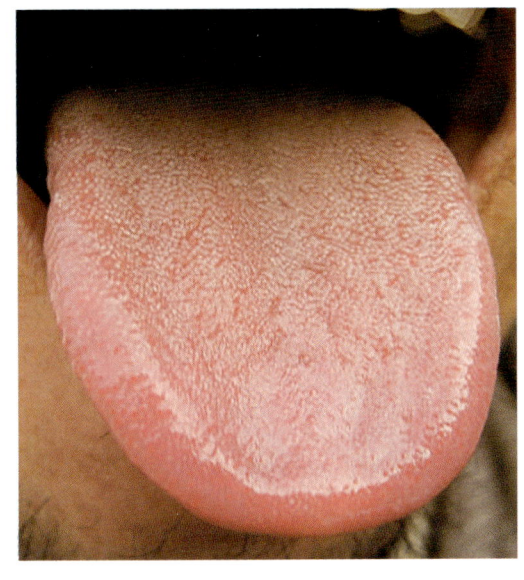

Fig 2.1-279

Patient, Male, 35years,

Case NO.: F118

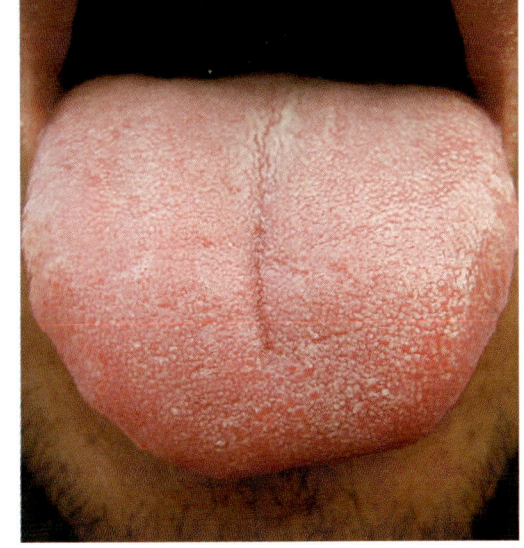

Red tongue

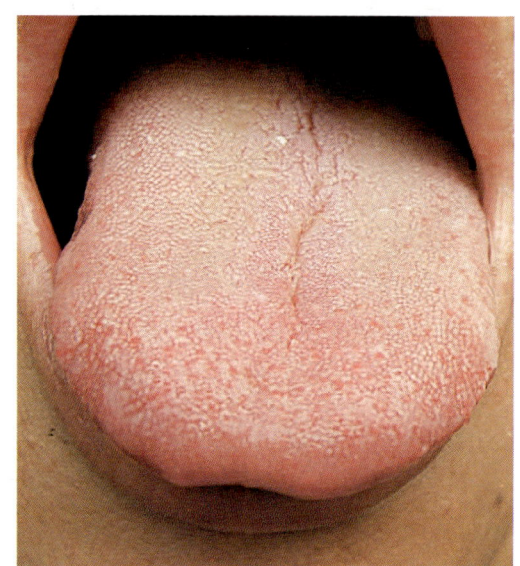

Fig 2.1-280

Patient, Female, 48years,

Case NO.: W275

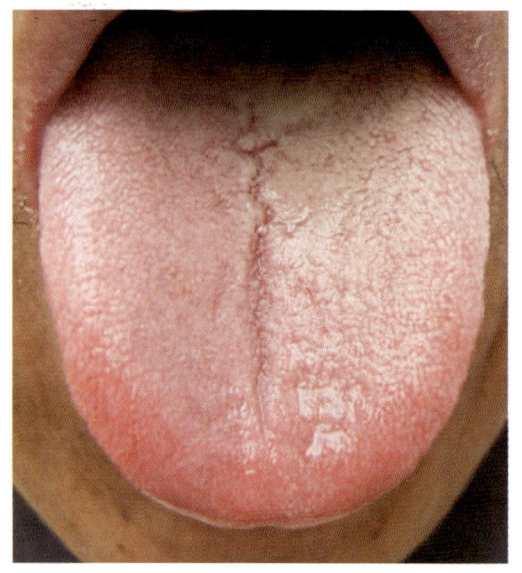

Fig 2.1-281

Patient, Male, 49years,

Case NO.: W105

Fig 2.1-282

Patient, Female, 50years,

Case NO.: W49

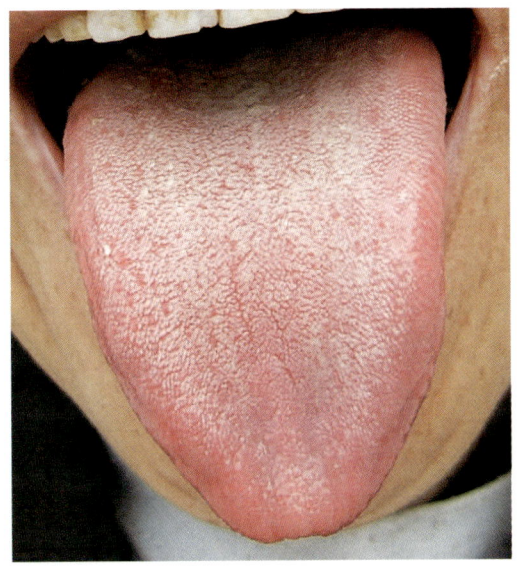

1.4 Crimson tongue

Infected with HIV yet clinically asymptomatic

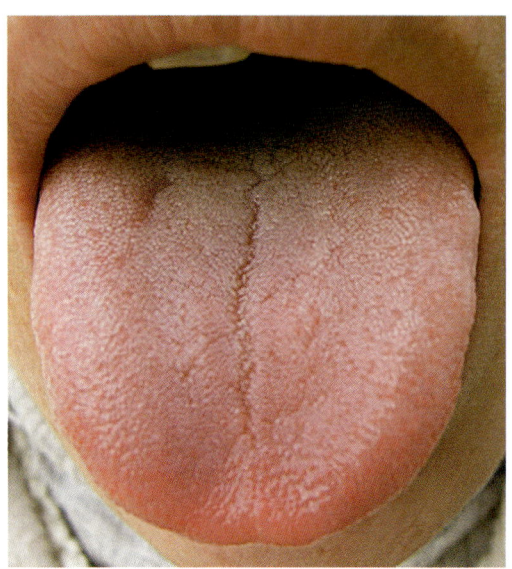

Fig 2.1-283

Patient, Female, 38years,

Case NO.: W200

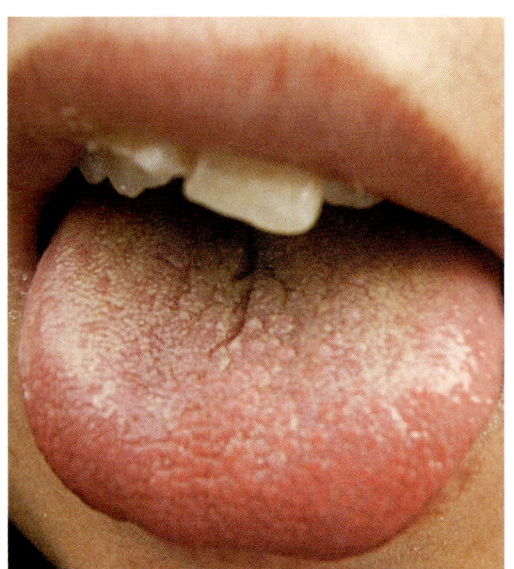

Fig 2.1-284

Patient, Female, 42years,

Case NO.: W650

Crimson tongue

Fig 2.1-285

Patient, Male, 35years,

Case NO.: W601

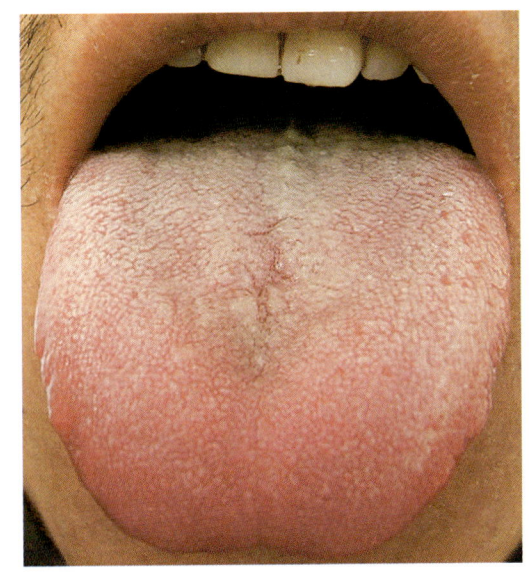

Fig 2.1-286

Patient, Male, 33years,

Case NO.: W158

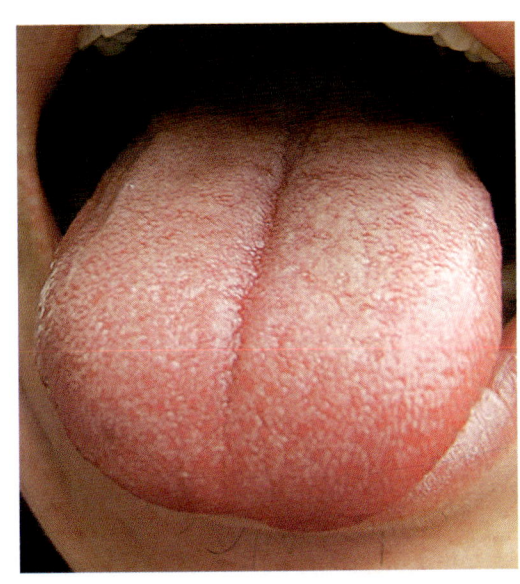

Crimson tongue

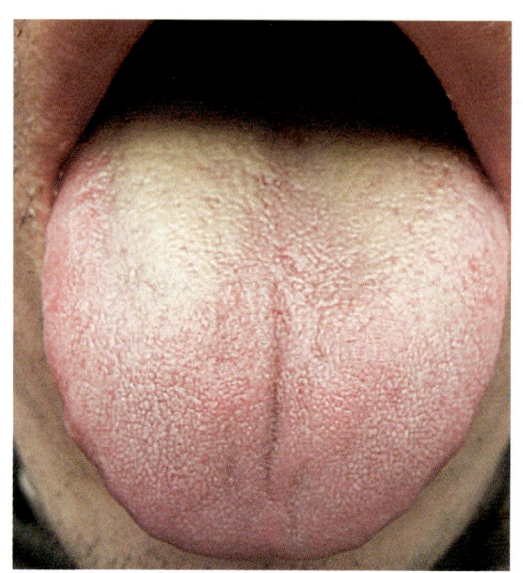

Fig 2.1-287

Patient, Male, 44years,

Case NO.: W663

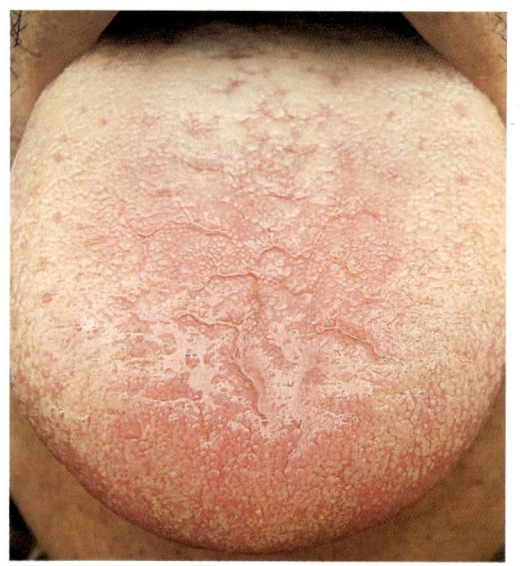

Fig 2.1-288

Patient, Male, 46years,

Case NO.: W306

Fig 2.1-289

Patient, Male, 31years,

Case NO.: W608

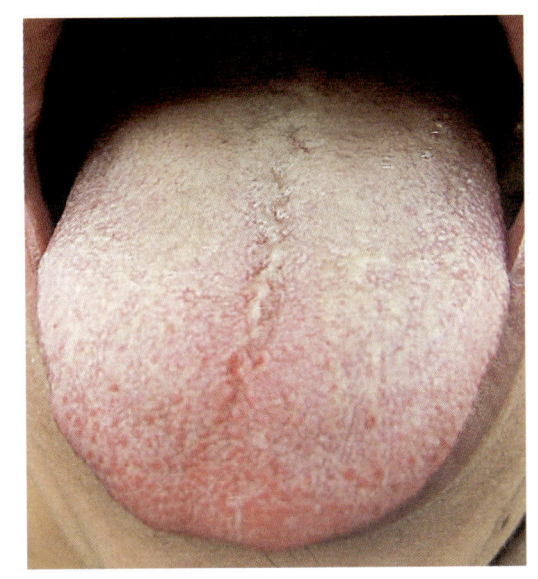

Fig 2.1-290

Patient, Male, 66years,

Case NO.: W132

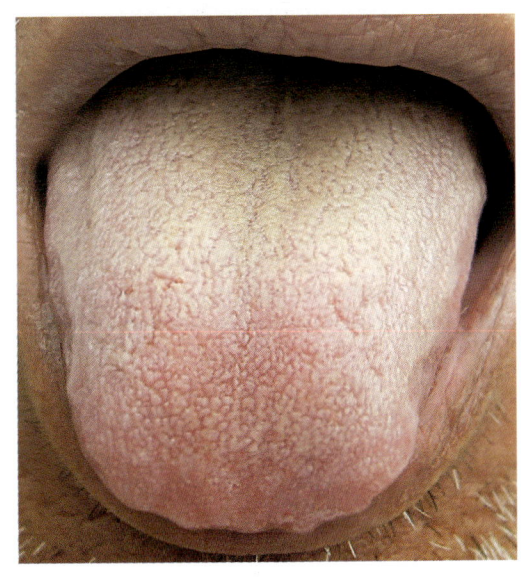

Crimson tongue

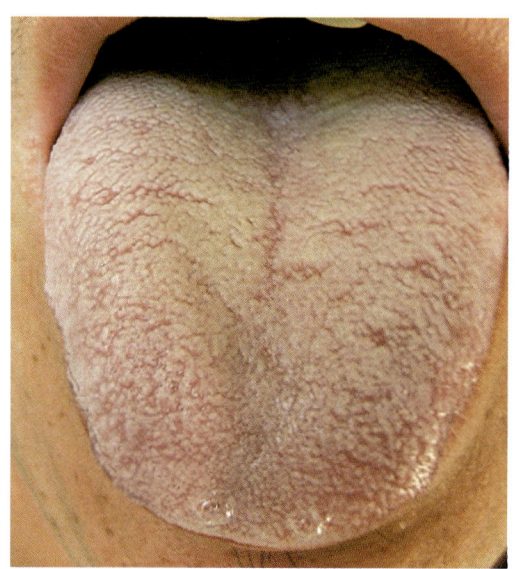

Fig 2.1-291

Patient, Male, 42years,

Case NO.: F29

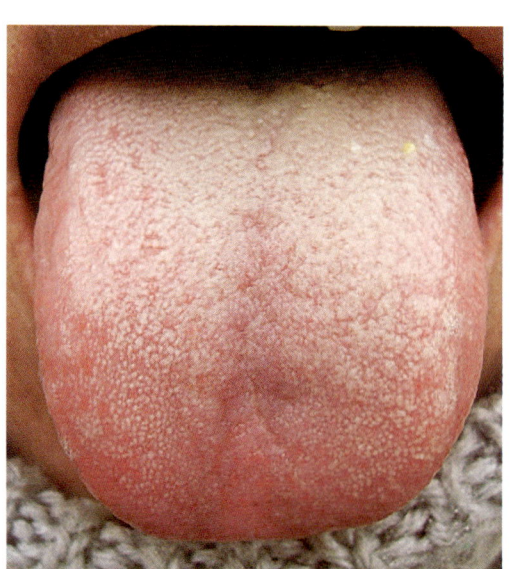

Fig 2.1-292

Patient, Female, 50years,

Case NO.: W661

Fig 2.1-293

Patient, Male, 49years,

Case NO.: W614

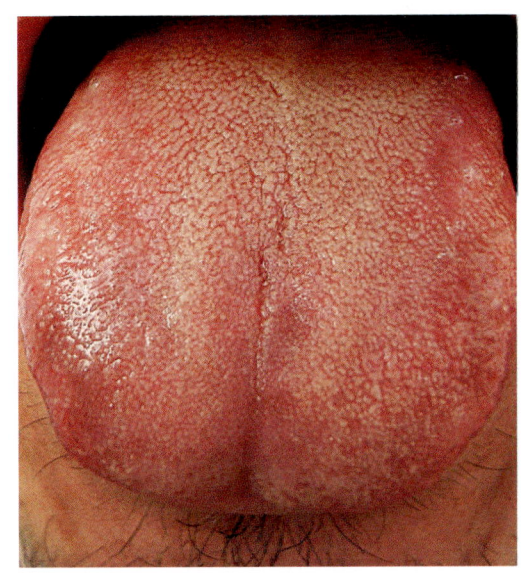

Fig 2.1-294

Patient, Male, 44years,

Case NO.: W671

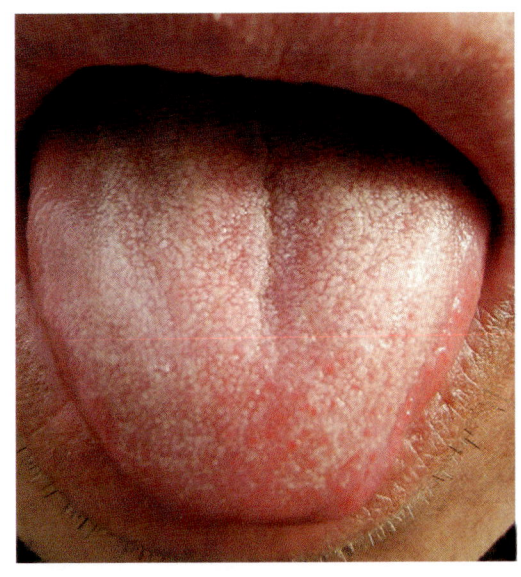

Crimson tongue

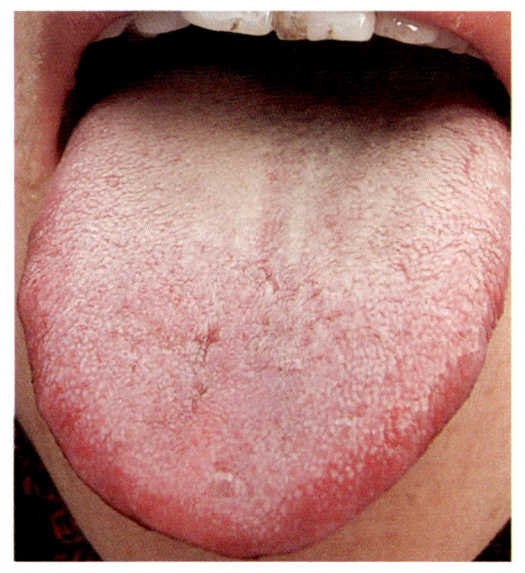

Fig 2.1-295

Patient, Female, 43years,

Case NO.: W646

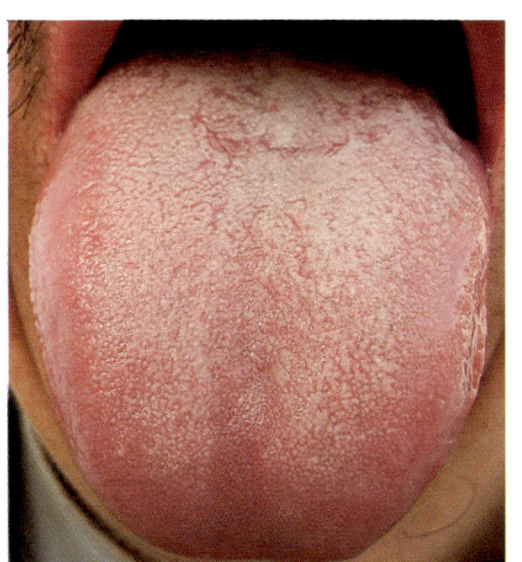

Fig 2.1-296

Patient, Male, 49years,

Case NO.: W613

Fig 2.1-297

Patient, Male, 39years,

Case NO.: W361

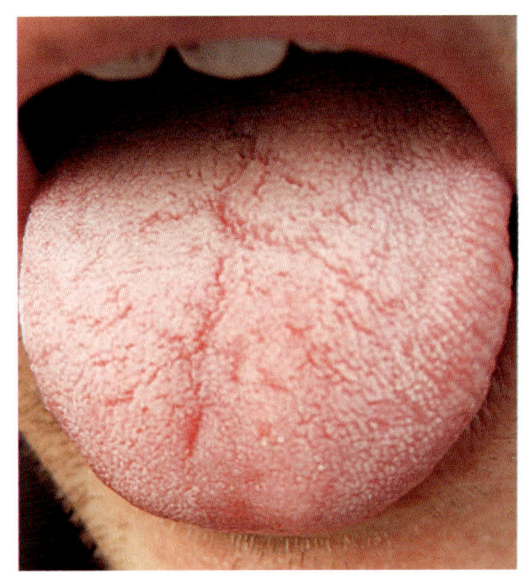

Fig 2.1-298

Patient, Female, 41years,

Case NO.: F61

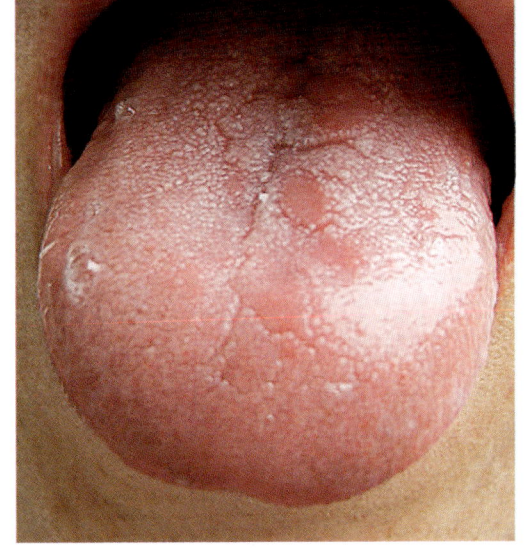

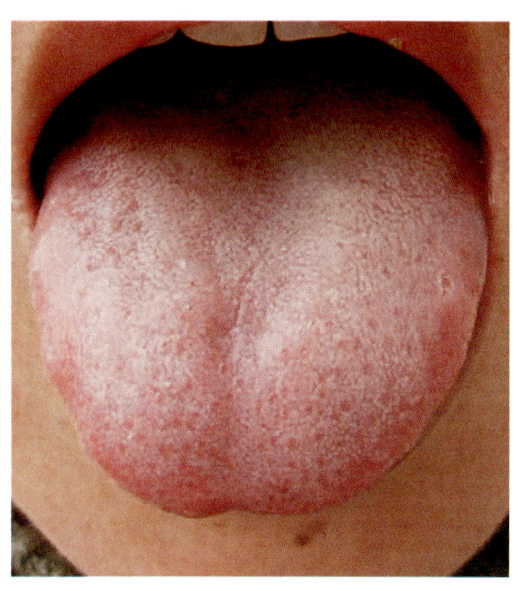

Fig 2.1-299

Patient, Female, 33years,

Case NO.: W14

Crimson tongue

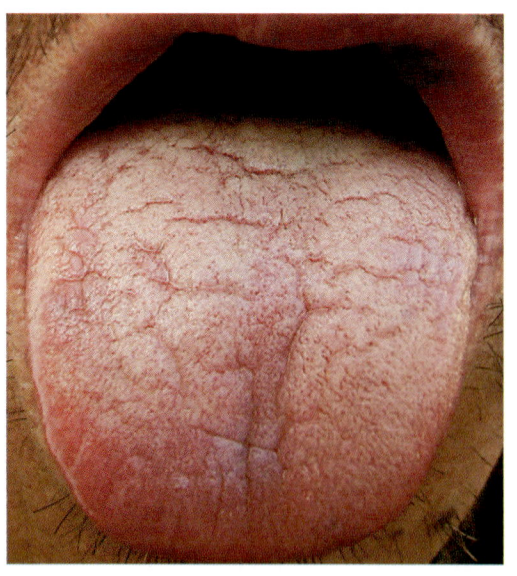

Fig 2.1-300

Patient, Male, 60years,

Case NO.: W600

Fig 2.1-301

Patient, Female, 52years,

Case NO.: F288

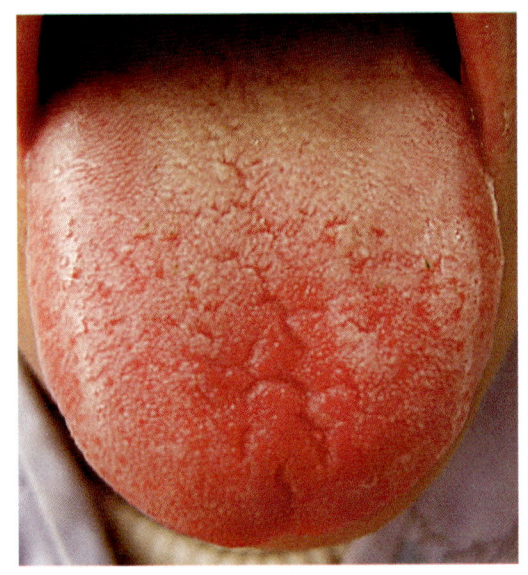

Fig 2.1-302

Patient, Male, 38years,

Case NO.: F2

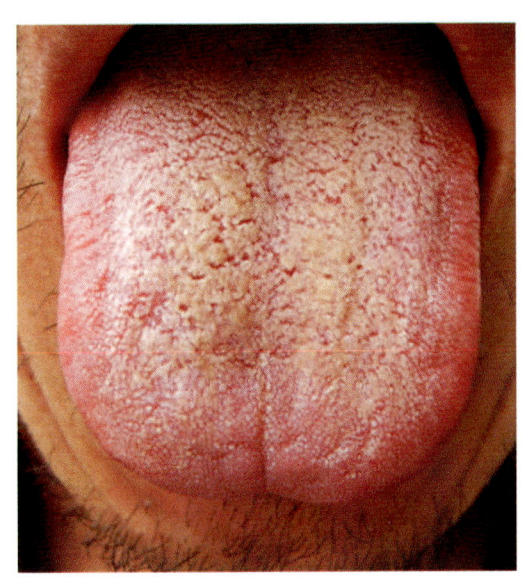

Crimson tongue

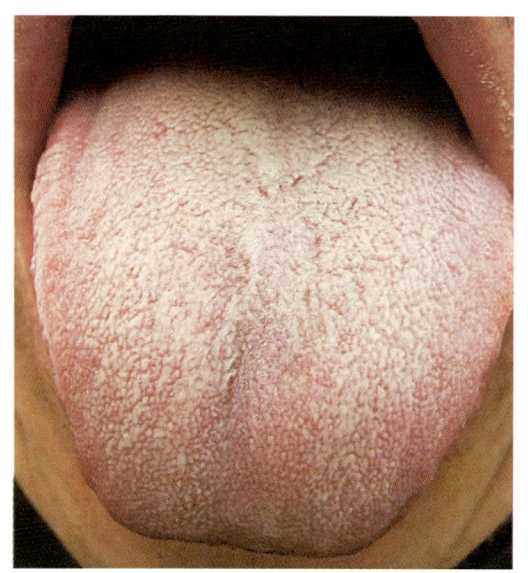

Fig 2.1-303

Patient, Male, 51years,

Case NO.: F233

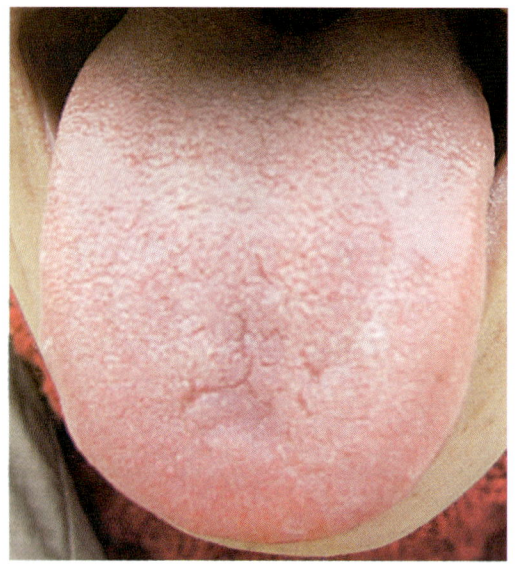

Fig 2.1-304

Patient, Female, 34years,

Case NO.: F141

Fig 2.1-305

Patient, Male, 42years,

Case NO.: F60

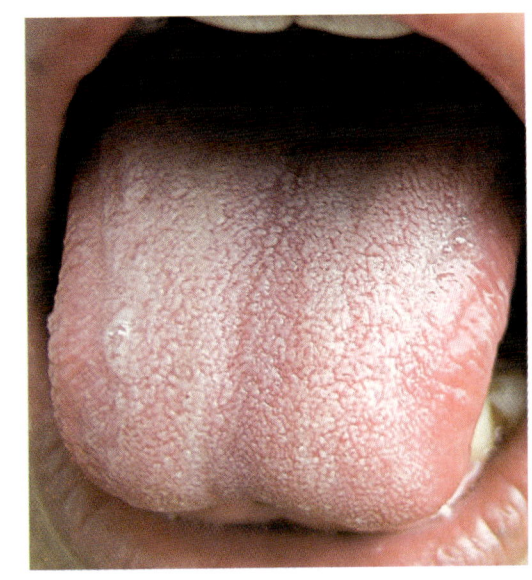

Fig 2.1-306

Patient, Male, 35years,

Case NO.: W352

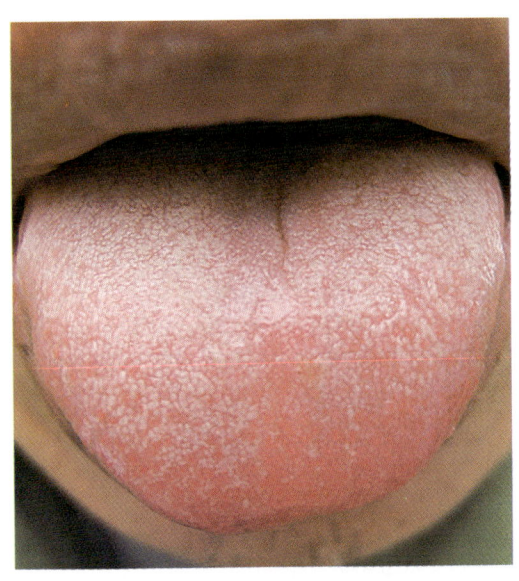

Crimson tongue

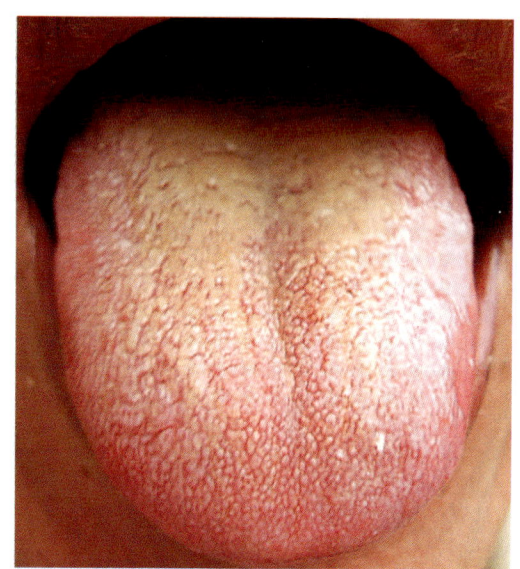

Fig 2.1-307

Patient, Male, 44years,

Case NO.: F67

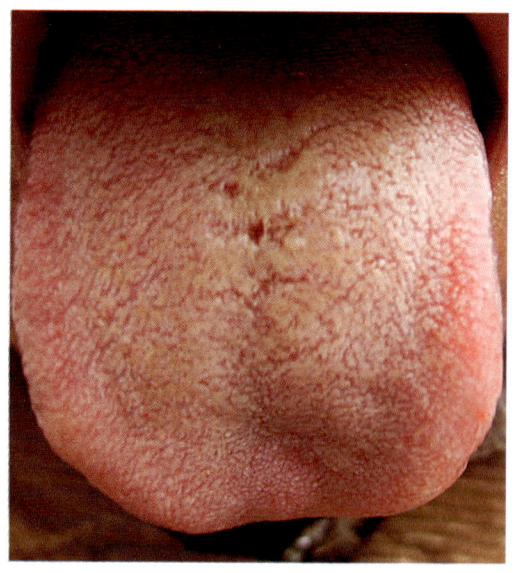

Fig 2.1-308

Patient, Male, 38years,

Case NO.: F287

Fig 2.1-309

Patient, Female, 50years,

Case NO.: F259

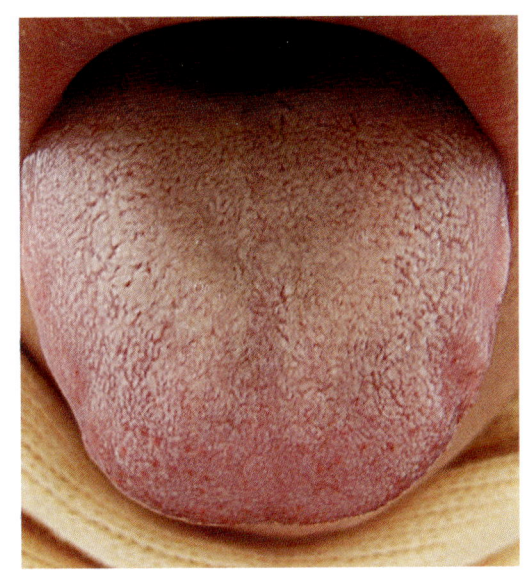

Fig 2.1-310

Patient, Male, 49years,

Case NO.: F110

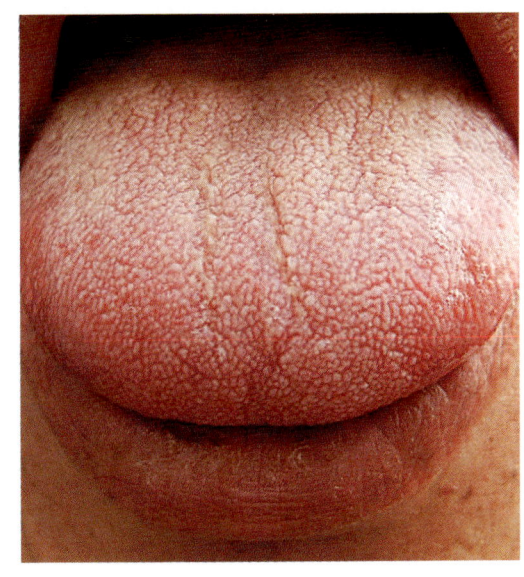

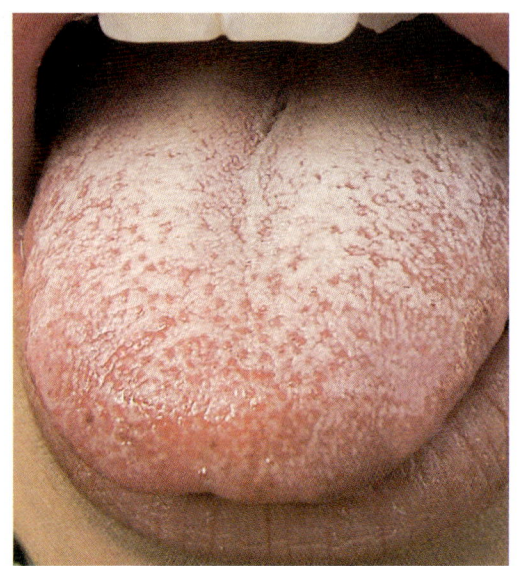

Fig 2.1-311

Patient, Female, 40years,

Case NO.: W603

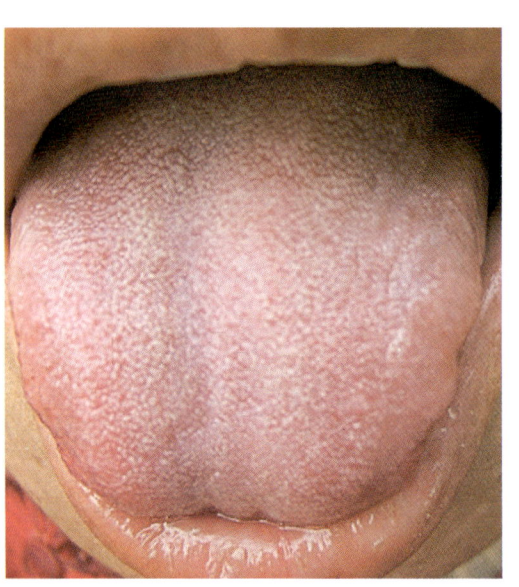

Fig 2.1-312

Patient, Female, 50years,

Case NO.: W693

Fig 2.1-313

Patient, Male, 40years,

Case NO.: W685

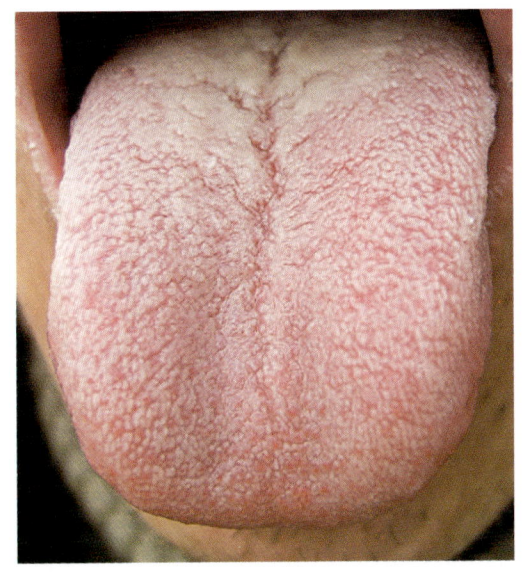

Fig 2.1-314

Patient, Female, 37years,

Case NO.: W695

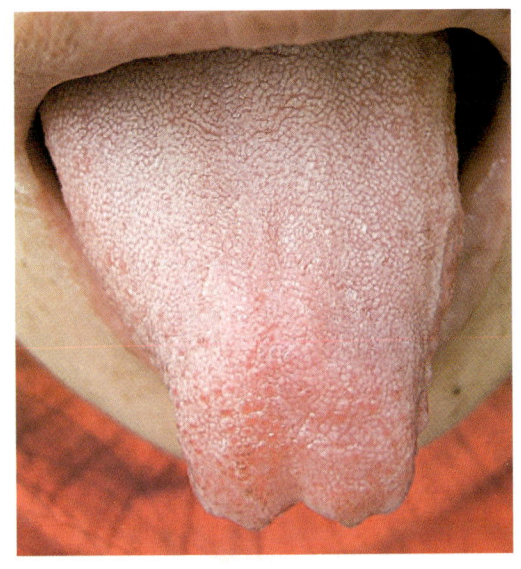

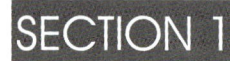
Crimson tongue

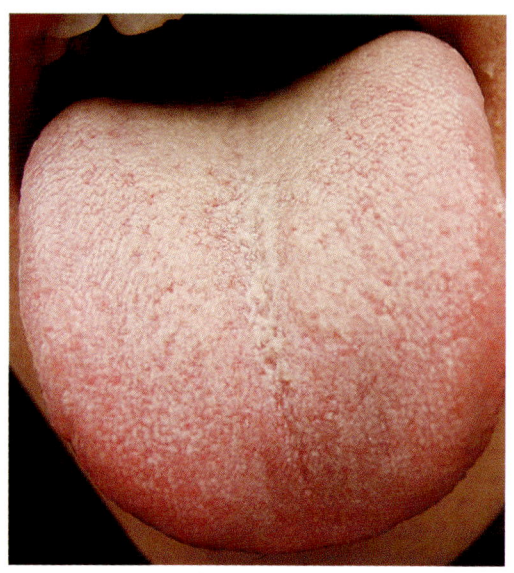

Fig 2.1-315

Patient, Male, 35years,

Case NO.: F155

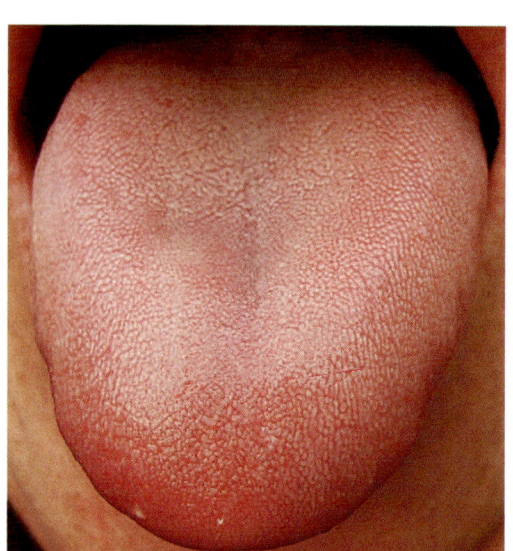

Fig 2.1-316

Patient, Female, 56years,

Case NO.: W388

Fig 2.1-317

Patient, Female, 36years,

Case NO.: W627

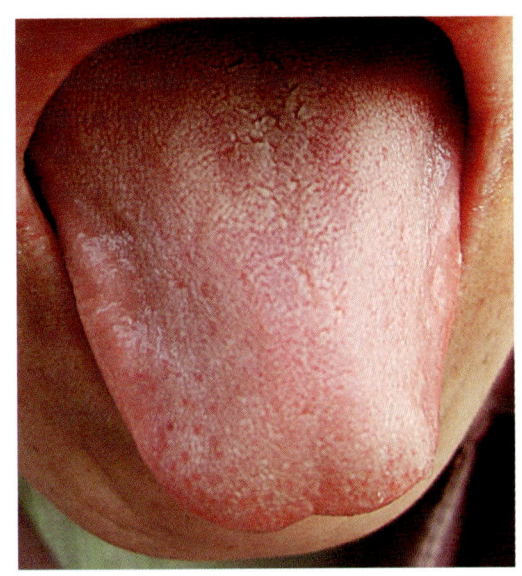

Fig 2.1-318

Patient, Female, 41years,

Case NO.: F8

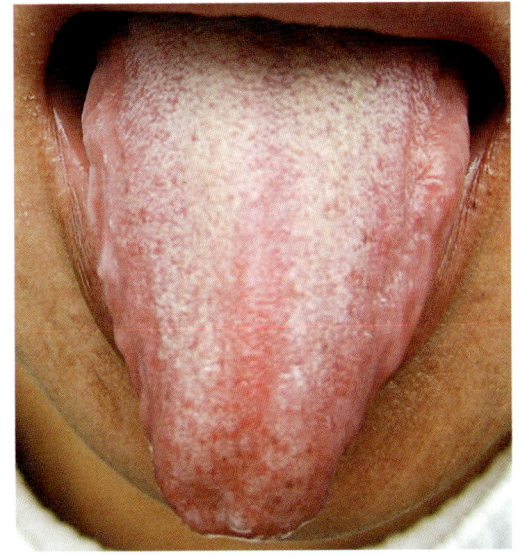

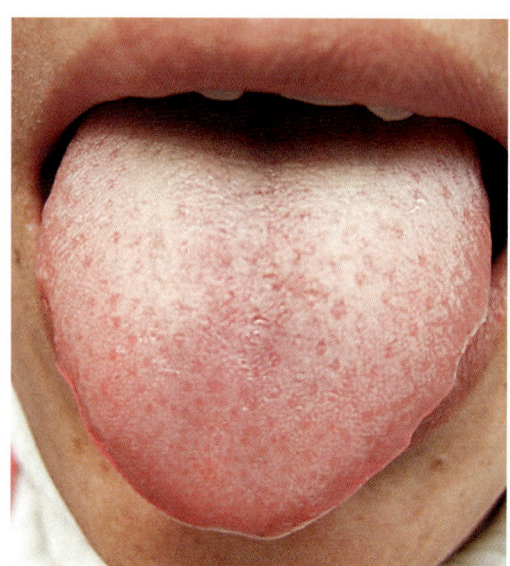

Fig 2.1-319

Patient, Female, 37years,

Case NO.: W138

Crimson tongue

1.5 Petechial tongue

Infected with HIV yet clinically asymptomatic

Fig 2.1-320

Patient, Female, 39years,

Case NO.: W124

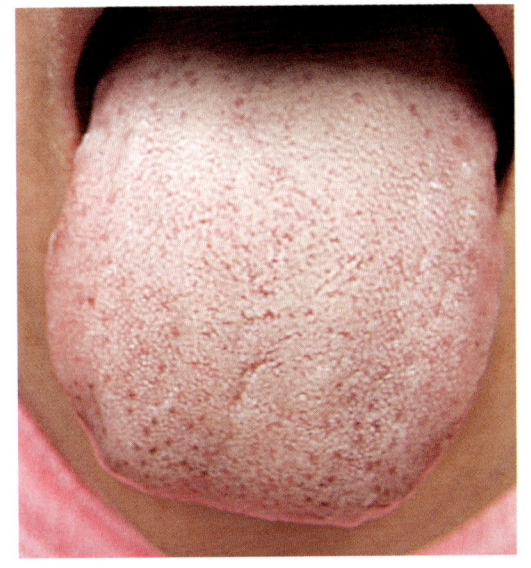

Fig 2.1-321

Patient, Female, 44years,

Case NO.: W684

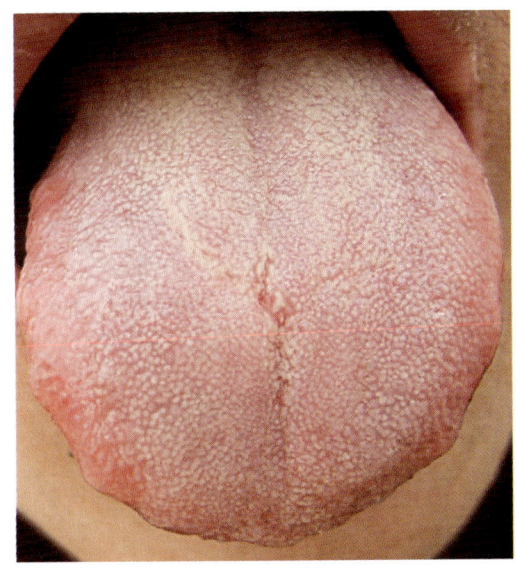

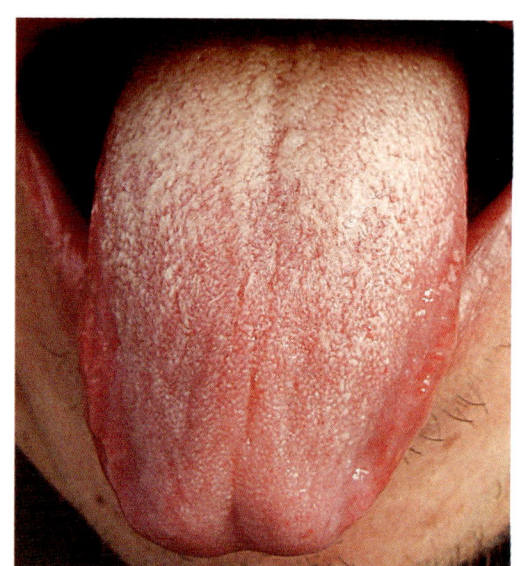

Fig 2.1-322

Patient, Male, 38years,

Case NO.: W640

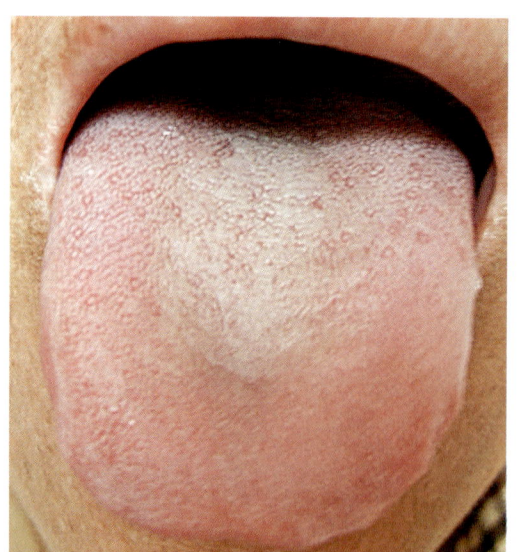

Fig 2.1-323

Patient, Female, 45years,

Case NO.: W129

Petechial tongue

2. *Tongue Shape*

2.1 Cracked tongue

Infected with HIV yet clinically asymptomatic

Fig 2.1-324

Patient, Male, 47years,

Case NO.: W549

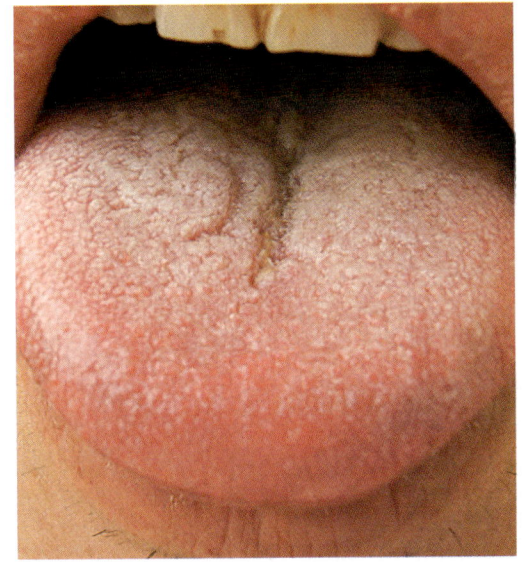

2.2 Tooth-marked tongue

Infected with HIV yet clinically asymptomatic

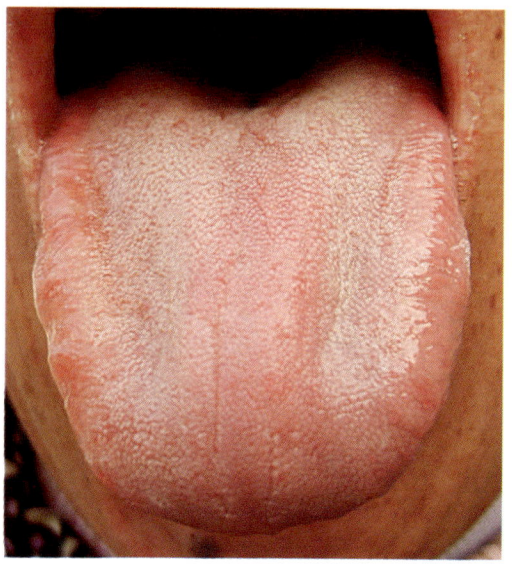

Fig 2.1-325

Patient, Female, 41years,

Case NO.: F122

3. *Tongue Coating*

3.1 Thick-yellow tongue coating

Infected with HIV yet clinically asymptomatic

Fig 2.1-326

Patient, Male, 41years,

Case NO.: F131

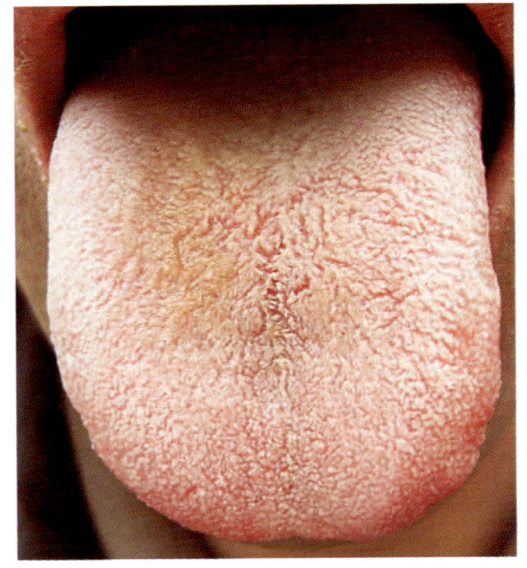

g 2.1-327

atient, Female, 49years,

ase NO.: W244

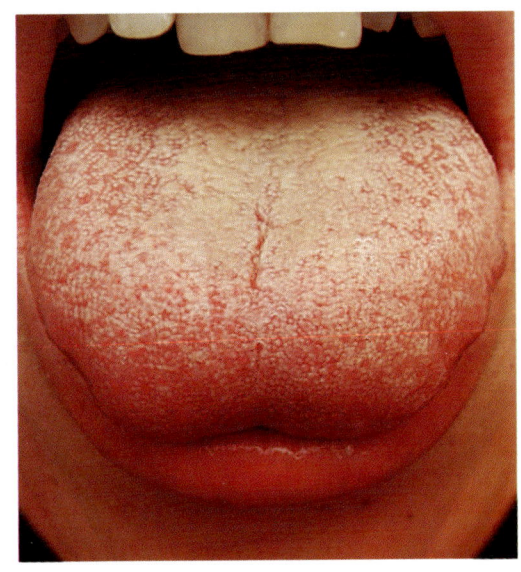

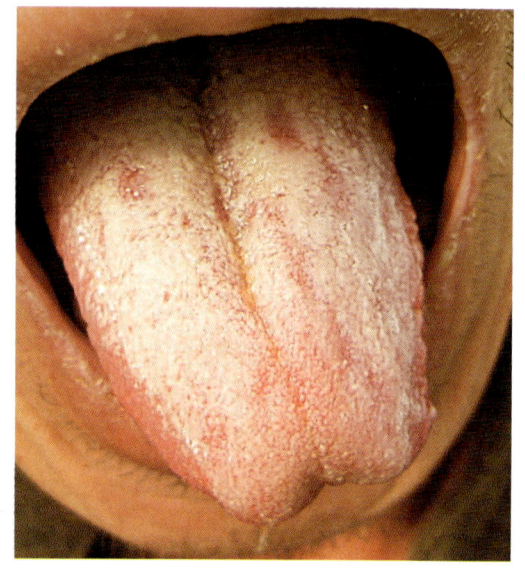

Fig 2.1-328

Patient, Male, 41years,

Case NO.: W220

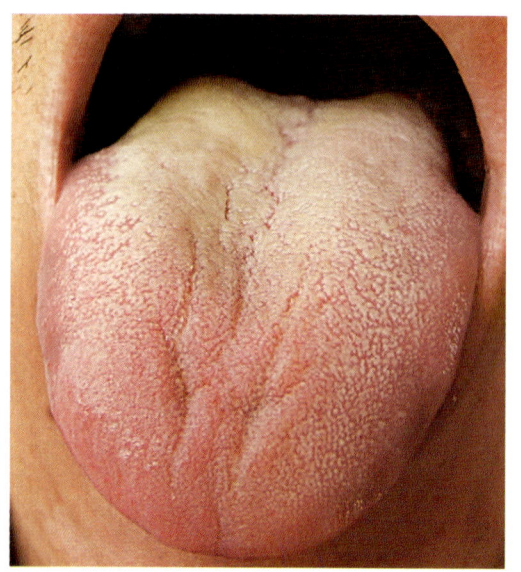

Fig 2.1-329

Patient, Male, 36years,

Case NO.: F27

3.2 Thick-white tongue coating

Infected with HIV yet clinically asymptomatic

Fig 2.1-330

Patient, Male, 32years,

Case NO.: W372

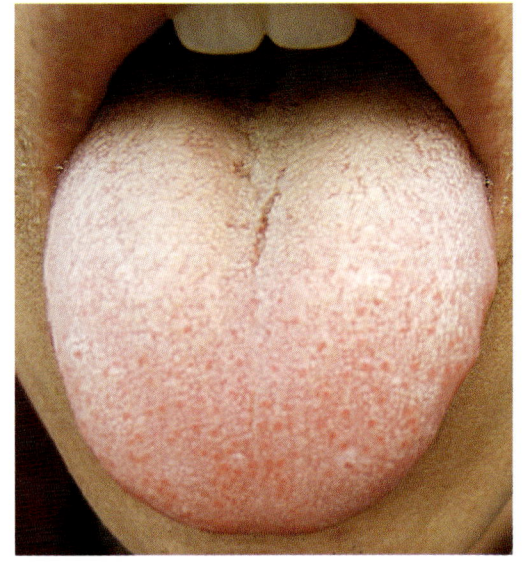

Fig 2.1-331

Patient, Male, 41years,

Case NO.: W288

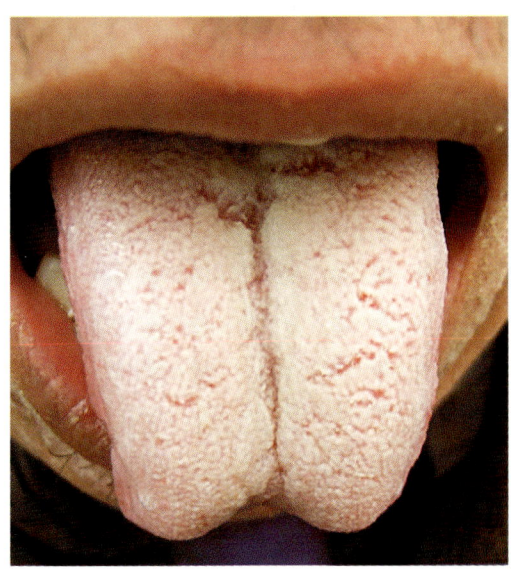

3.3 Greasy tongue coating

Infected with HIV yet clinically asymptomatic

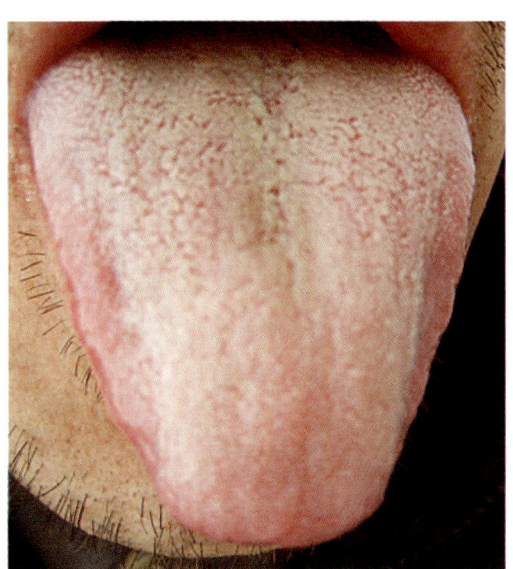

Fig 2.1-332

Patient, Male, 42years,

Case NO.: F358

3.4 Slippery and greasy tongue coating

Infected with HIV yet clinically asymptomatic

Fig 2.1-333

Patient, Female, 44years,

Case NO.: W67

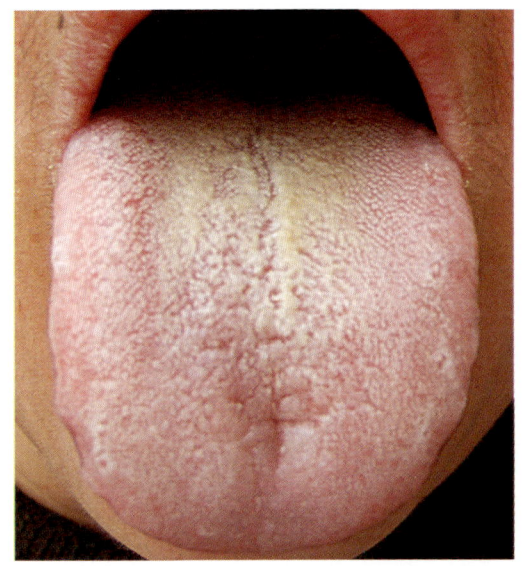

1. *Tongue Color*

1.1 Pale tongue

AIDS stage

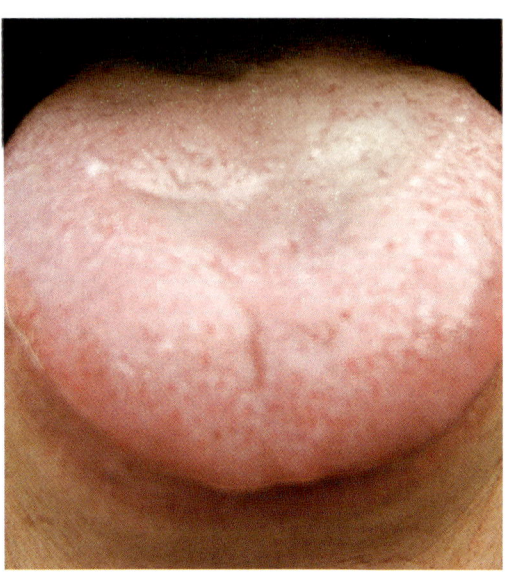

Fig 2.2-1

Patient, Female, 45years,

Case NO.: W319

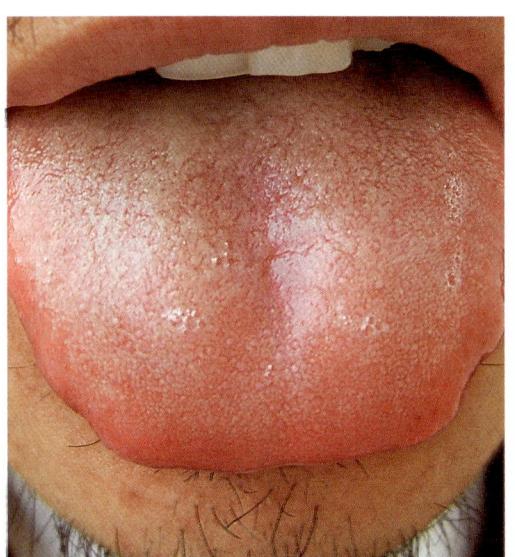

Fig 2.2-2

Patient, Male, 32years,

Case NO.: W22

Fig 2.2-3

Patient, Female, 47years,

Case NO.: W384

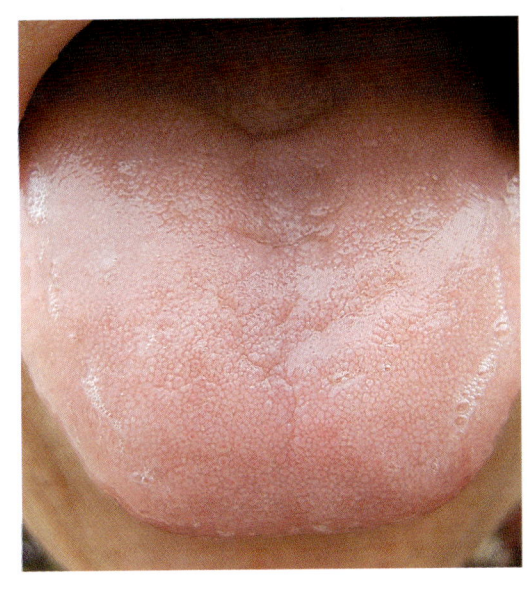

Fig 2.2-4

Patient, Female, 50years,

Case NO.: W20

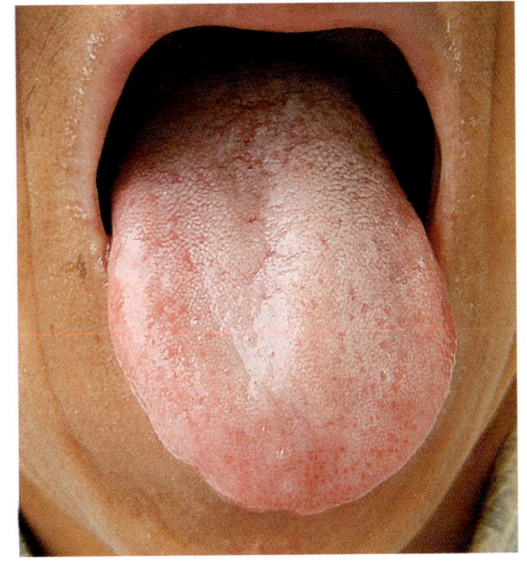

Pale tongue

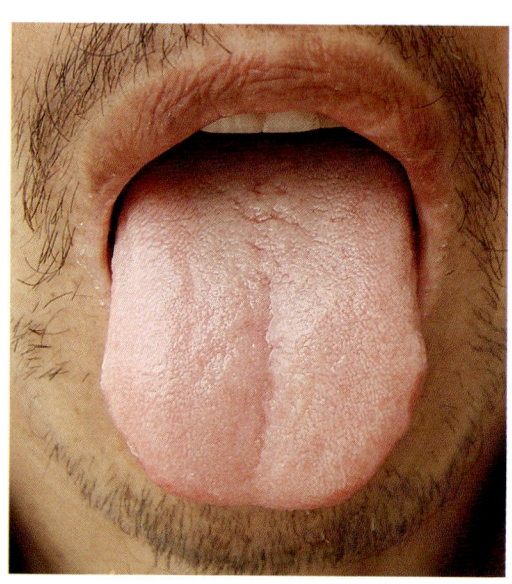

Fig 2.2-5

Patient, Male, 44years,

Case NO.: W75

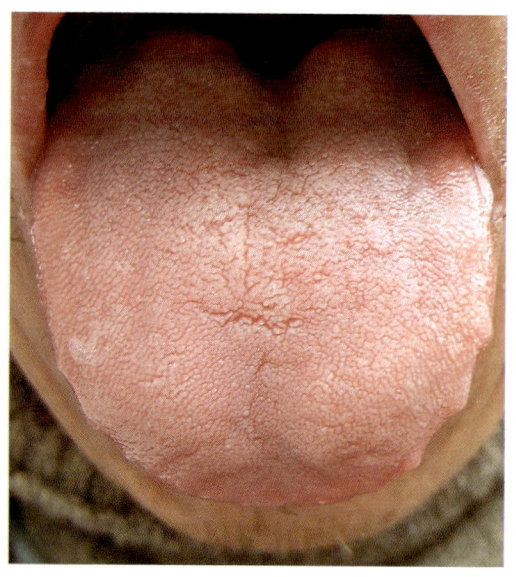

Fig 2.2-6

Patient, Male, 51years,

Case NO.: W98

Fig 2.2-7

Patient, Male, 54years,

Case NO.: W316

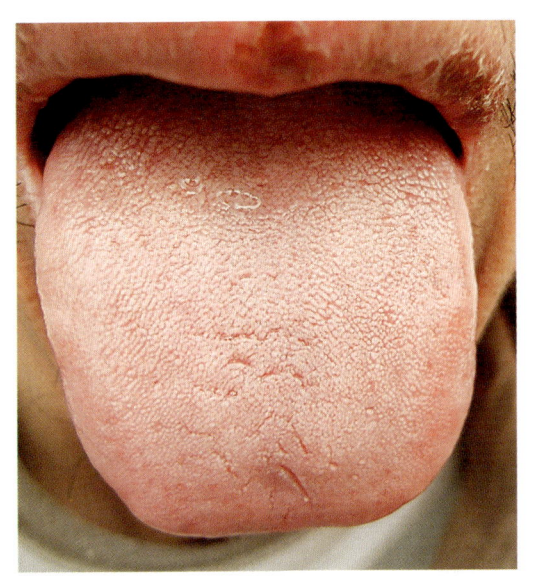

Fig 2.2-8

Patient, Male, 54years,

Case NO.: W137

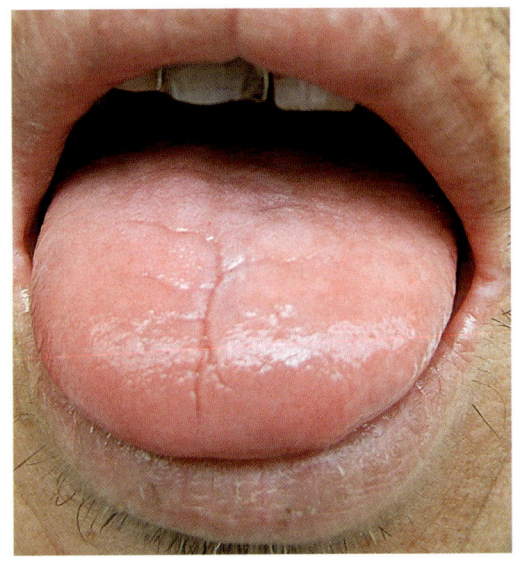

Pale tongue

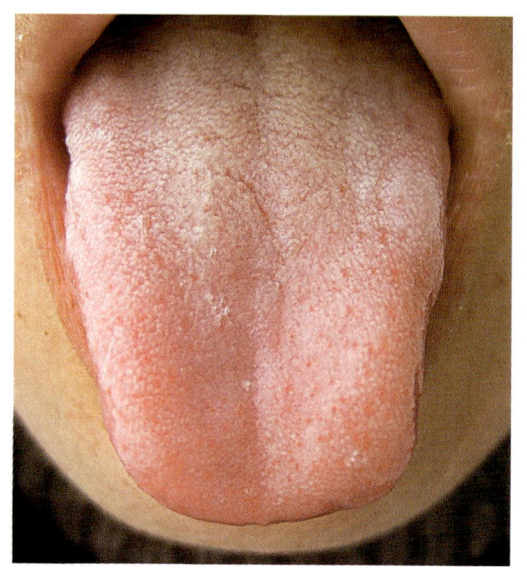

Fig 2.2-9

Patient, Female, 28years,

Case NO.: W743

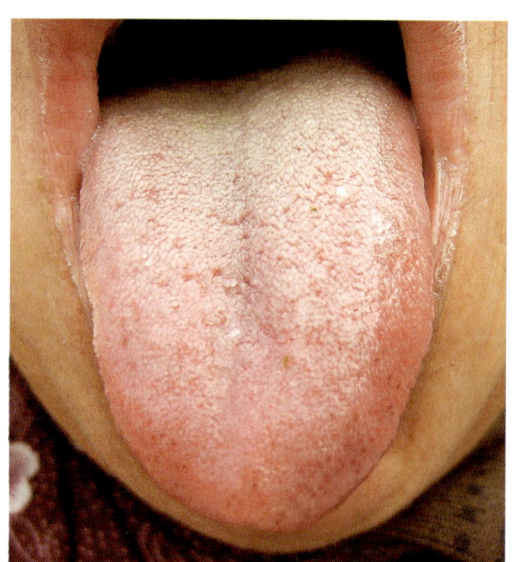

Fig 2.2-10

Patient, Female, 56years,

Case NO.: W305

Fig 2.2-11

Patient, Male, 51years,

Case NO.: W370

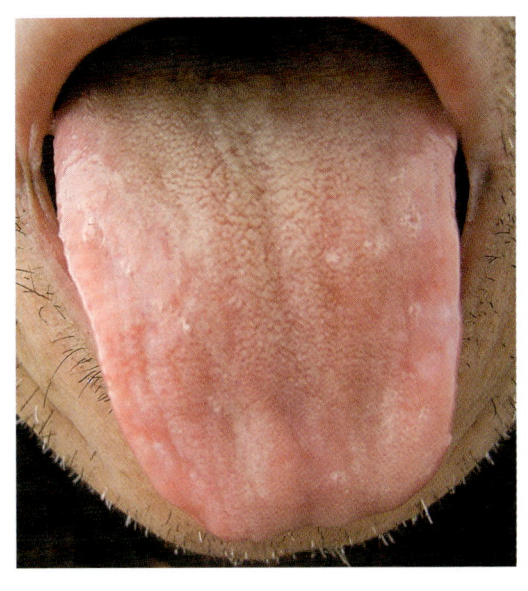

Fig 2.2-12

Patient, Male, 41years,

Case NO.: W78

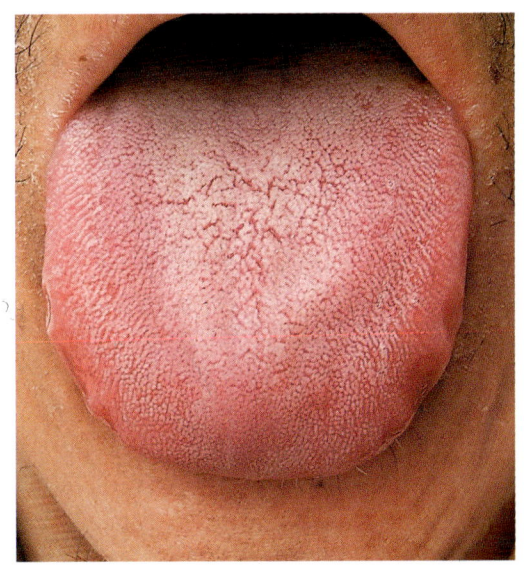

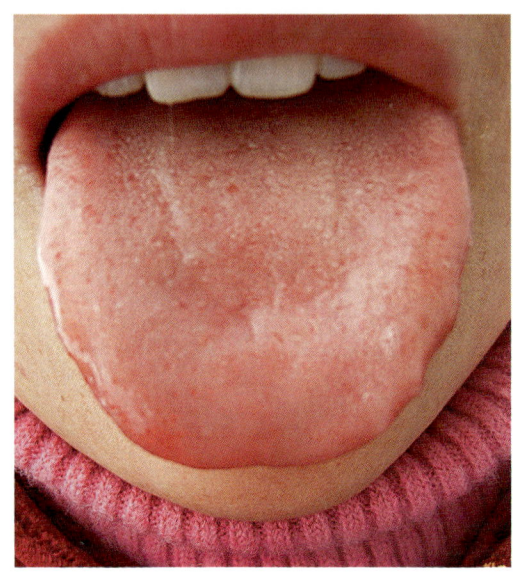

Fig 2.2-13

Patient, Female, 35years,

Case NO.: W745

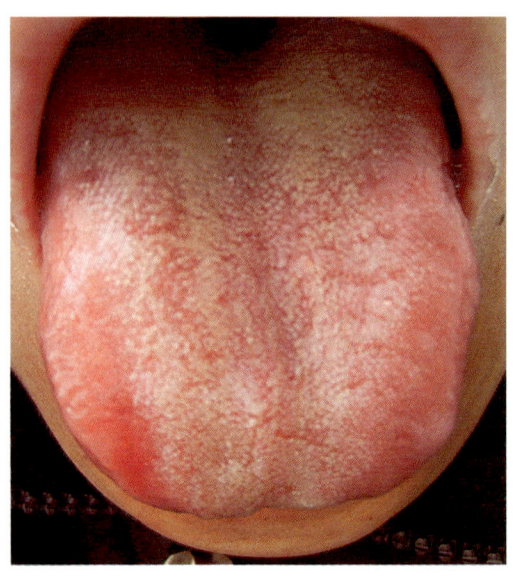

Fig 2.2-14

Patient, Male, 33years,

Case NO.: W364

Fig 2.2-15

Patient, Female, 60years,

Case NO.: W304

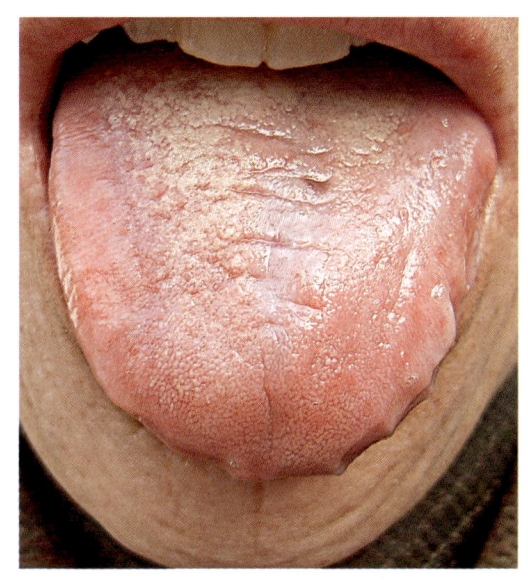

Fig 2.2-16

Patient, Male, 52years,

Case NO.: W428

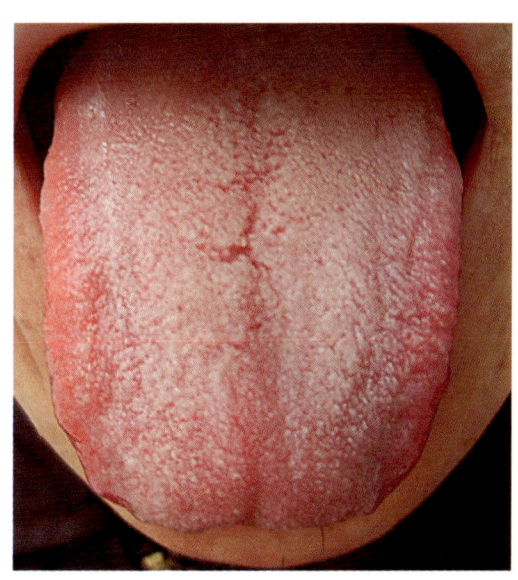

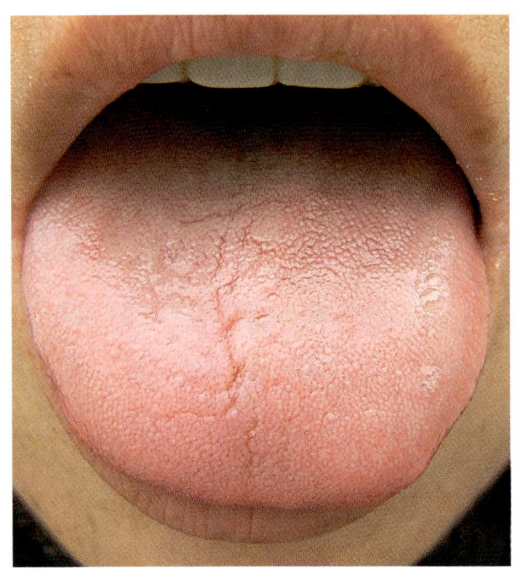

Fig 2.2-17

Patient, Female, 41years,

Case NO.: W48

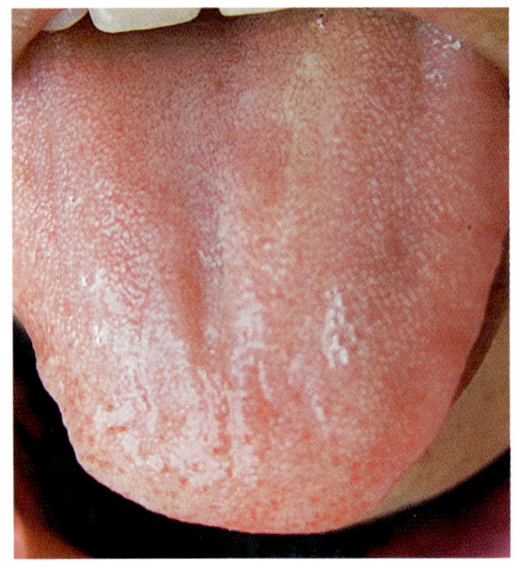

Fig 2.2-18

Patient, Female, 41years,

Case NO.: F320

Pale tongue

Fig 2.2-19

Patient, Female, 43years,

Case NO.: F139

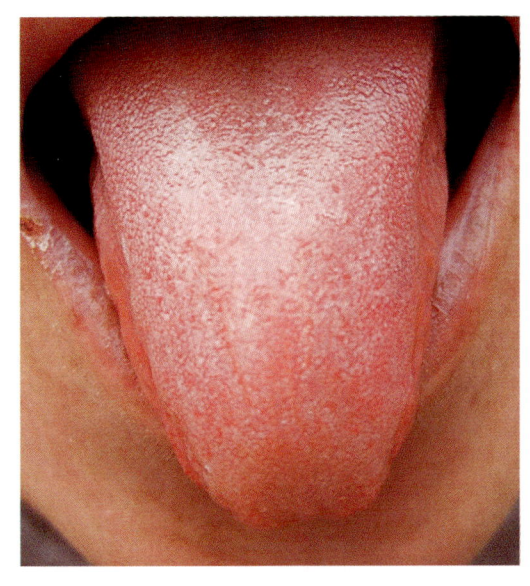

Fig 2.2-20

Patient, Female, 44years,

Case NO.: F209

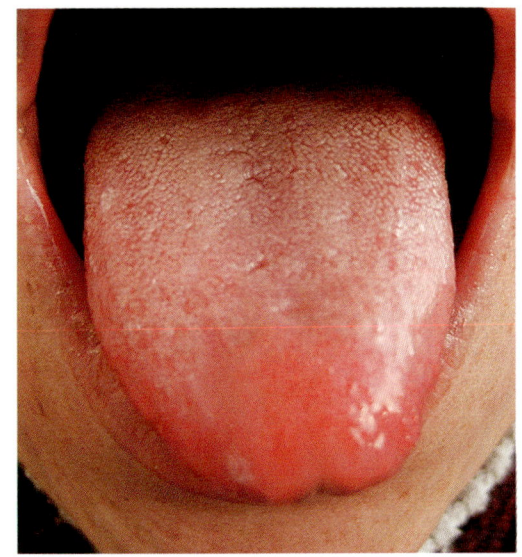

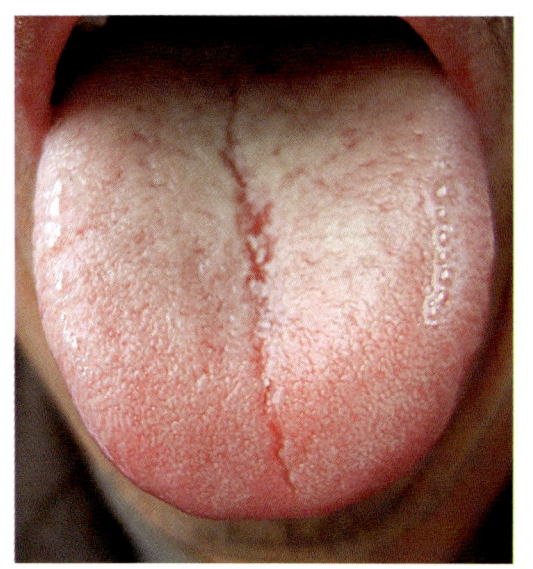

Fig 2.2-21

Patient, Male, 48years,

Case NO.: W414

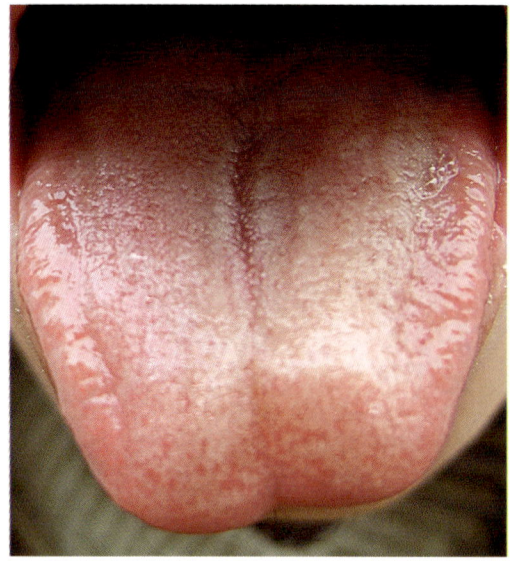

Fig 2.2-22

Patient, Male, 28years,

Case NO.: F72

Fig 2.2-23

Patient, Male, 35years,

Case NO.: F129

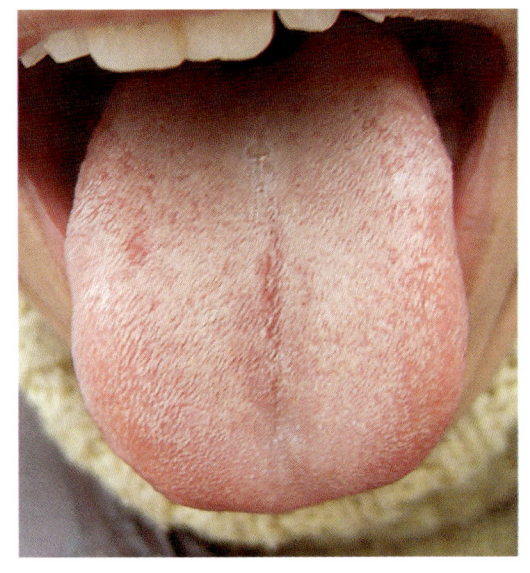

Fig 2.2-24

Patient, Female, 43years,

Case NO.: W507

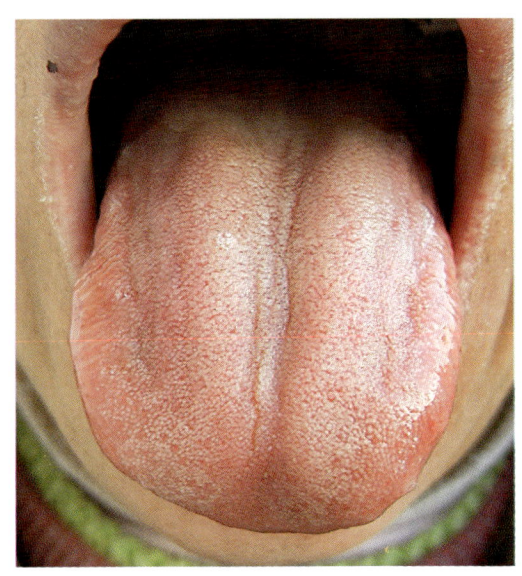

Pale tongue

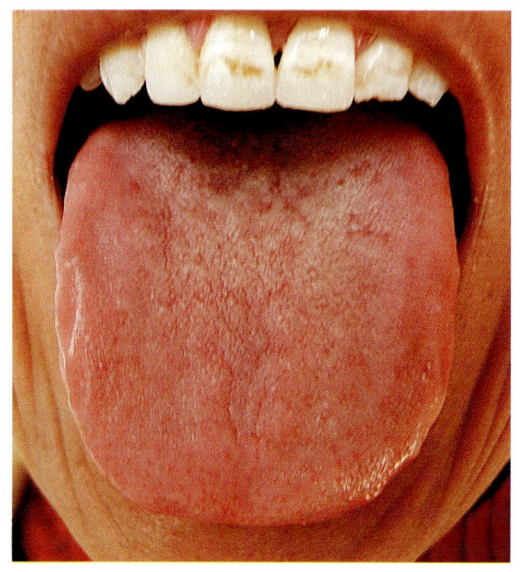

Fig 2.2-25

Patient, Female, 42years,

Case NO.: F81

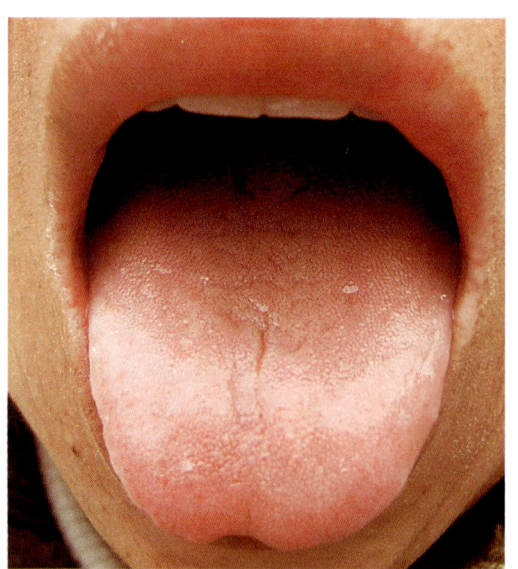

Fig 2.2-26

Patient, Female, 35years,

Case NO.: W45

Fig 2.2-27

Patient, Female, 56years,

Case NO.: W50

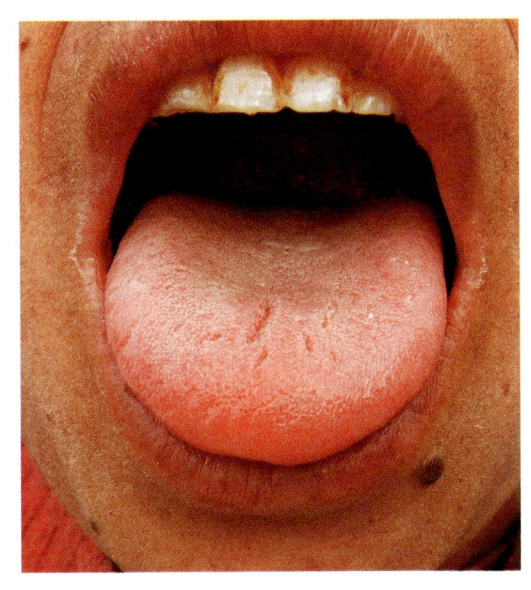

Fig 2.2-28

Patient, Female, 43years,

Case NO.: F308

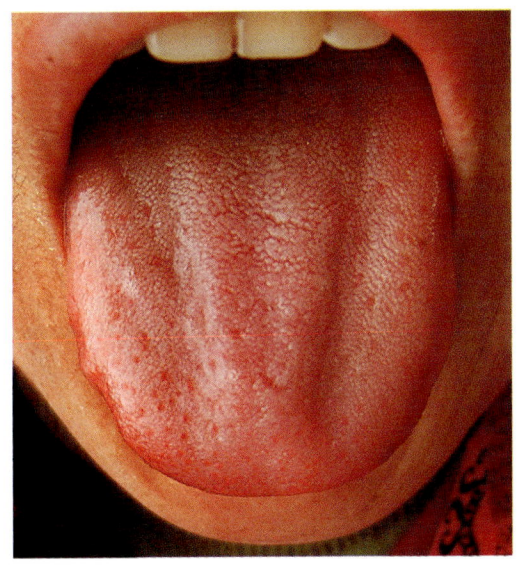

Pale tongue

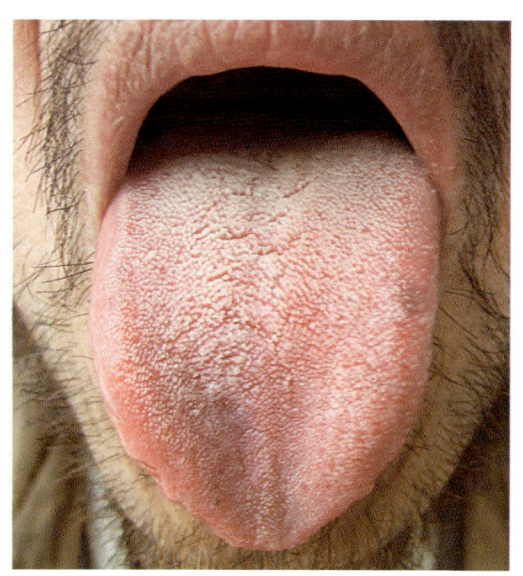

Fig 2.2-29

Patient, Male, 37years,

Case NO.: W424

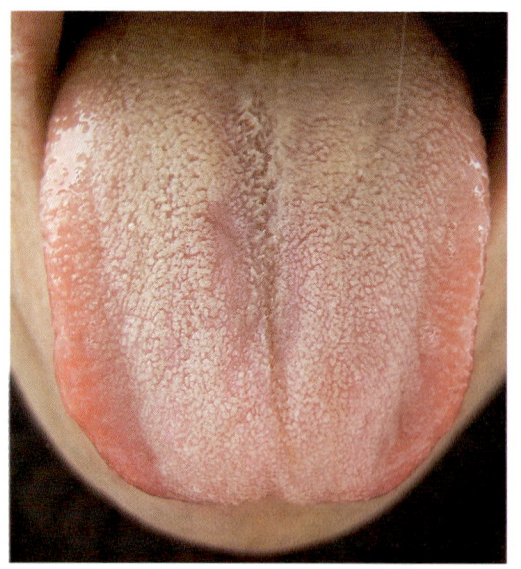

Fig 2.2-30

Patient, Male, 42years,

Case NO.: F261

Fig 2.2-31

Patient, Female, 40years,

Case NO.: W280

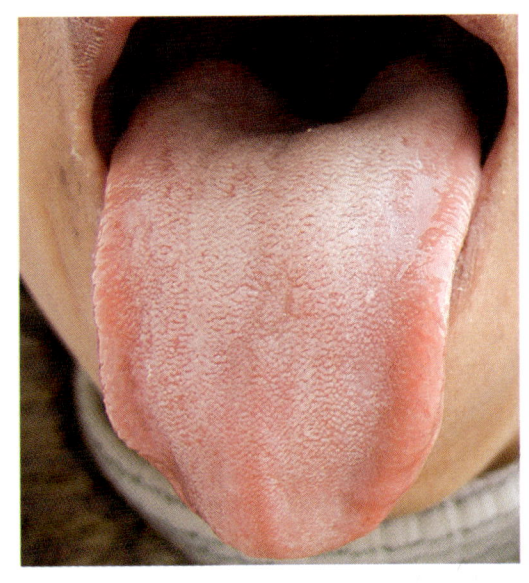

Fig 2.2-32

Patient, Female, 57years,

Case NO.: F304

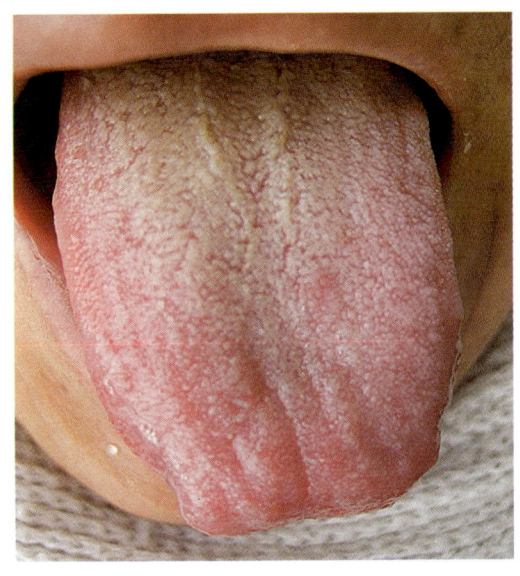

1.2 Light red tongue

AIDS stage

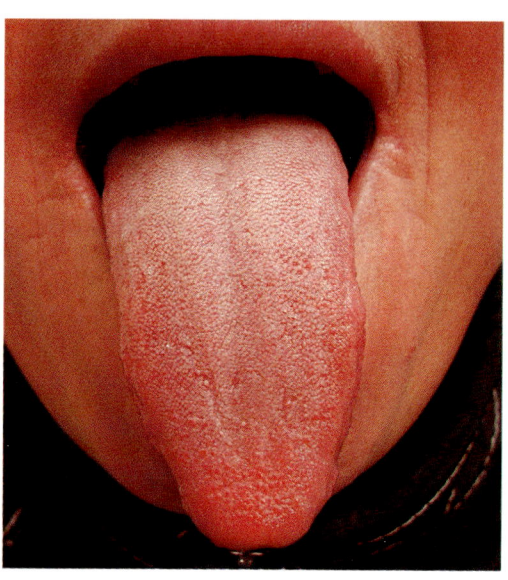

Fig 2.2-33

Patient, Female, 44years,

Case NO.: W529

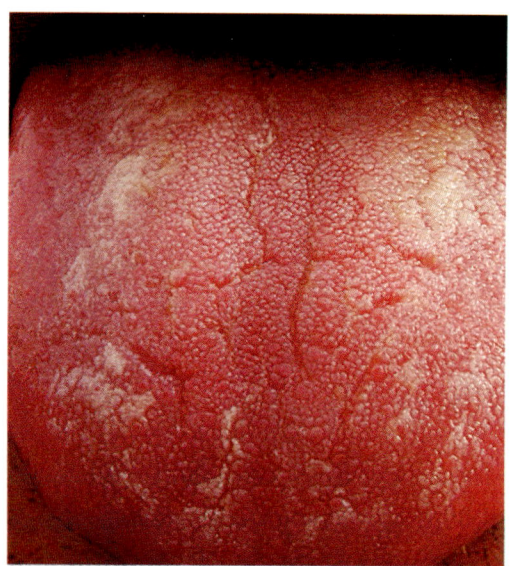

Fig 2.2-34

Patient, Male, 45years,

Case NO.: W648

Light red tongue

Fig 2.2-35

Patient, Female, 40years,

Case NO.: F150

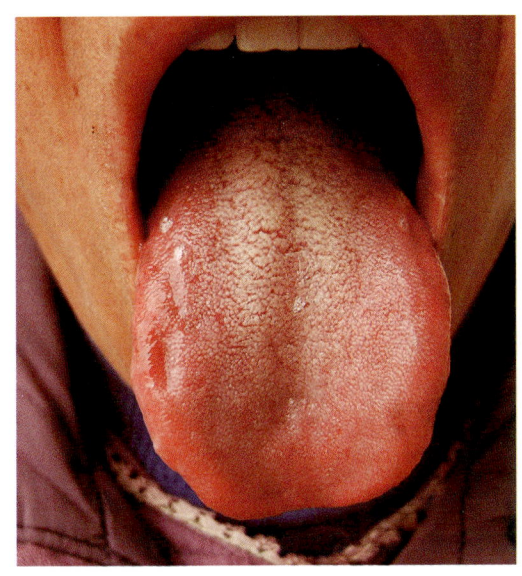

Fig 2.2-36

Patient, Female, 29years,

Case NO.: 247

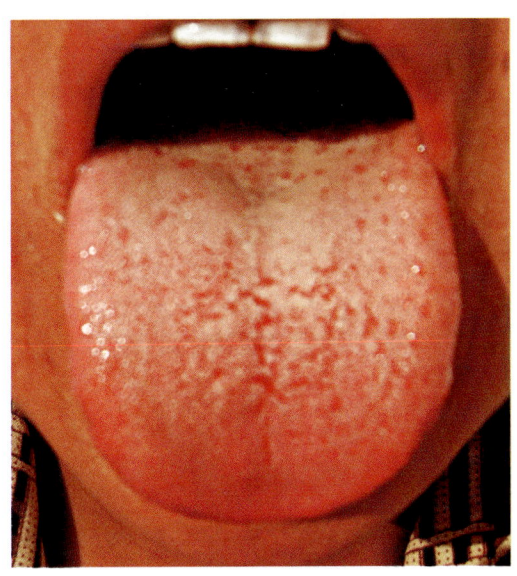

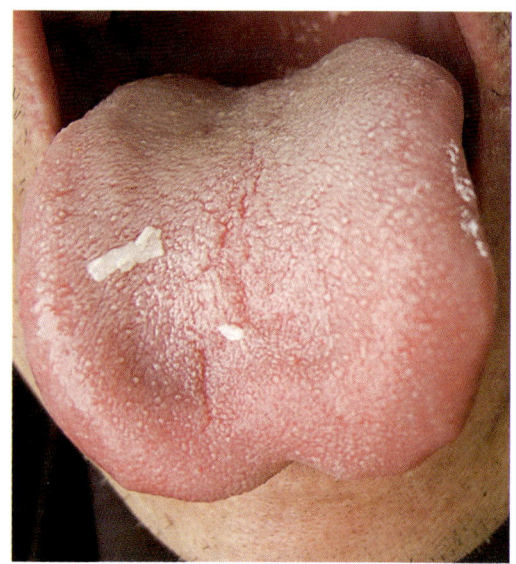

Fig 2.2-37

Patient, Male, 46years,

Case NO.: W728

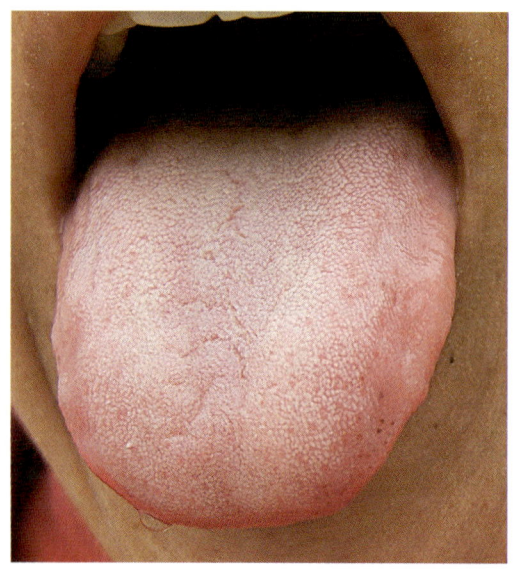

Fig 2.2-38

Patient, Female, 35years,

Case NO.: W402

Fig 2.2-39

Patient, Female, 46years,

Case NO.: W442

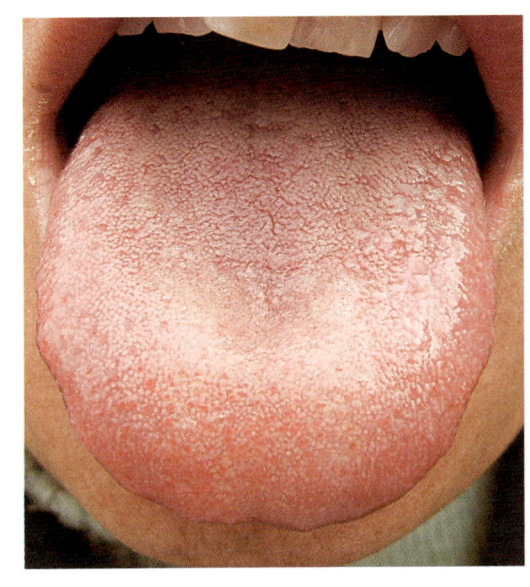

Fig 2.2-40

Patient, Male, 31years,

Case NO.: W662

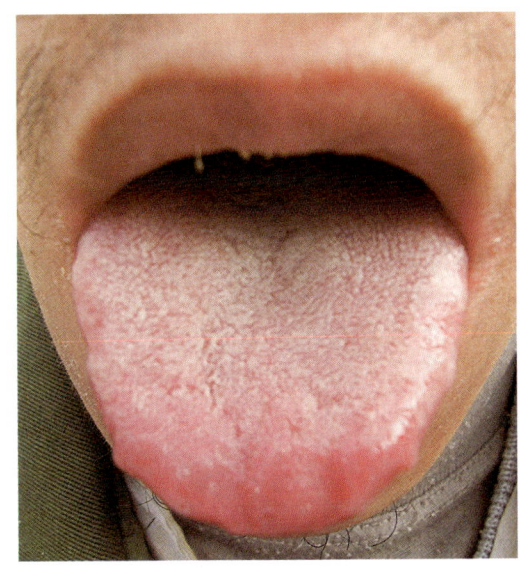

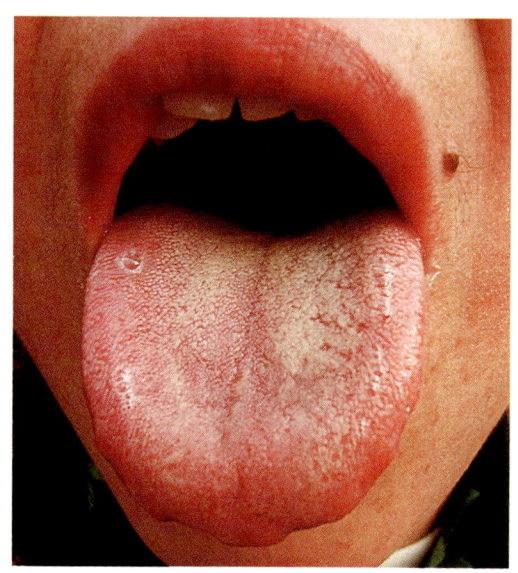

Fig 2.2-41

Patient, Female, 42years,

Case NO.: W651

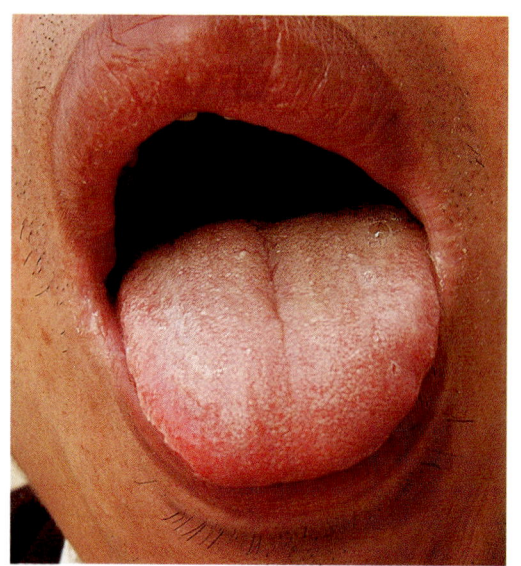

Fig 2.2-42

Patient, Male, 36years,

Case NO.: W199

Light red tongue

Fig 2.2-43

Patient, Male, 50years,

Case NO.: W187

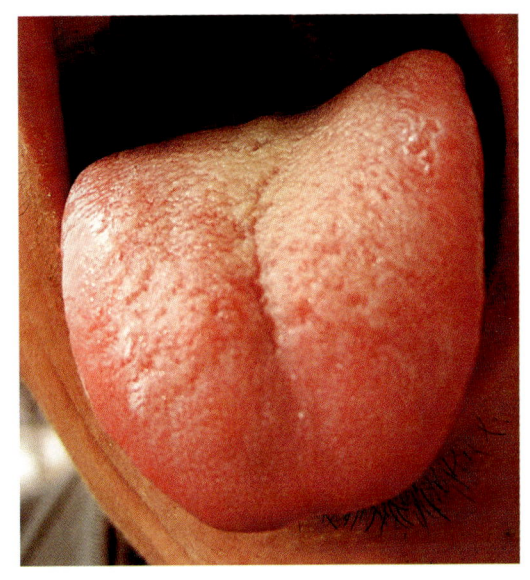

Fig 2.2-44

Patient, Female, 36years,

Case NO.: W410

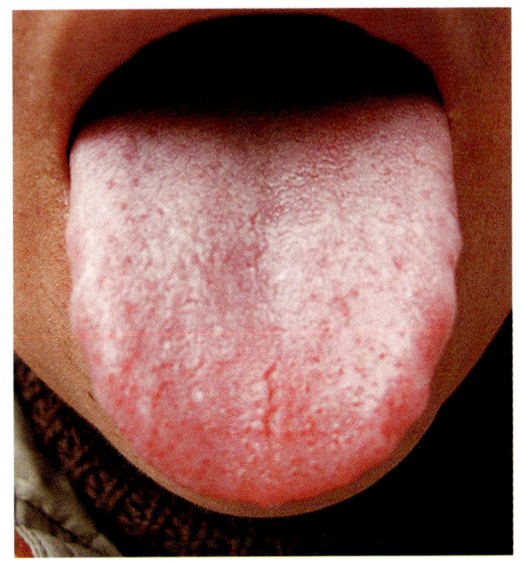

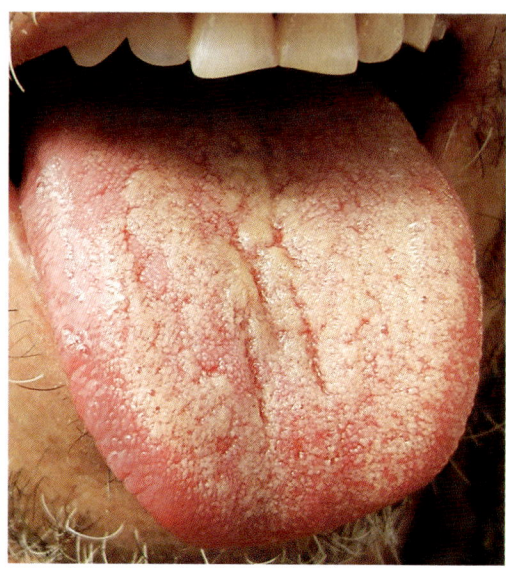

Fig 2.2-45

Patient, Male, 61years,

Case NO.: W252

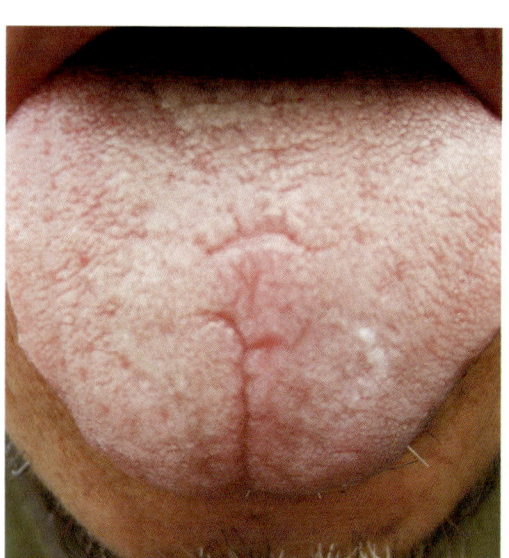

Fig 2.2-46

Patient, Male, 55years,

Case NO.: W351

Light red tongue

Fig 2.2-47

Patient, Female, 39years,

Case NO.: W309

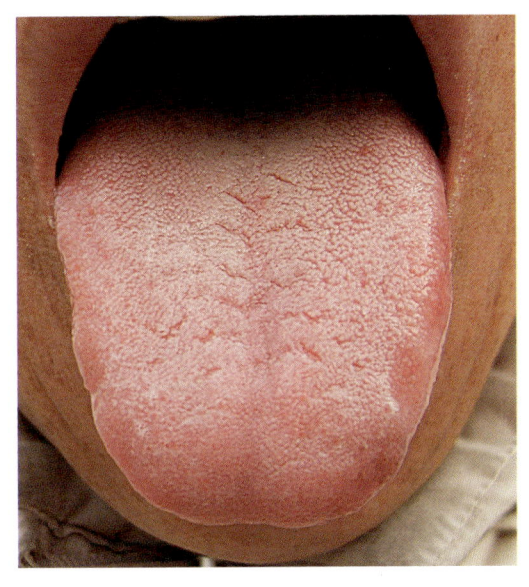

Fig 2.2-48

Patient, Male, 52years,

Case NO.: W367

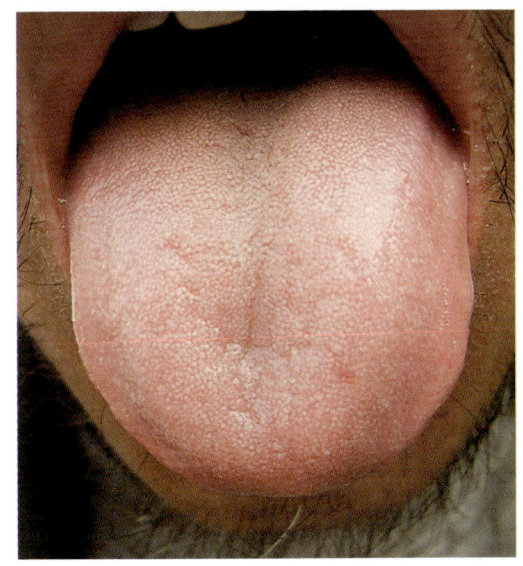

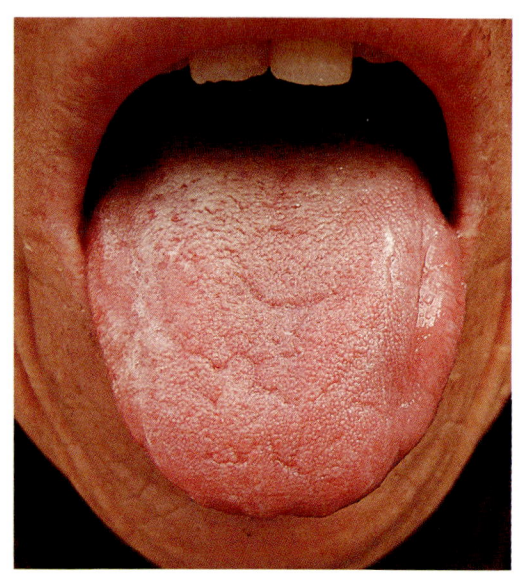

Fig 2.2-49

Patient, Female, 68years,

Case NO.: F99

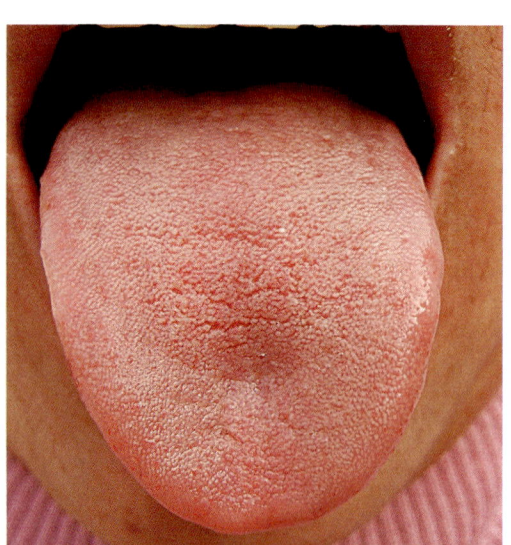

Fig 2.2-50

Patient, Female, 44years,

Case NO.: F117

Fig 2.2-51

Patient, Female, 36years,

Case NO.: W314

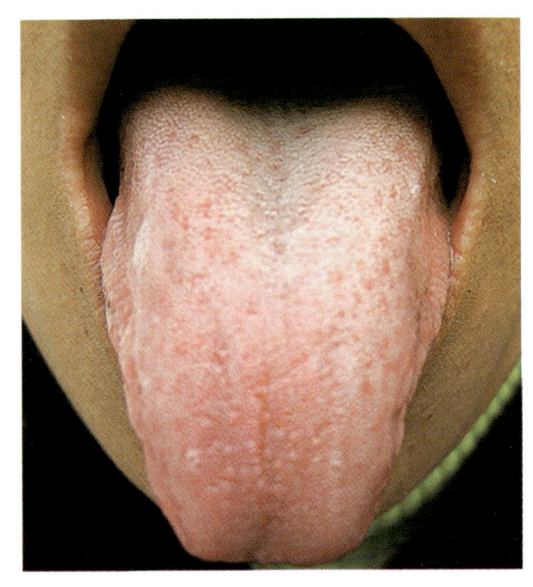

Fig 2.2-52

Patient, Female, 59years,

Case NO.: F92

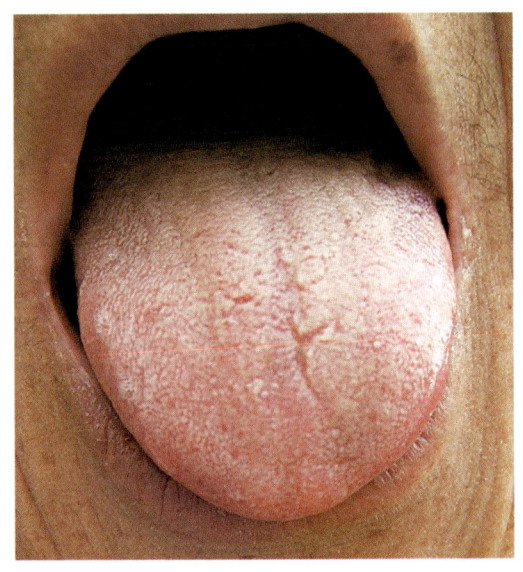

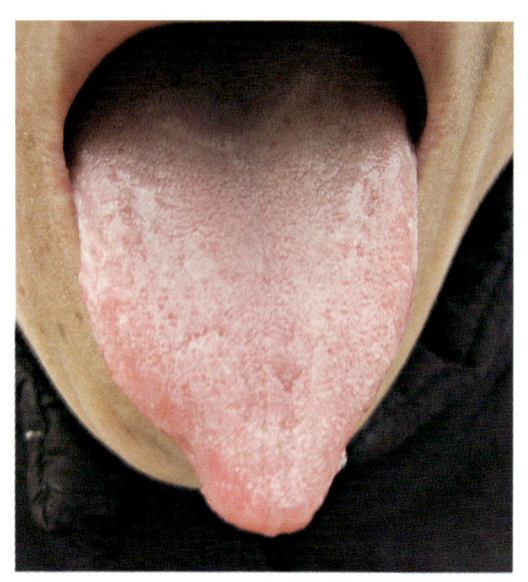

Fig 2.2-53

Patient, Female, 38years,

Case NO.: W381

Light red tongue

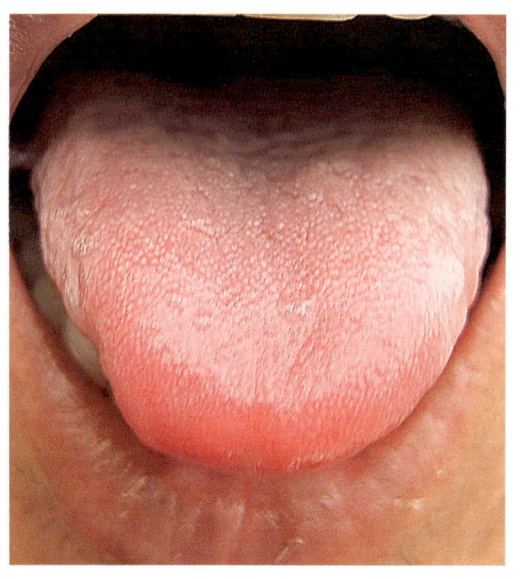

Fig 2.2-54

Patient, Female, 50years,

Case NO.: W126

Fig 2.2-55

Patient, Female, 39years,

Case NO.: W413

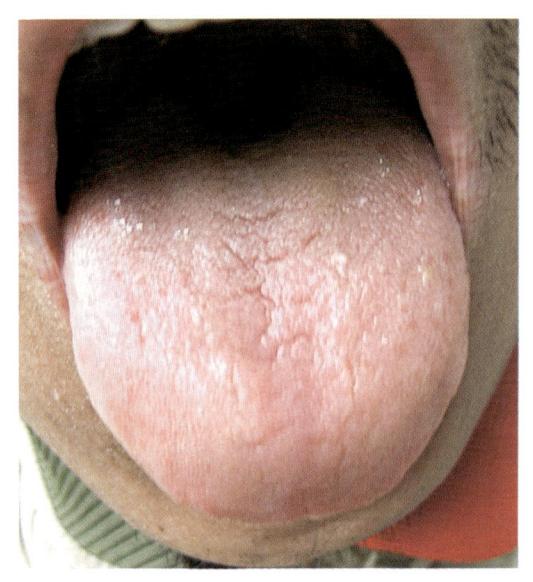

Fig 2.2-56

Patient, Male, 40years,

Case NO.: W53

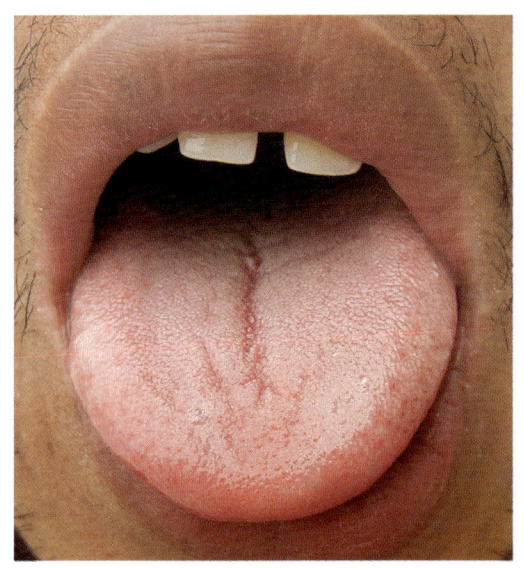

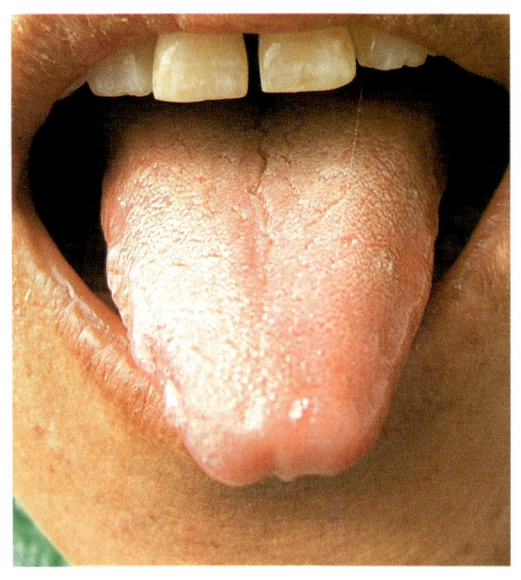

Fig 2.2-57

Patient, Female, 47years,

Case NO.: W204

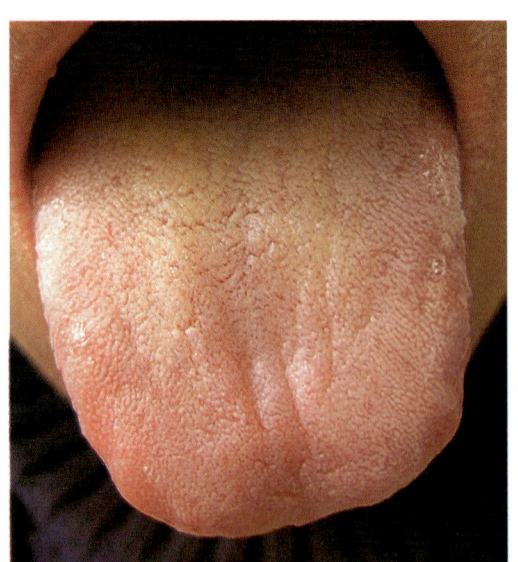

Fig 2.2-58

Patient, Female, 42years,

Case NO.: W194

Fig 2.2-59

Patient, Female, 46years,

Case NO.: F239

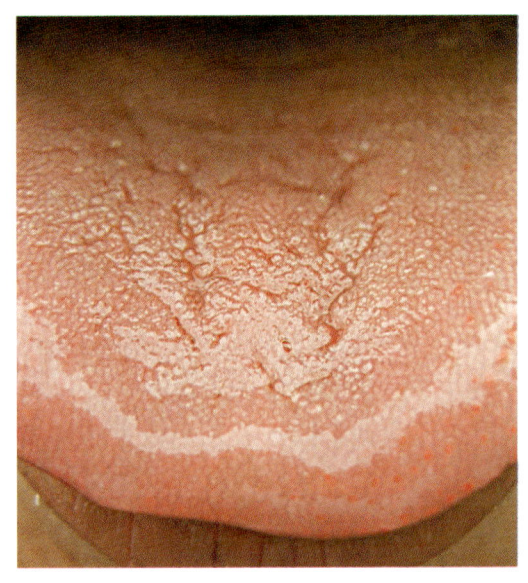

Fig 2.2-60

Patient, Male, 33years,

Case NO.: W230

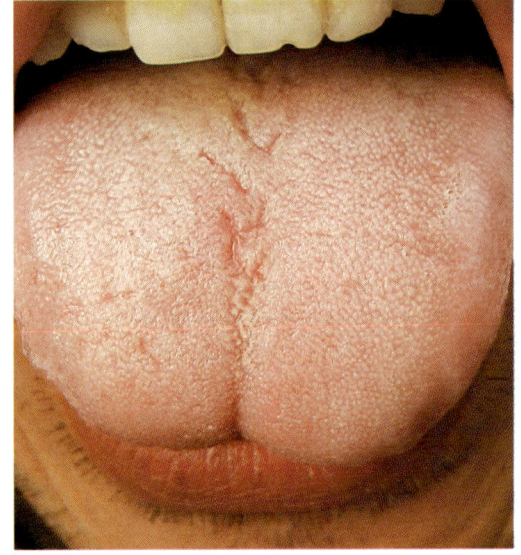

Light red tongue

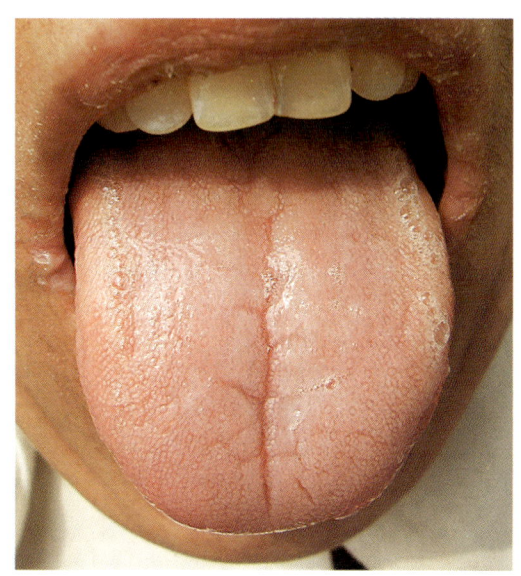

Fig 2.2-61

Patient, Female, 45years,

Case NO.: W182

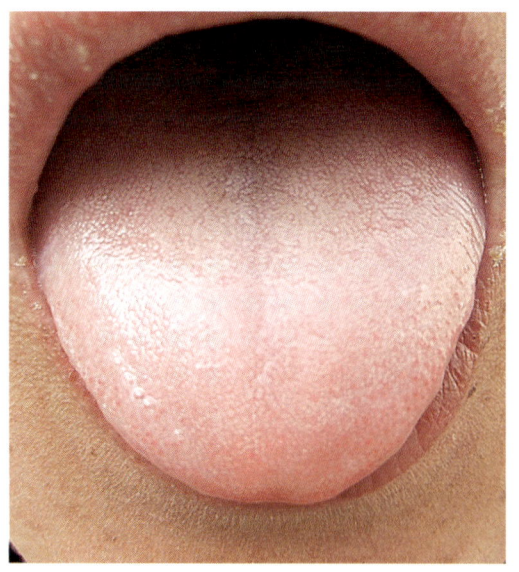

Fig 2.2-62

Patient, Female, 40years,

Case NO.: F95

Fig 2.2-63

Patient, Female, 64years,

Case NO.: F240

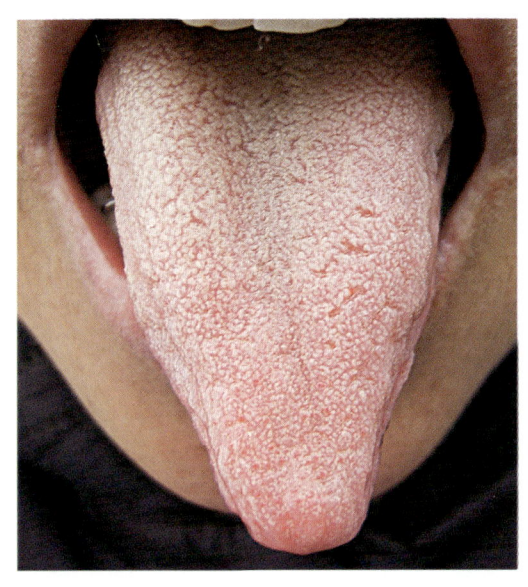

Fig 2.2-64

Patient, Female, 42years,

Case NO.: W747

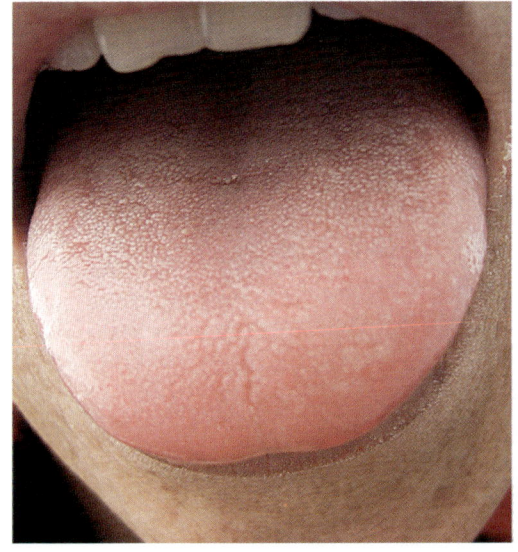

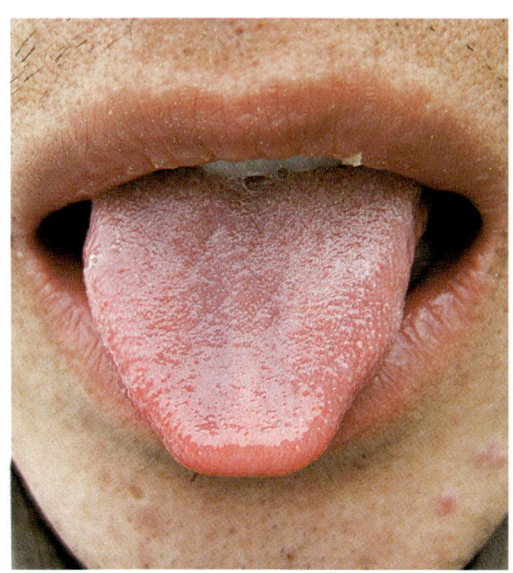

Fig 2.2-65

Patient, Male, 34years,

Case NO.: F255

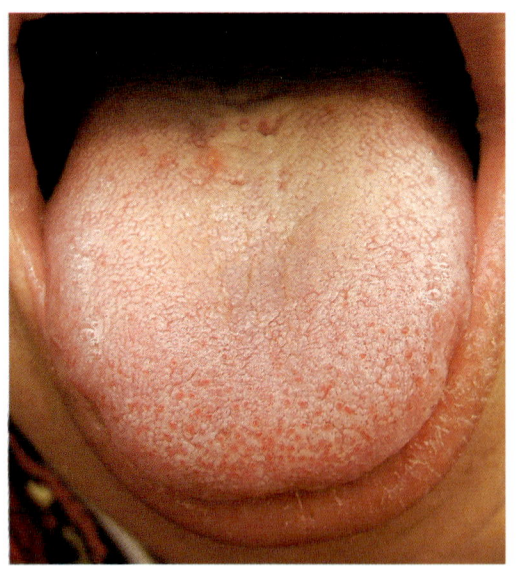

Fig 2.2-66

Patient, Female, 47years,

Case NO.: W343

Fig 2.2-67

Patient, Female, 39years,

Case NO.: W286

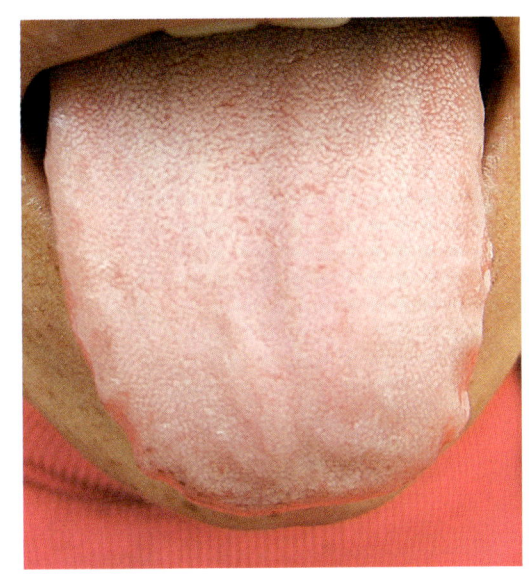

Fig 2.2-68

Patient, Female, 55years,

Case NO.: W592

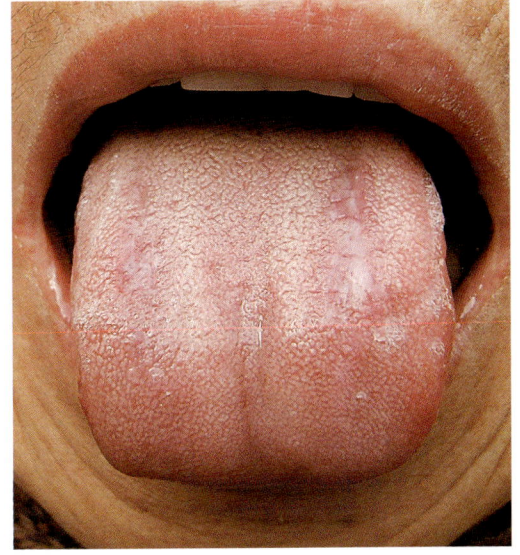

Light red tongue

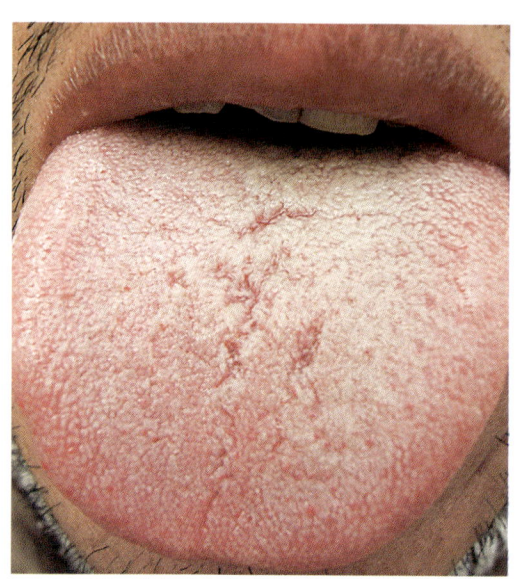

Fig 2.2-69

Patient, Male, 54years,

Case NO.: W593

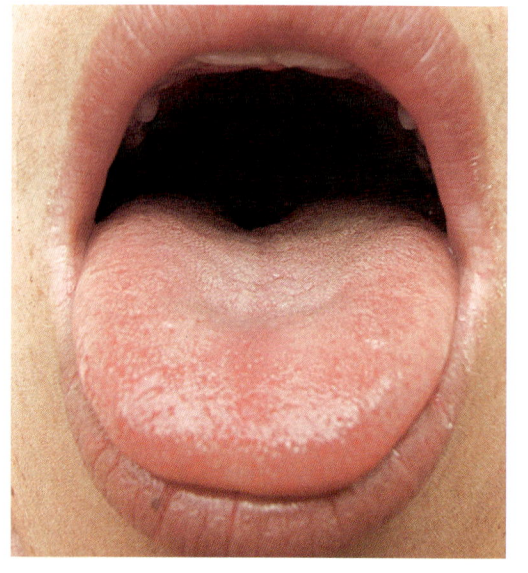

Fig 2.2-70

Patient, Female, 36years,

Case NO.: W546

Fig 2.2-71

Patient, Male, 35years,

Case NO.: W84

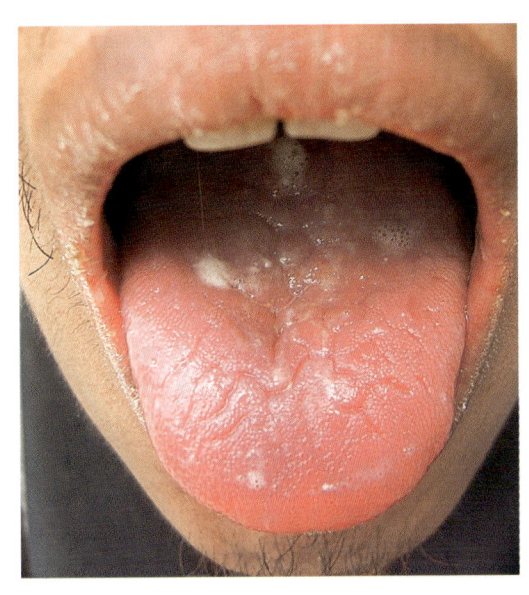

Fig 2.2-72

Patient, Female, 38years,

Case NO.: W83

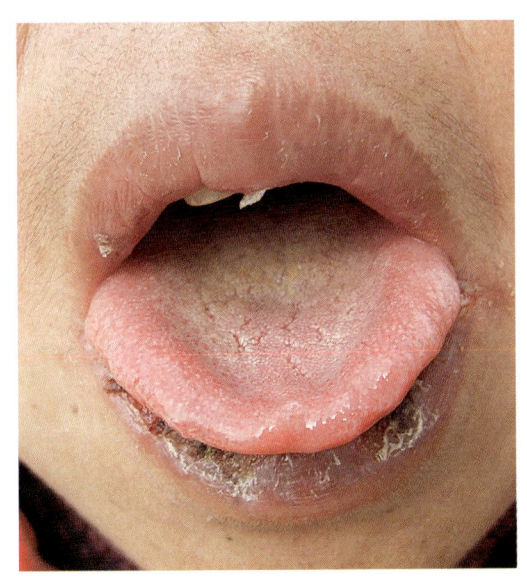

Light red tongue

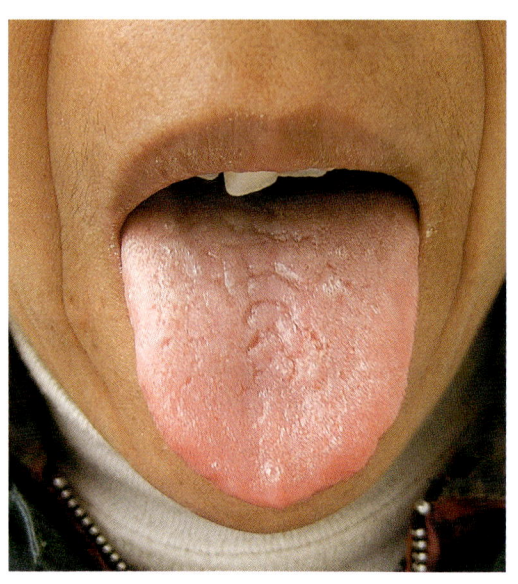

Fig 2.2-73

Patient, Female, 47years,

Case NO.: W19

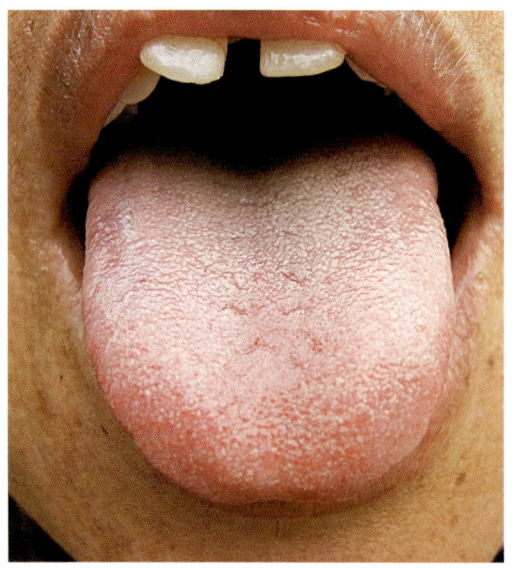

Fig 2.2-74

Patient, Female, 49years,

Case NO.: W552

Fig 2.2-75

Patient, Male, 35years,

Case NO.: W587

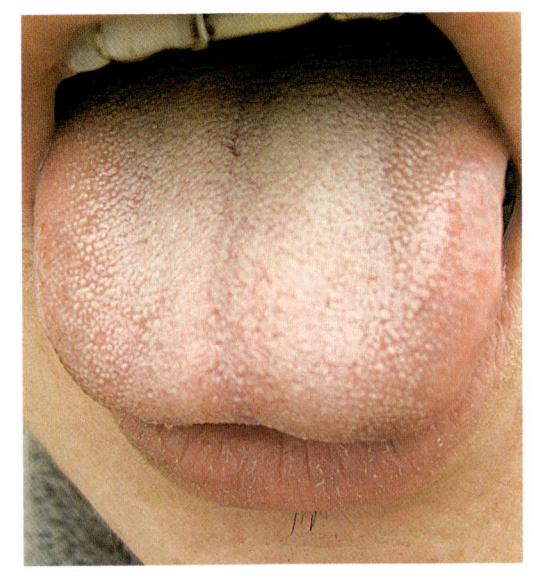

Fig 2.2-76

Patient, Female, 43years,

Case NO.: W202

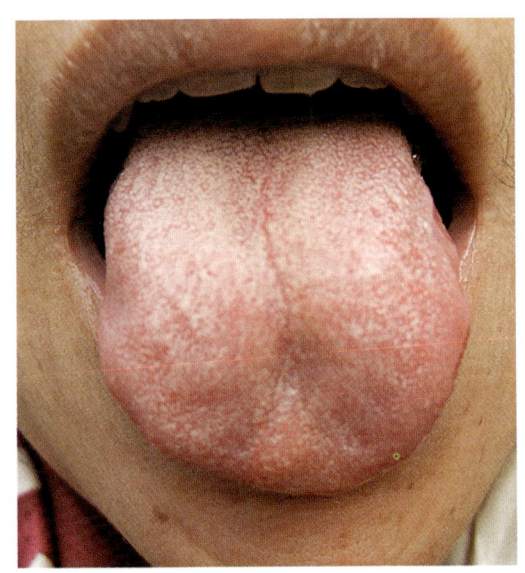

Light red tongue

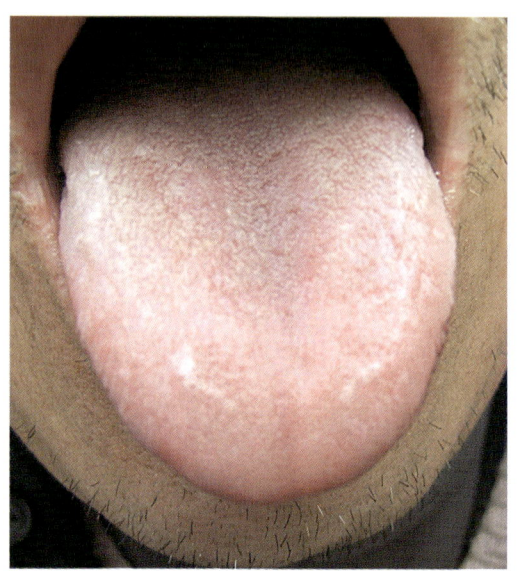

Fig 2.2-77

Patient, Male, 50years,

Case NO.: F199

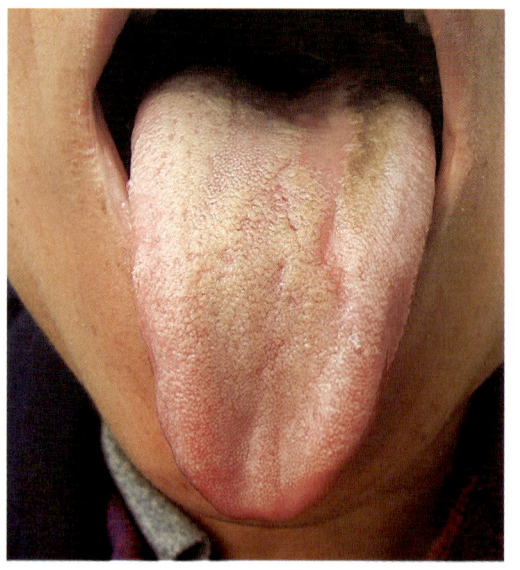

Fig 2.2-78

Patient, Female, 51years,

Case NO.: W183

Fig 2.2-79

Patient, Male, 47years,

Case NO.: W239

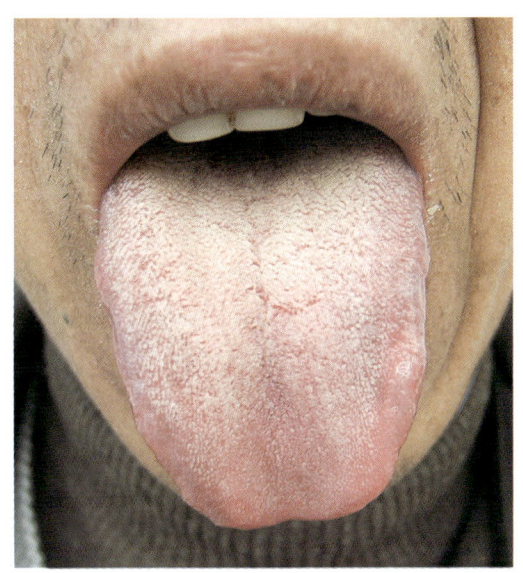

Fig 2.2-80

Patient, Female, 53years,

Case NO.: F200

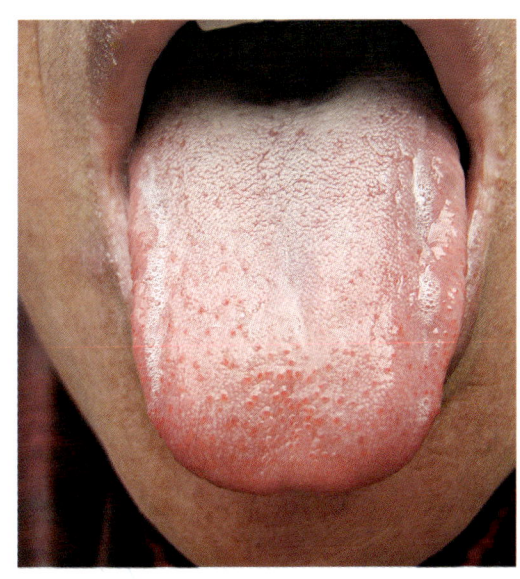

Light red tongue

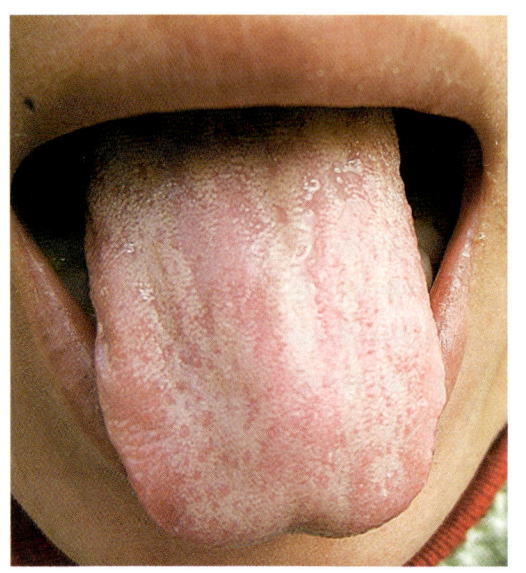

Fig 2.2-81

Patient, Female, 39years,

Case NO.: W625

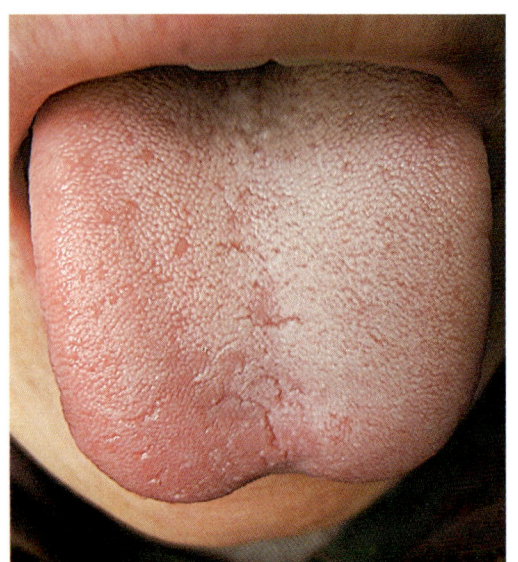

Fig 2.2-82

Patient, Female, 48years,

Case NO.: W517

Fig 2.2-83

Patient, Male, 48years,

Case NO.: W509

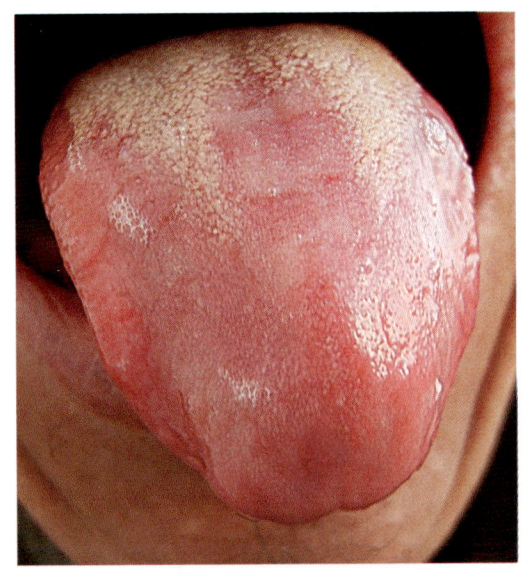

Fig 2.2-84

Patient, Male, 33years,

Case NO.: F71

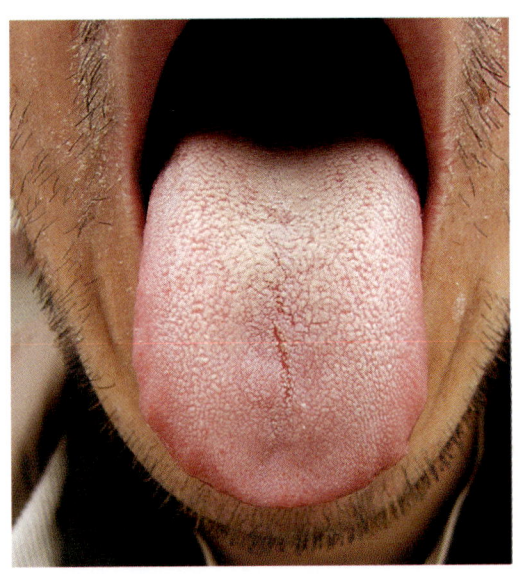

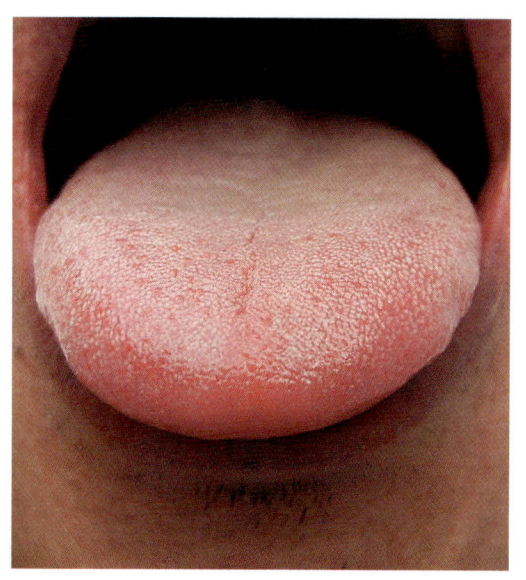

Fig 2.2-85

Patient, Male, 38years,

Case NO.: W100

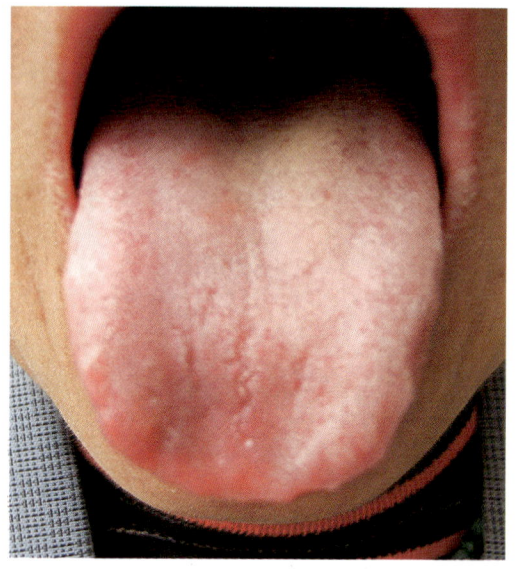

Fig 2.2-86

Patient, Female, 52years,

Case NO.: F3

Fig 2.2-87

Patient, Male, 48years,

Case NO.: W60

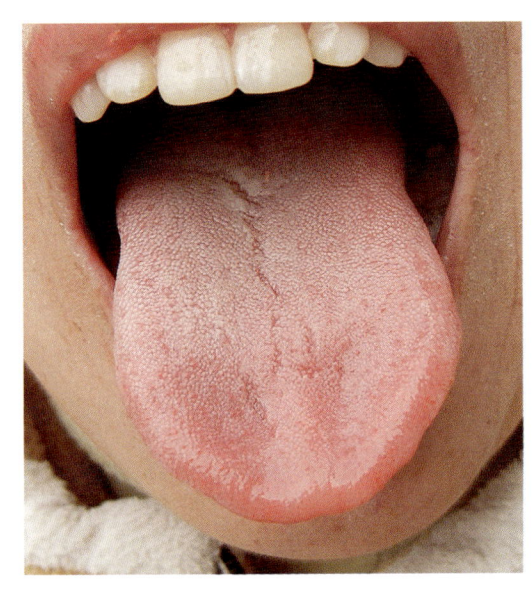

Fig 2.2-88

Patient, Male, 49years,

Case NO.: W80

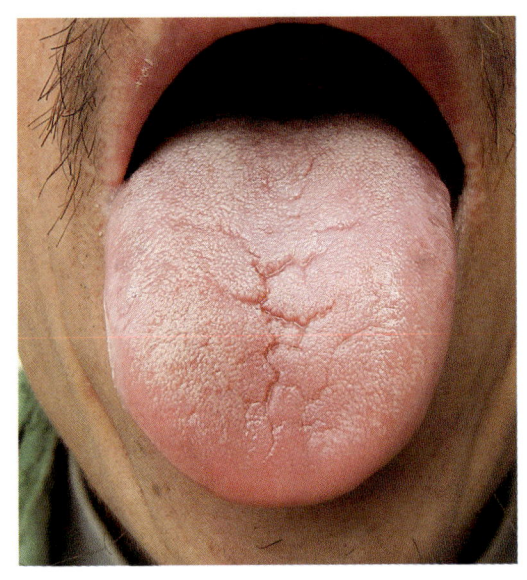

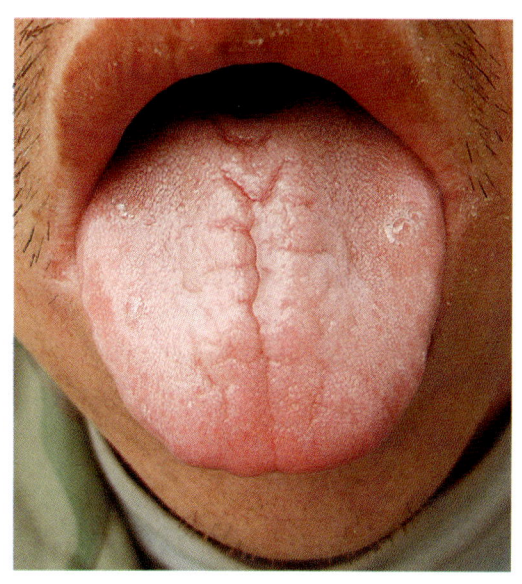

Fig 2.2-89

Patient, Male, 38years,

Case NO.: W77

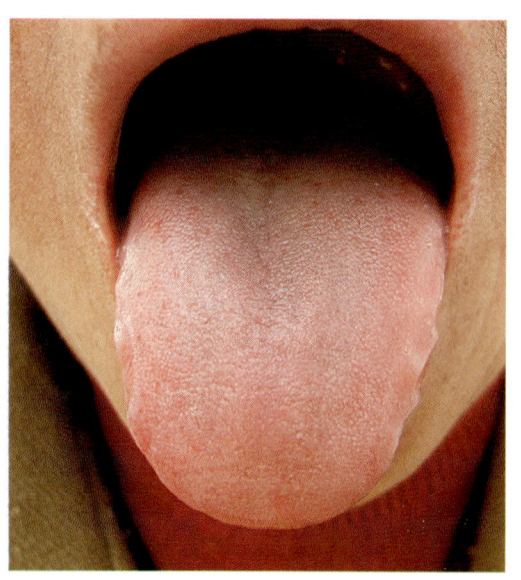

Fig 2.2-90

Patient, Female, 36years,

Case NO.: W91

Fig 2.2-91

Patient, Male, 34years,

Case NO.: W89

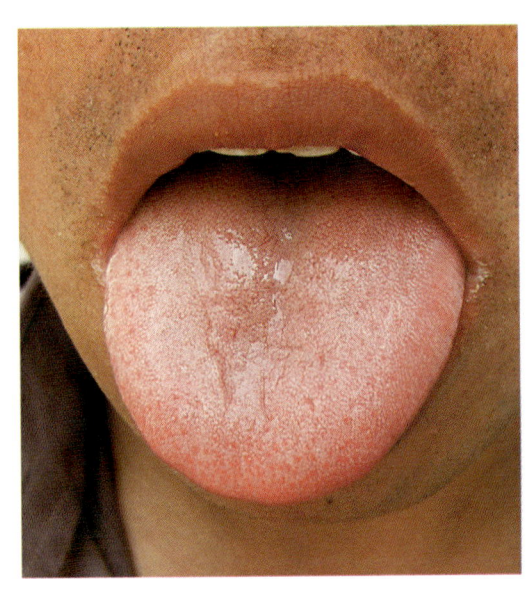

Fig 2.2-92

Patient, Female, 32years,

Case NO.: F85

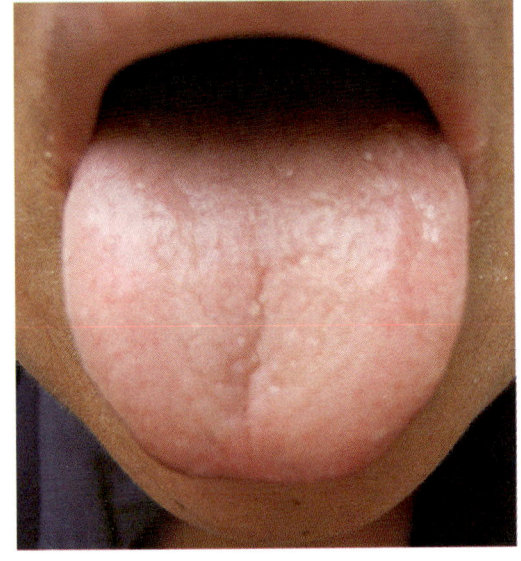

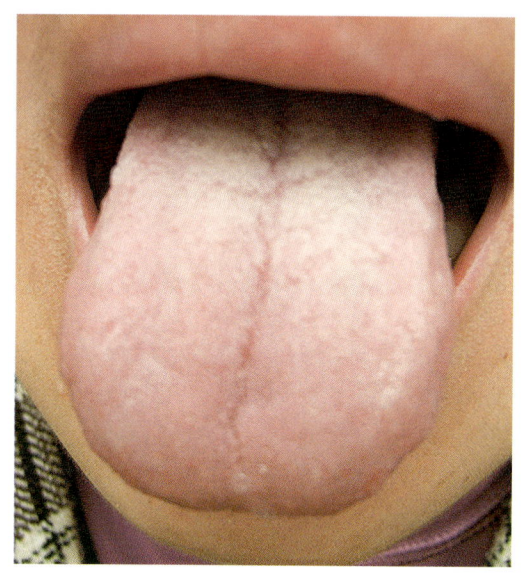

Fig 2.2-93

Patient, Female, 38years,

Case NO.: F72

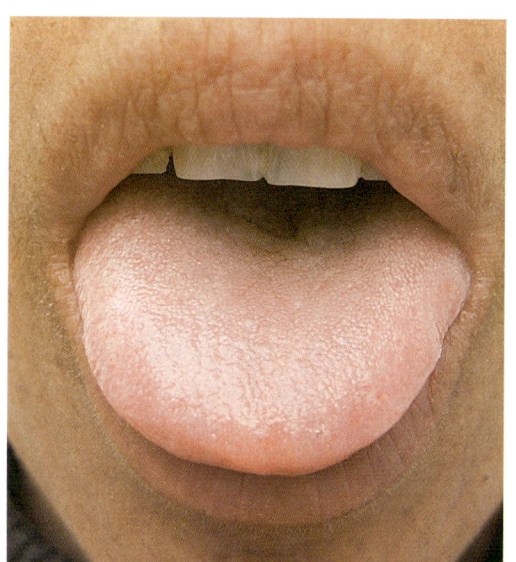

Fig 2.2-94

Patient, Female, 51years,

Case NO.: W103

Fig 2.2-95

Patient, Female, 40years,

Case NO.: F76

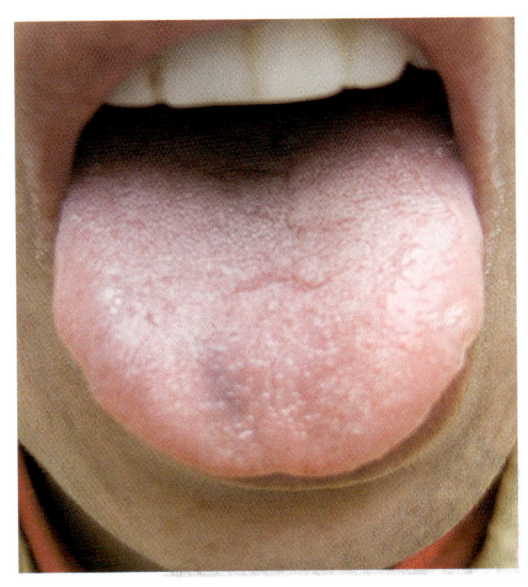

Fig 2.2-96

Patient, Female, 37years,

Case NO.: F19

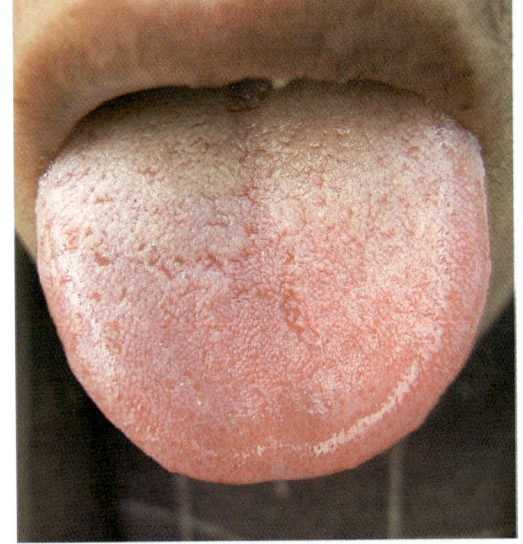

Light red tongue

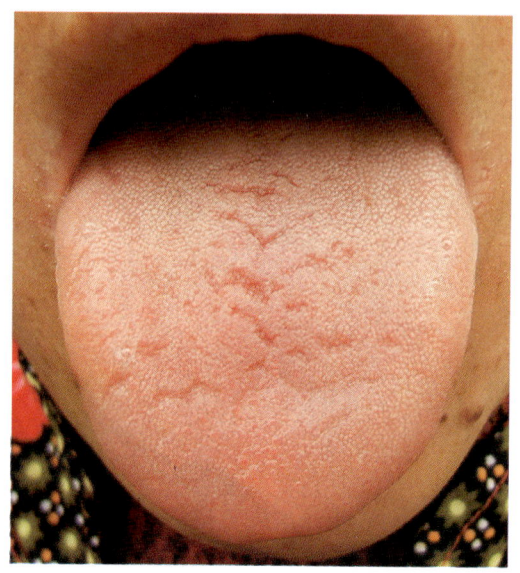

Fig 2.2-97

Patient, Female, 40years,

Case NO.: W329

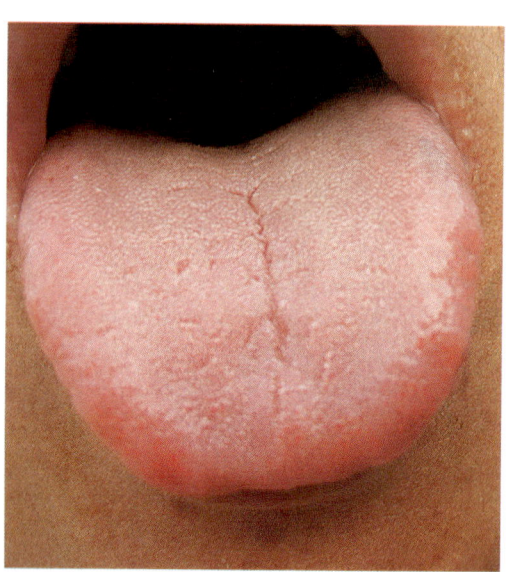

Fig 2.2-98

Patient, Female, 44years,

Case NO.: W370

Fig 2.2-99

Patient, Female, 48years,

Case NO.: W399

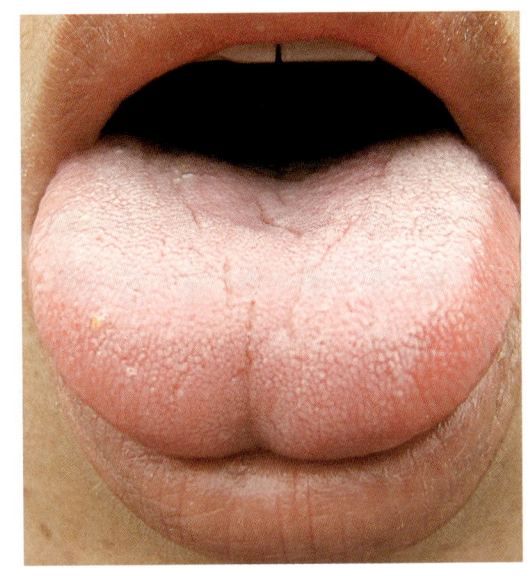

Fig 2.2-100

Patient, Female, 54years,

Case NO.: W125

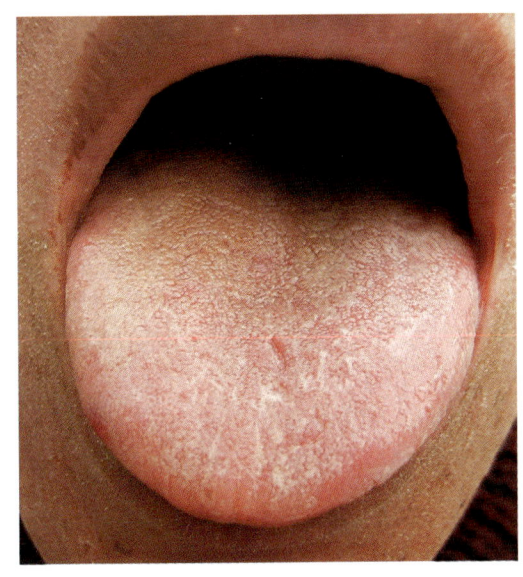

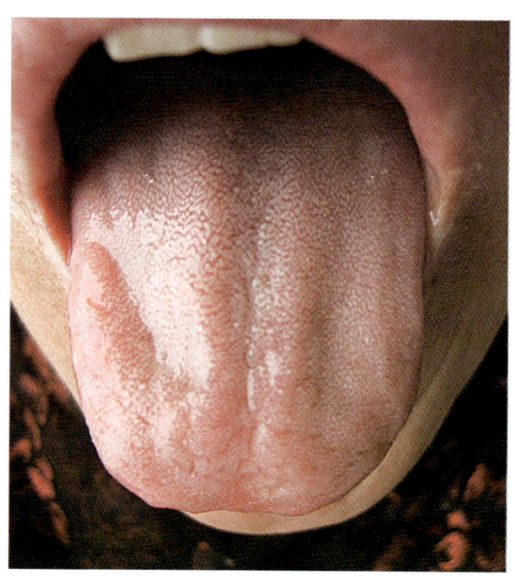

Fig 2.2-101

Patient, Female, 51years,

Case NO.: W735

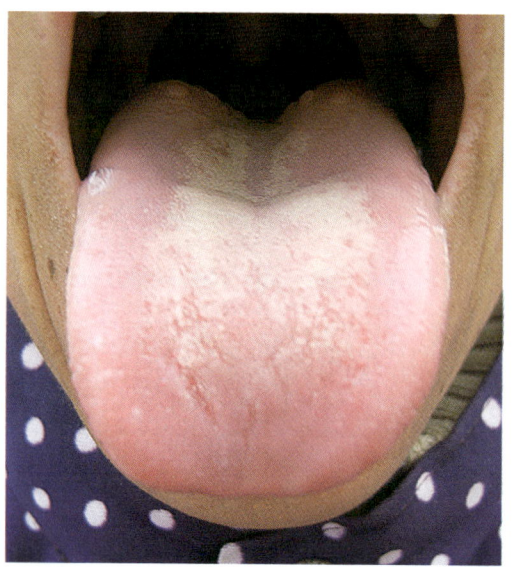

Fig 2.2-102

Patient, Female, 42years,

Case NO.: F90

Fig 2.2-103

Patient, Female, 48years,

Case NO.: W447

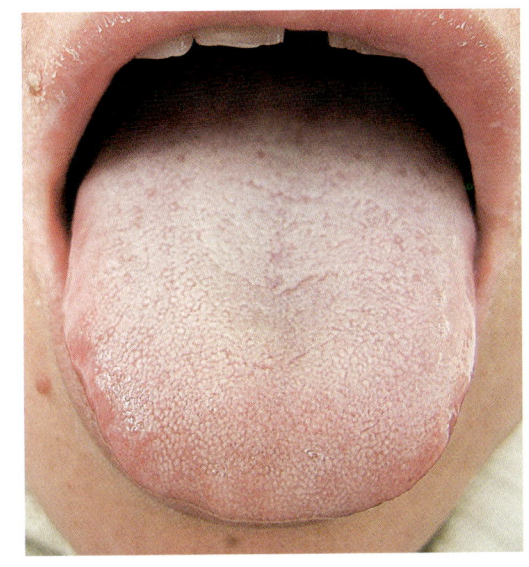

Fig 2.2-104

Patient, Female, 64years,

Case NO.: F289

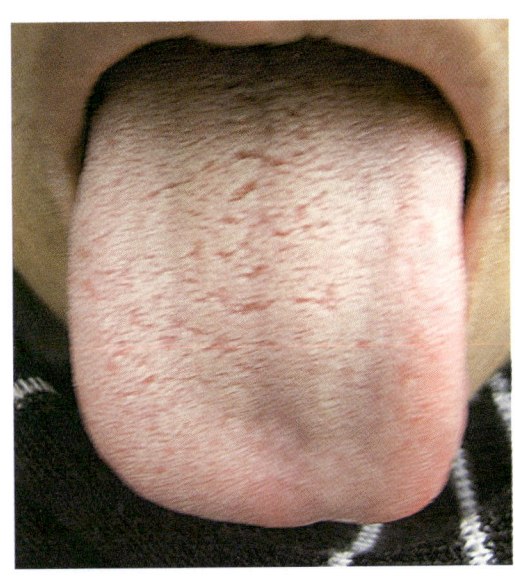

Light red tongue

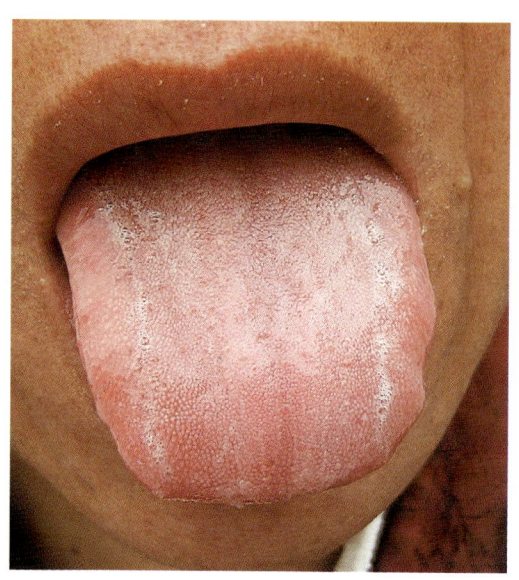

Fig 2.2-105

Patient, Female, 46years,

Case NO.: W47

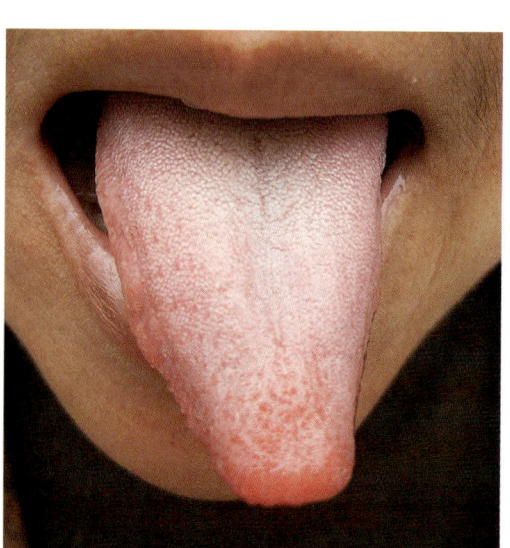

Fig 2.2-106

Patient, Female, 42years,

Case NO.: F7

Fig 2.2-107

Patient, Female, 37years,

Case NO.: F123

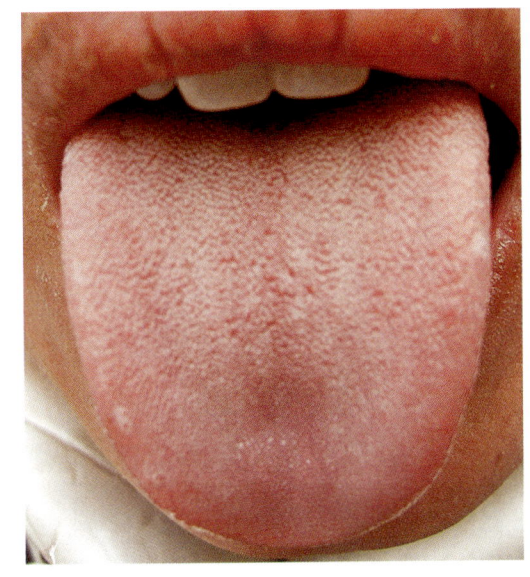

Fig 2.2-108

Patient, Female, 40years,

Case NO.: W21

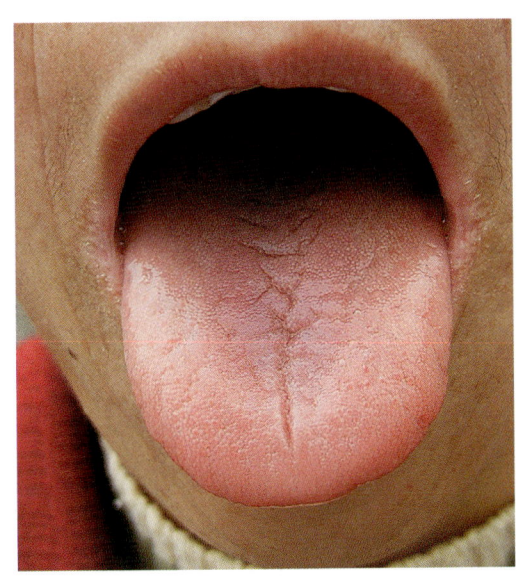

Light red tongue

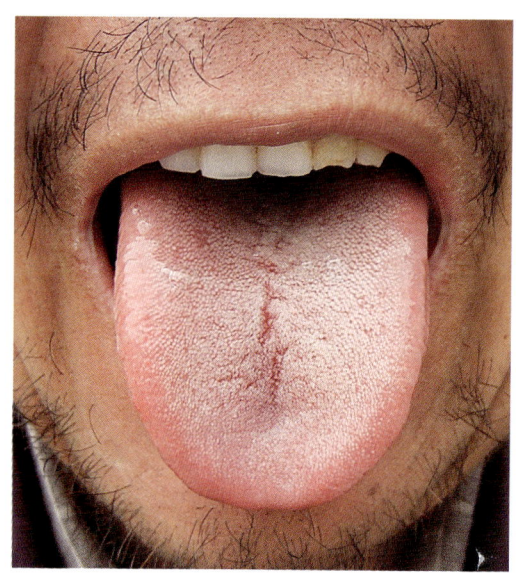

Fig 2.2-109

Patient, Male, 46years,

Case NO.: W29

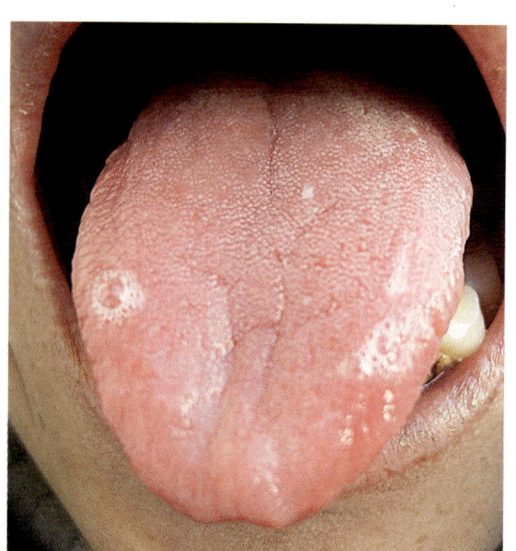

Fig 2.2-110

Patient, Female, 50years,

Case NO.: W503

Fig 2.2-111

Patient, Male, 50years,

Case NO.: W512

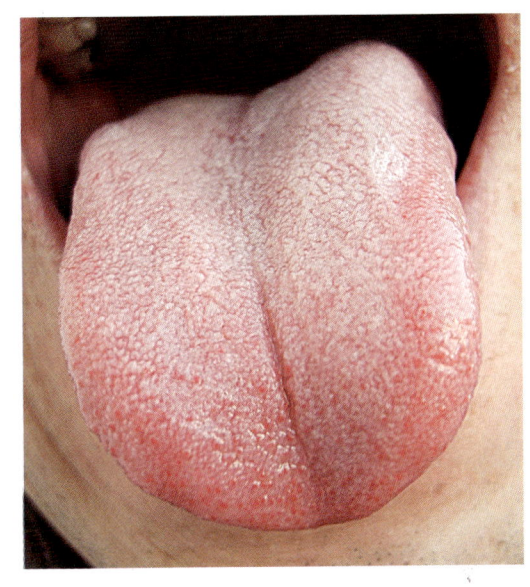

Fig 2.2-112

Patient, Male, 49years,

Case NO.: F350

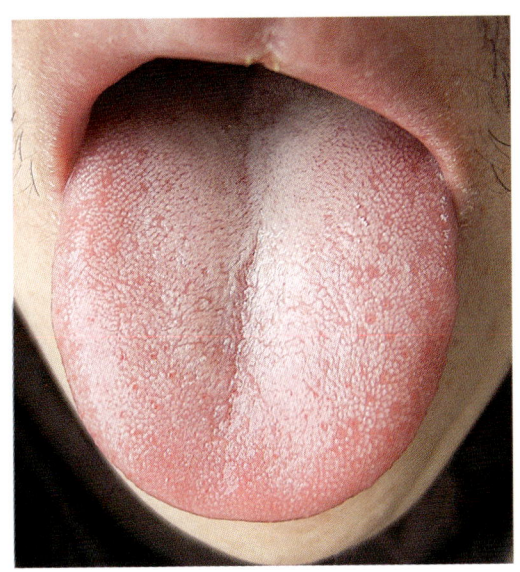

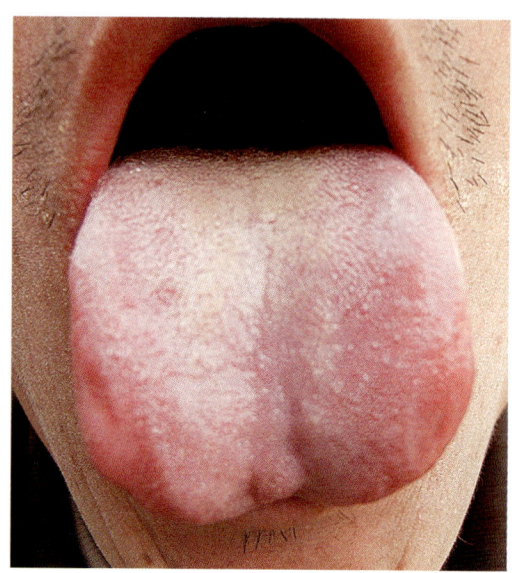

Fig 2.2-113

Patient, Male, 39years,

Case NO.: W626

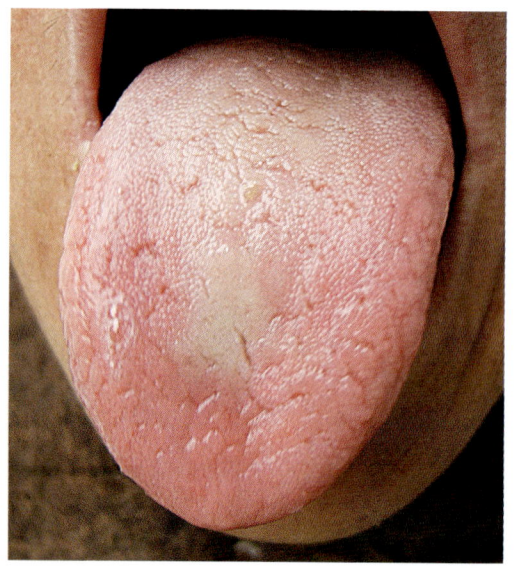

Fig 2.2-114

Patient, Female, 74years,

Case NO.: F132

Fig 2.2-115

Patient, Male, 38years,

Case NO.: W52

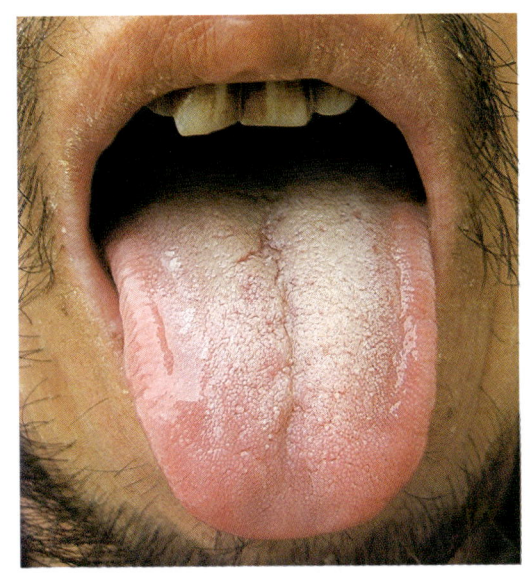

Fig 2.2-116

Patient, Female, 50years,

Case NO.: W318

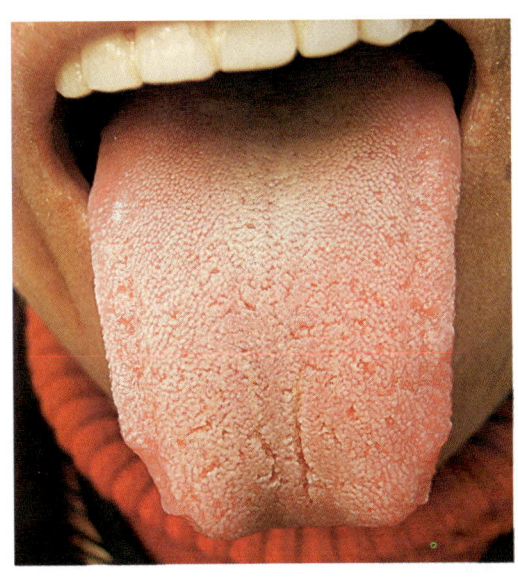

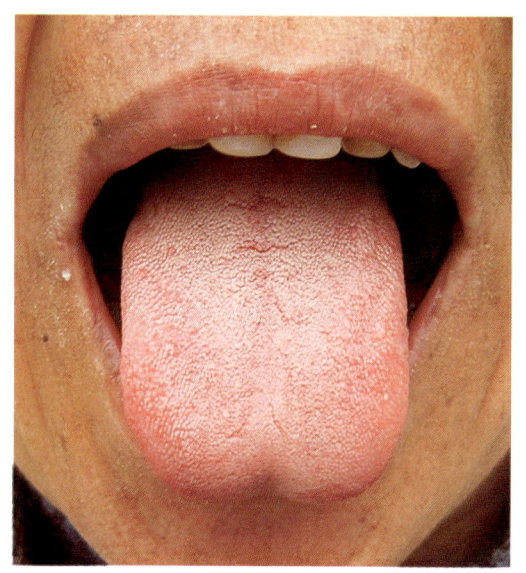

Fig 2.2-117

Patient, Female, 47years,

Case NO.: W44

Light red tongue

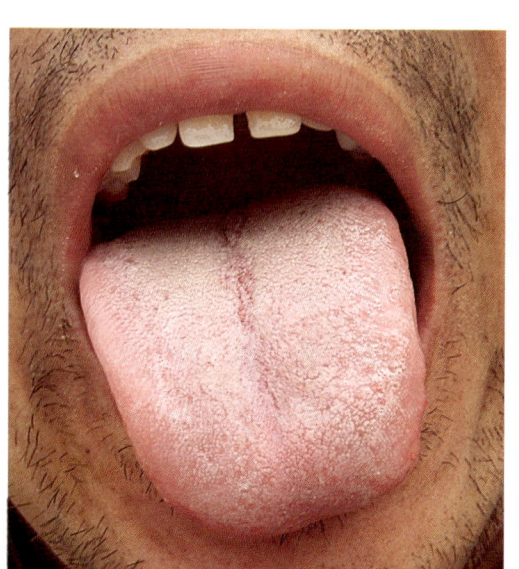

Fig 2.2-118

Patient, Female, 43years,

Case NO.: W40

Fig 2.2-119

Patient, Male, 36years,

Case NO.: W199

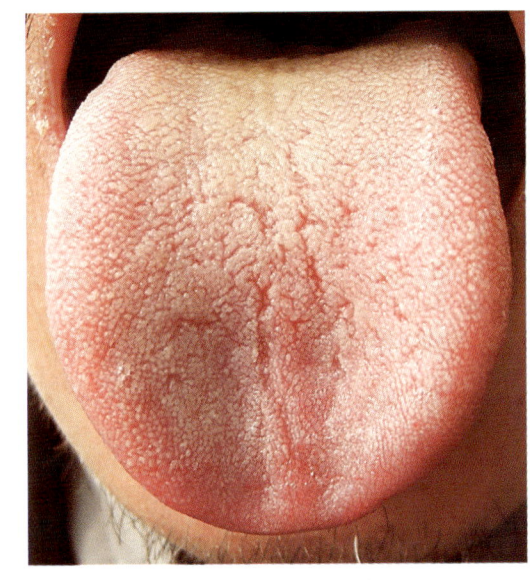

Fig 2.2-120

Patient, Female, 42years,

Case NO.: W247

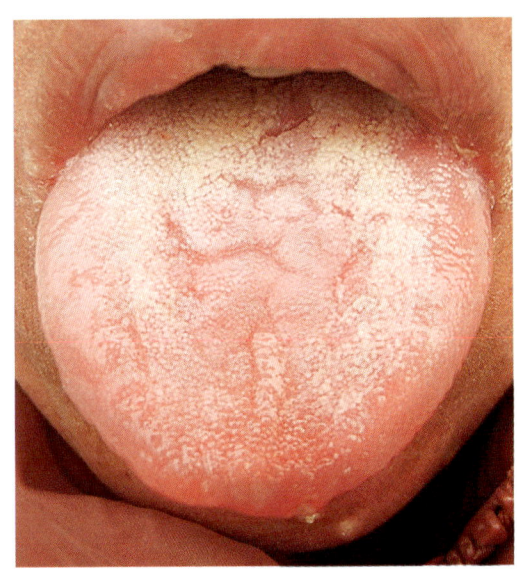

Light red tongue

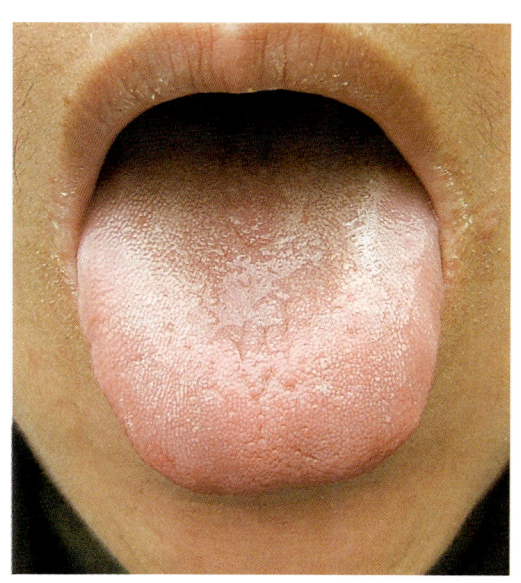

Fig 2.2-121

Patient, Female, 51years,

Case NO.: W24

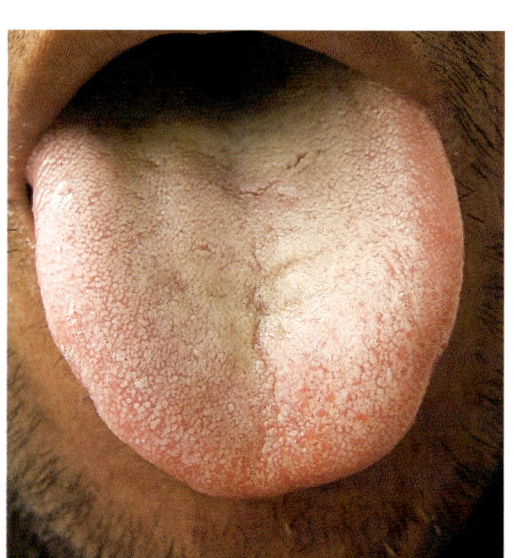

Fig 2.2-122

Patient, Male, 46years,

Case NO.: W181

Fig 2.2-123

Patient, Male, 48years,

Case NO.: W32

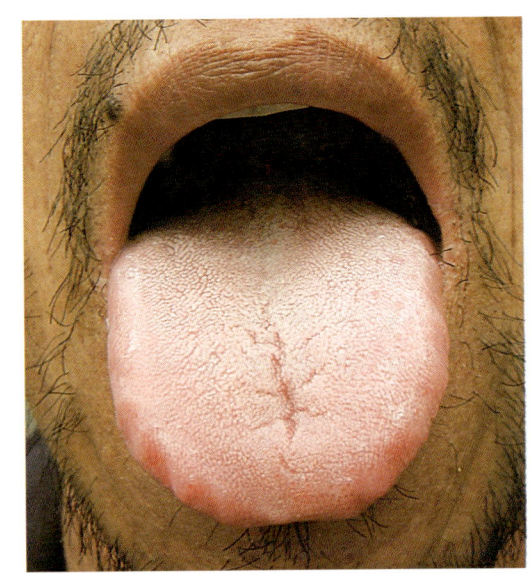

Fig 2.2-124

Patient, Male, 34years,

Case NO.: F135

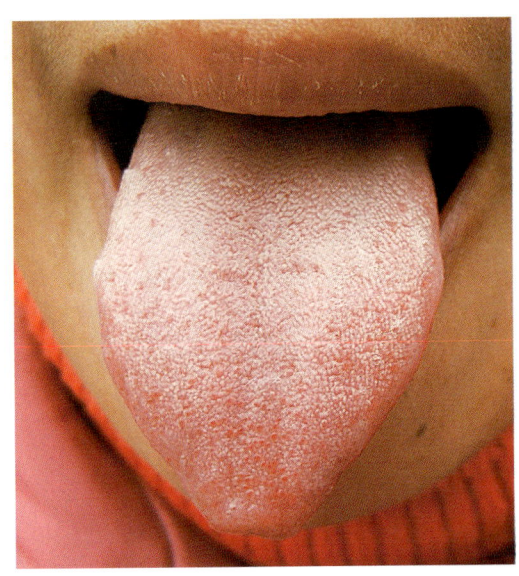

Light red tongue

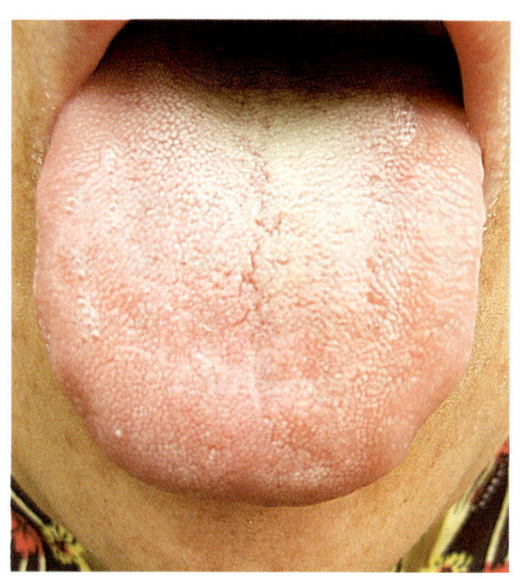

Fig 2.2-125

Patient, Female, 38years,

Case NO.: W248

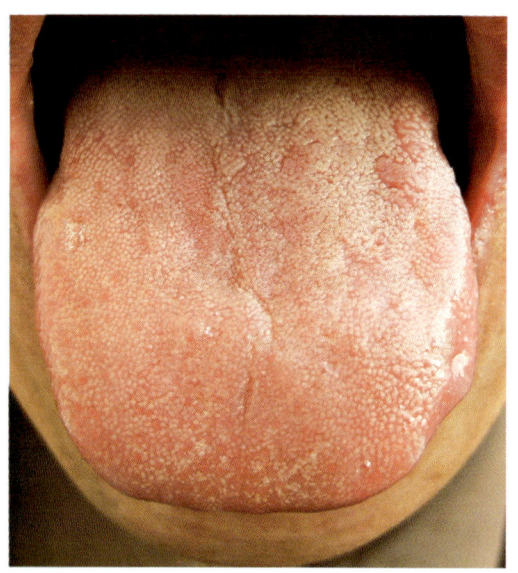

Fig 2.2-126

Patient, Male, 40years,

Case NO.: W495

Fig 2.2-127

Patient, Female, 46years,

Case NO.: F326

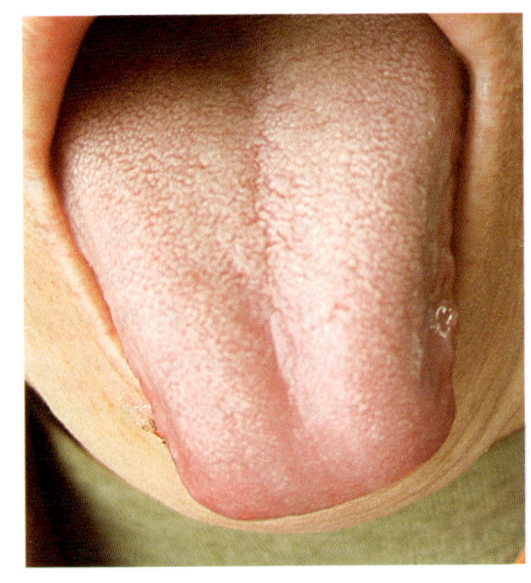

Fig 2.2-128

Patient, Female, 43years,

Case NO.: F198

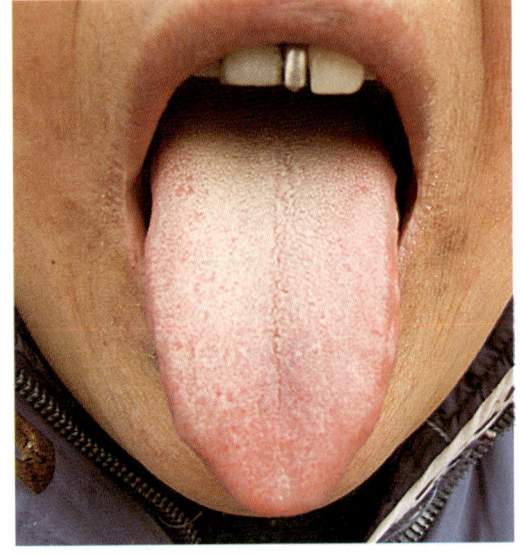

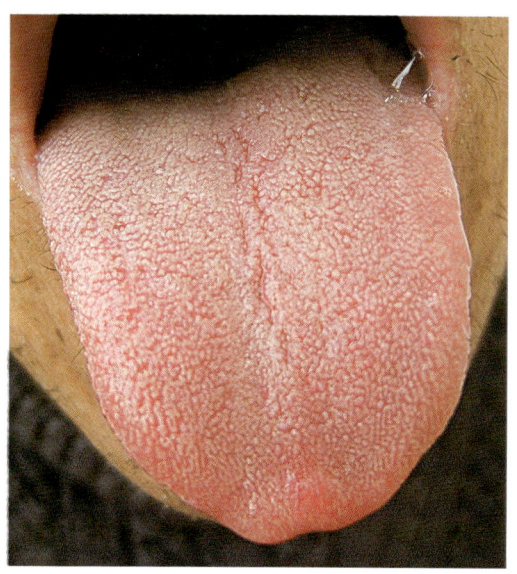

Fig 2.2-129

Patient, Male, 41years,

Case NO.: W696

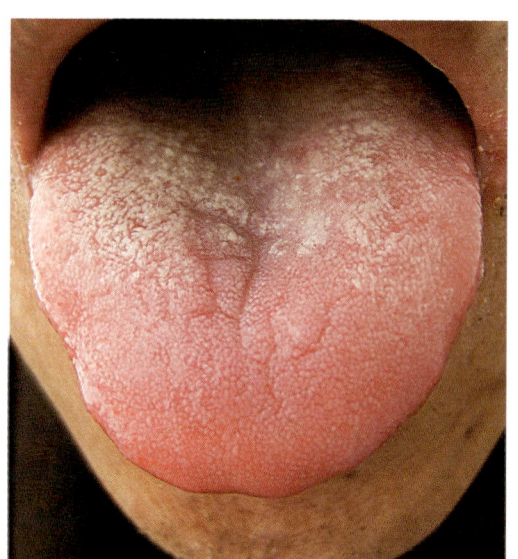

Fig 2.2-130

Patient, Male, 51years,

Case NO.: F357

Fig 2.2-131

Patient, Female, 37years,

Case NO.: W734

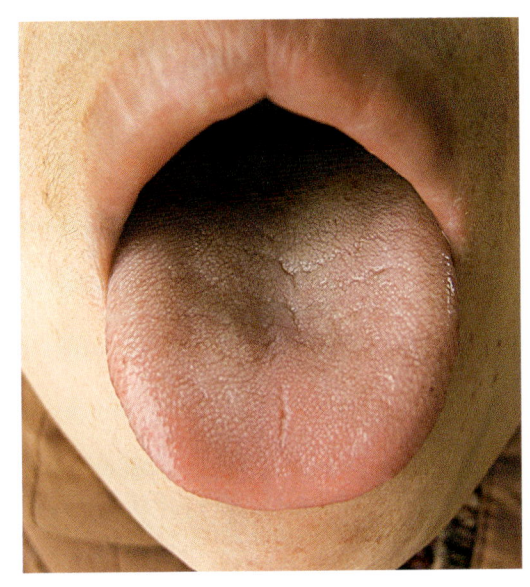

Fig 2.2-132

Patient, Female, 43years,

Case NO.: F341

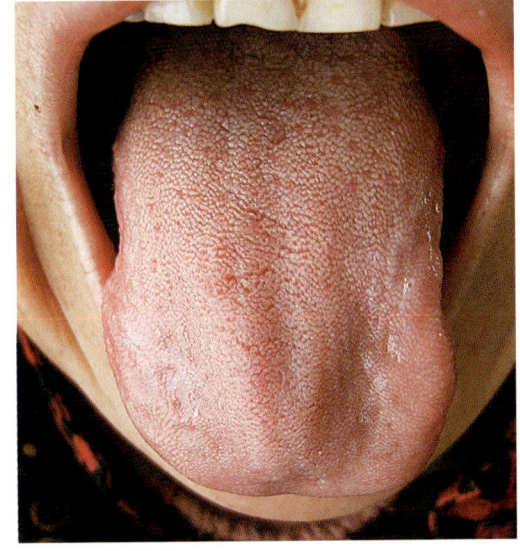

Light red tongue

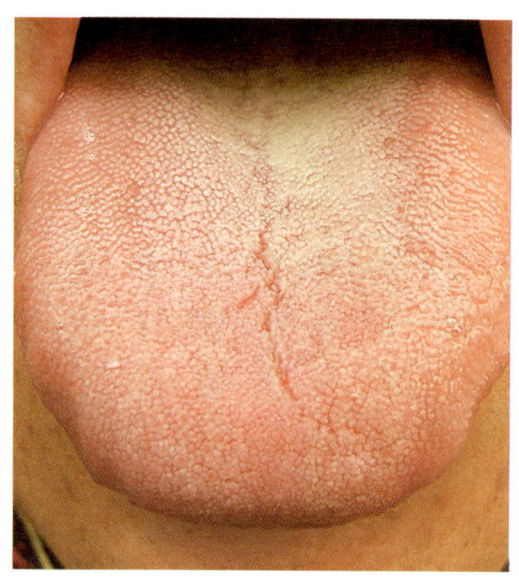

Fig 2.2-133

Patient, Female, 38years,

Case NO.: W248

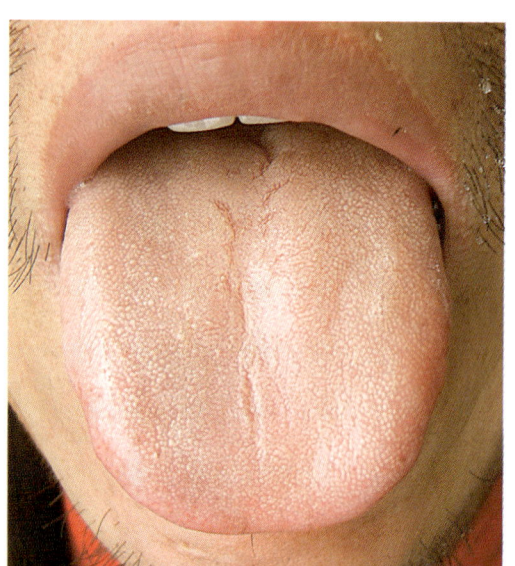

Fig 2.2-134

Patient, Male, 35years,

Case NO.: F337

Fig 2.2-135

Patient, Male, 42years,

Case NO.: W733

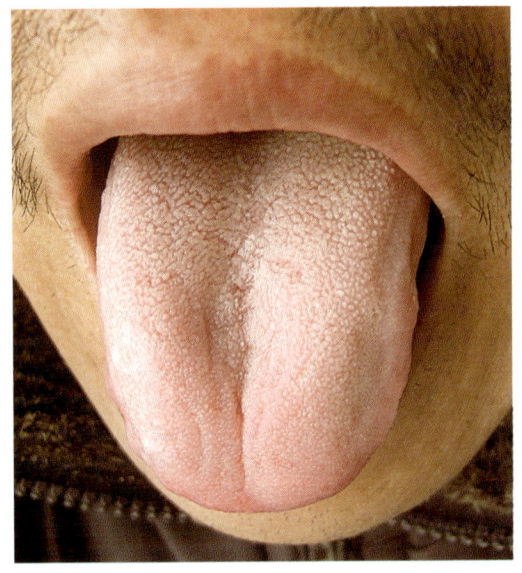

Fig 2.2-136

Patient, Female, 53years,

Case NO.: W292

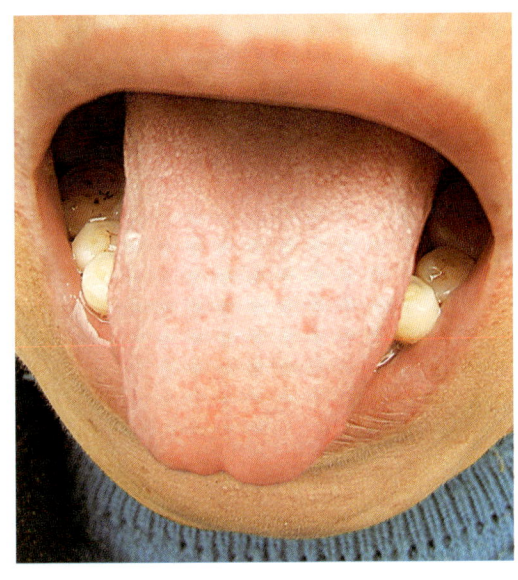

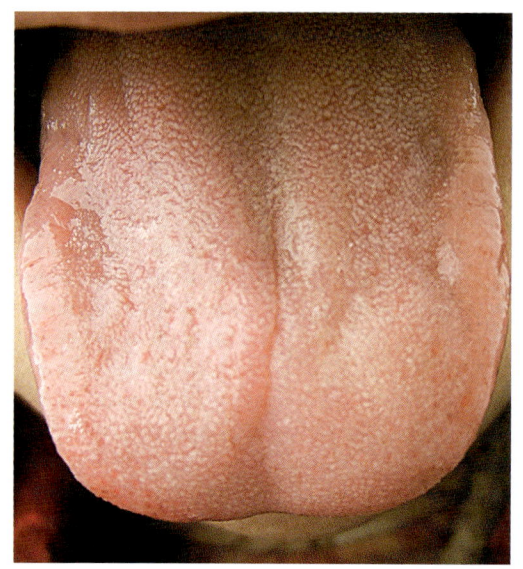

Fig 2.2-137

Patient, Female, 32years,

Case NO.: F367

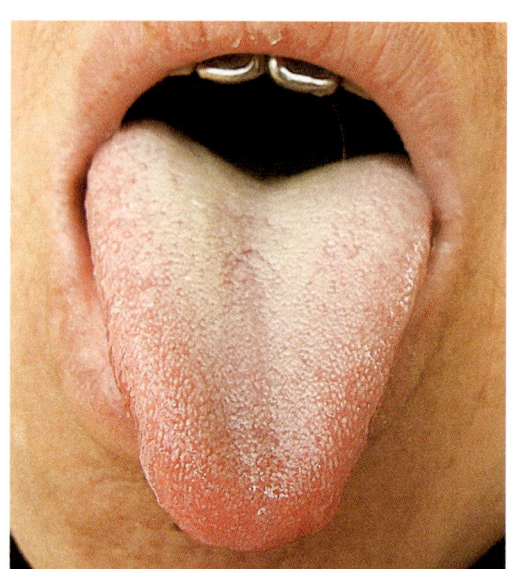

Fig 2.2-138

Patient, Female, 50years,

Case NO.: W573

Fig 2.2-139

Patient, Female, 36years,

Case NO.: W550

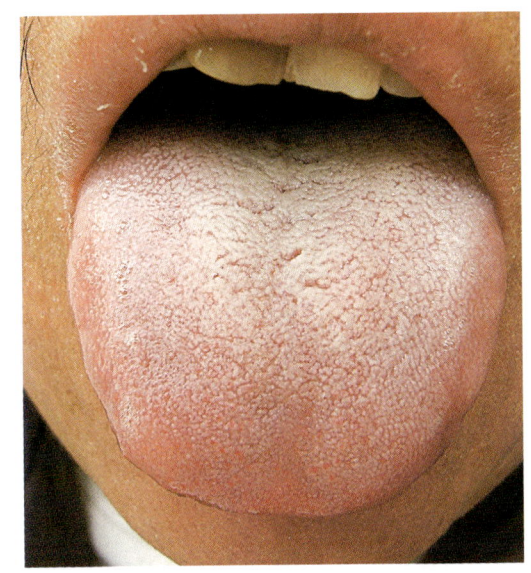

Fig 2.2-140

Patient, Female, 55years,

Case NO.: F164

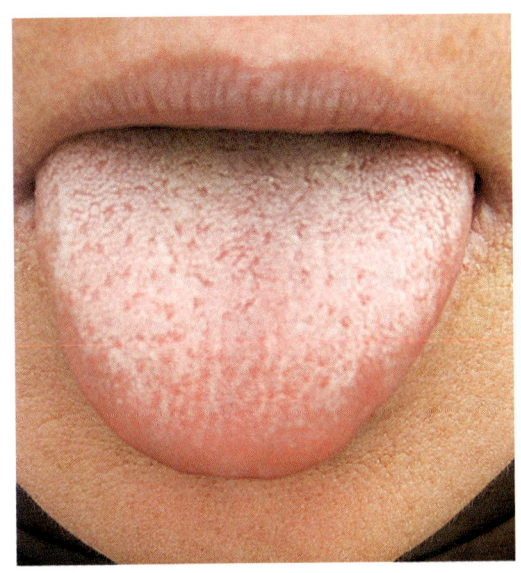

Light red tongue

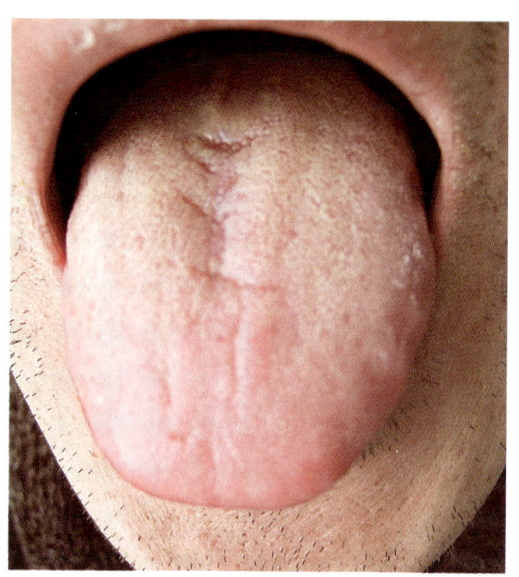

Fig 2.2-141

Patient, Male, 40years,

Case NO.: F302

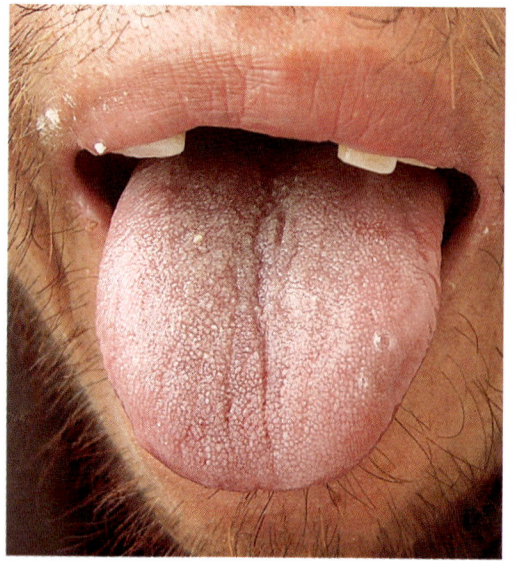

Fig 2.2-142

Patient, Male, 44years,

Case NO.: W5

Fig 2.2-143

Patient, Female, 33years,

Case NO.: F119

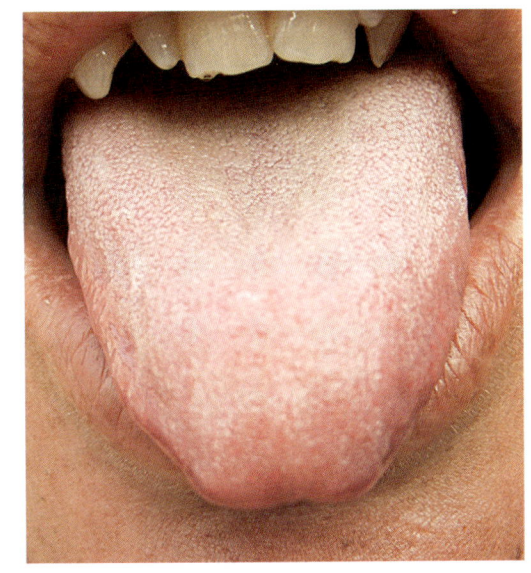

Fig 2.2-144

Patient, Female, 42years,

Case NO.: W499

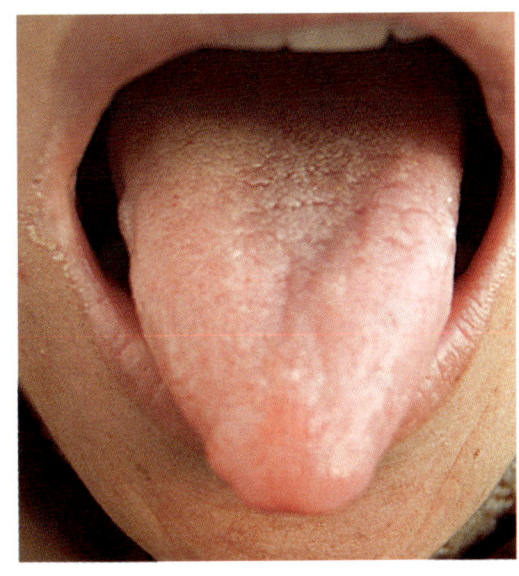

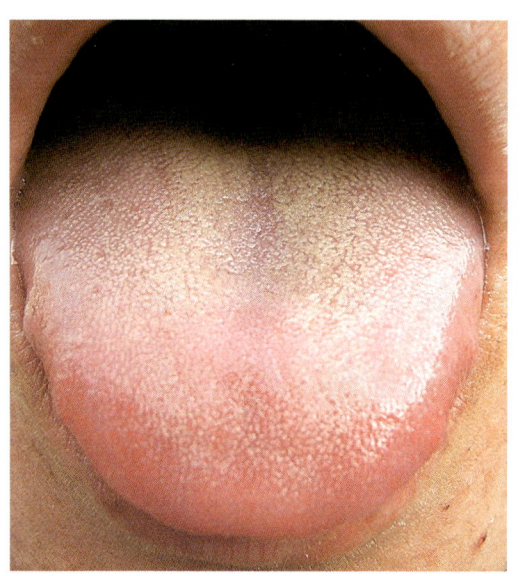

Fig 2.2-145

Patient, Male, 42years,

Case NO.: W649

Light red tongue

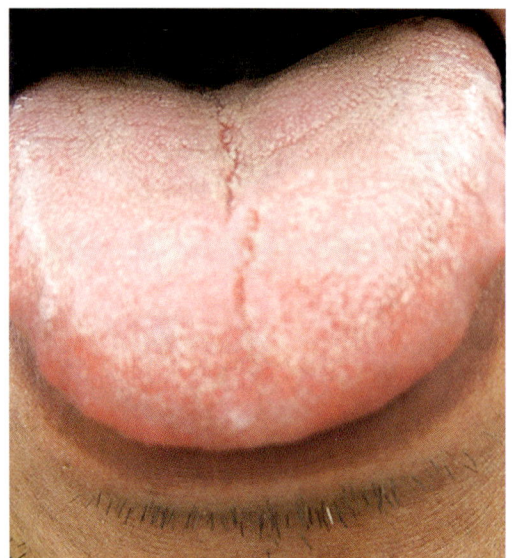

Fig 2.2-146

Patient, Male, 54years,

Case NO.: F205

Fig 2.2-147

Patient, Female, 50years,

Case NO.: W242

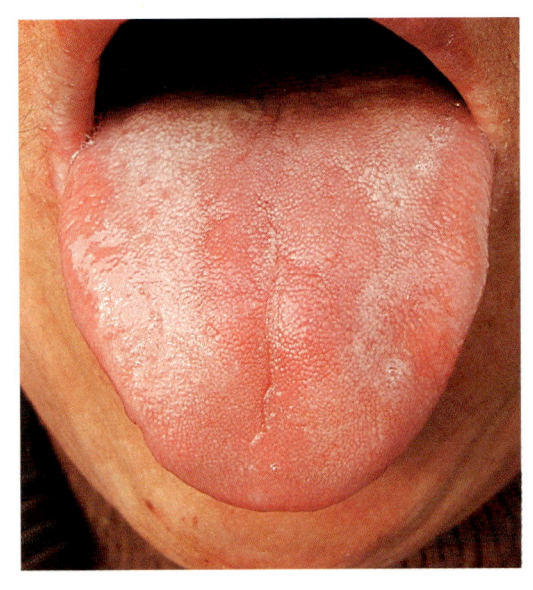

Fig 2.2-148

Patient, Female, 35years,

Case NO.: W6

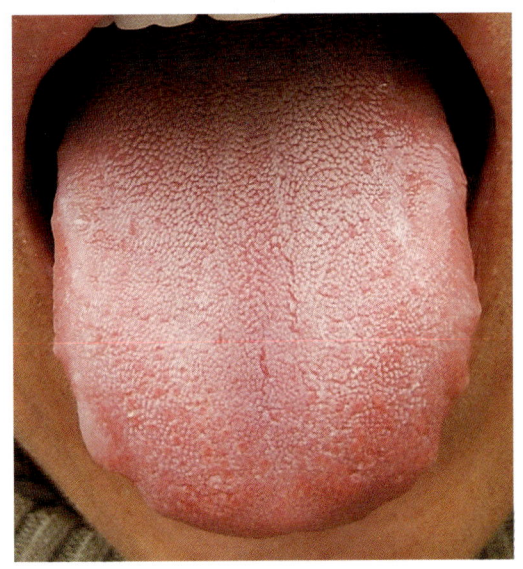

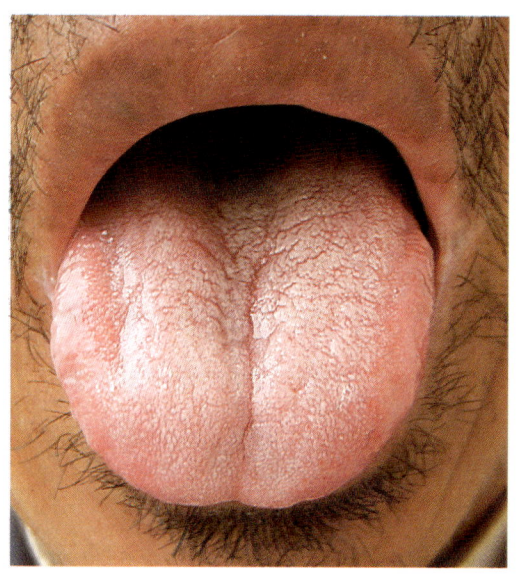

Fig 2.2-149

Patient, Male, 51years,

Case NO.: W15

Light red tongue

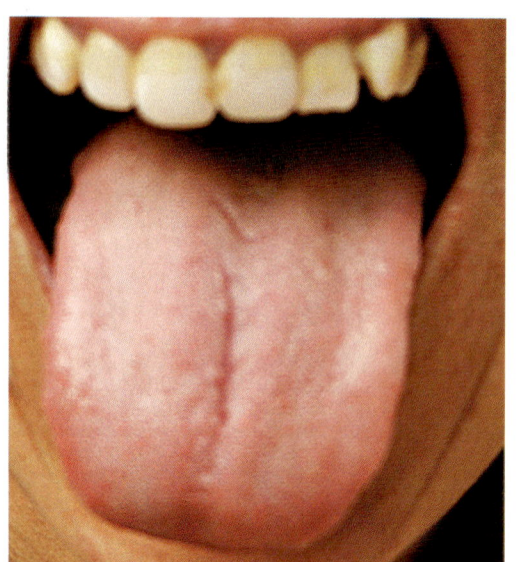

Fig 2.2-150

Patient, Female, 32years,

Case NO.: 300

Fig 2.2-151

Patient, Female, 51years,

Case NO.: W406

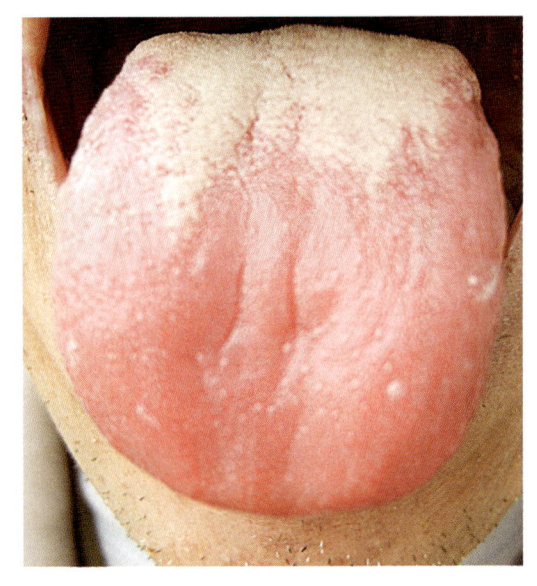

Fig 2.2-152

Patient, Male, 30years,

Case NO.: 328

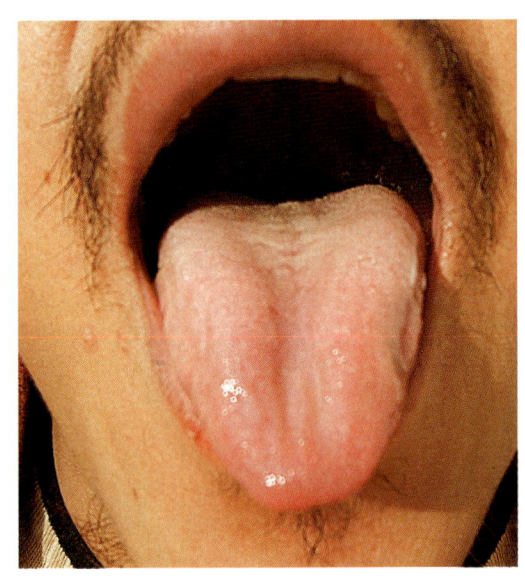

Light red tongue

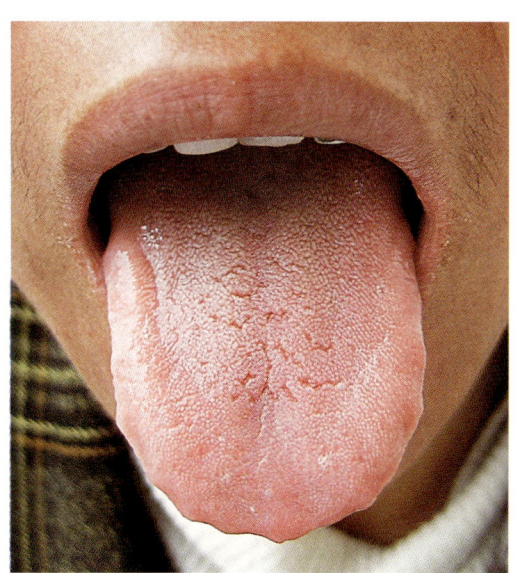

Fig 2.2-153

Patient, Female, 41years,

Case NO.: W17

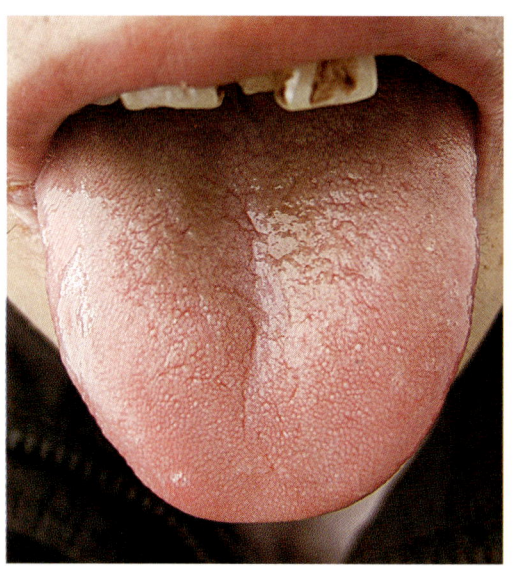

Fig 2.2-154

Patient, Male, 34years,

Case NO.: W750

Fig 2.2-155

Patient, Female, 53years,

Case NO.: F228

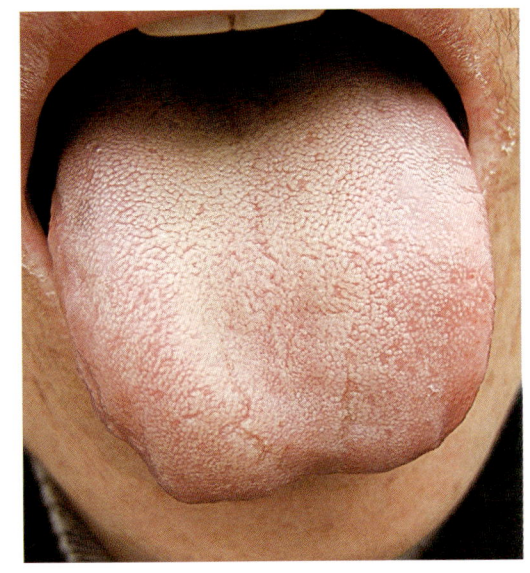

Fig 2.2-156

Patient, Female, 44years,

Case NO.: W518

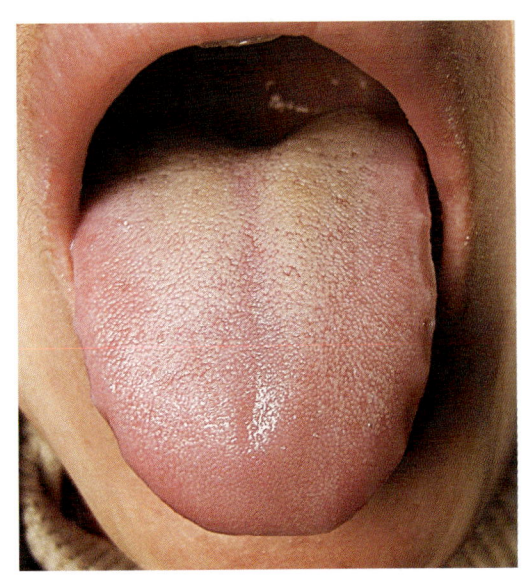

Light red tongue

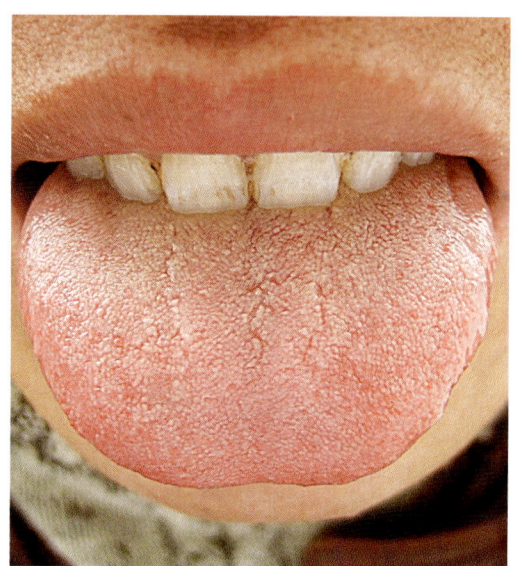

Fig 2.2-157

Patient, Female, 37years,

Case NO.: F264

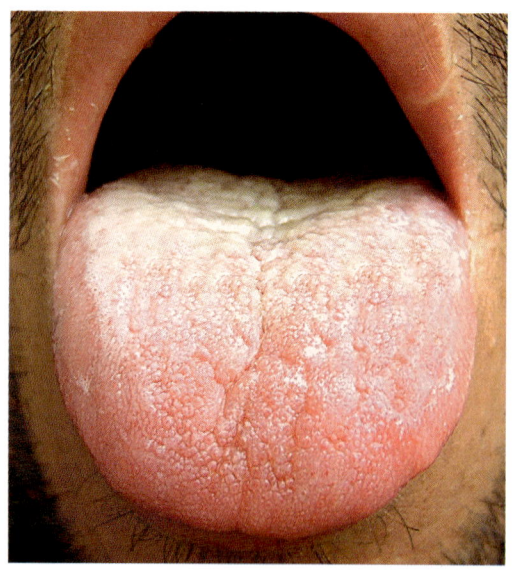

Fig 2.2-158

Patient, Male, 43years,

Case NO.: F63

Fig 2.2-159

Patient, Male, 39years,

Case NO.: W697

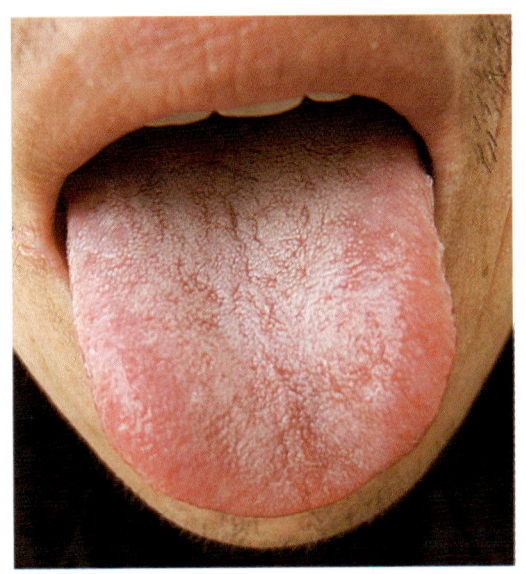

1.3 Red tongue

AIDS stage

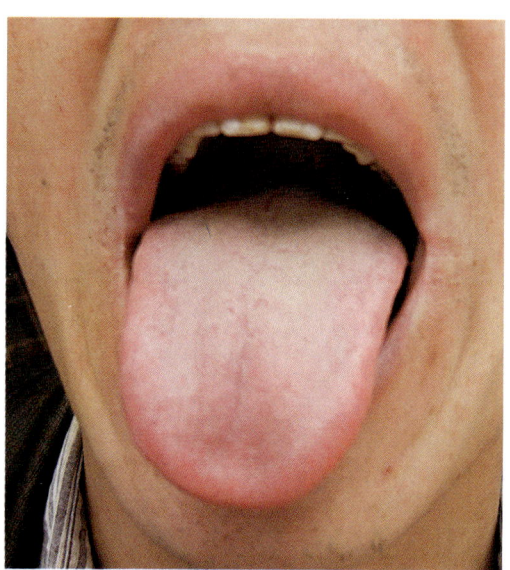

Fig 2.2-160

Patient, Male, 31years,

Case NO.: 317

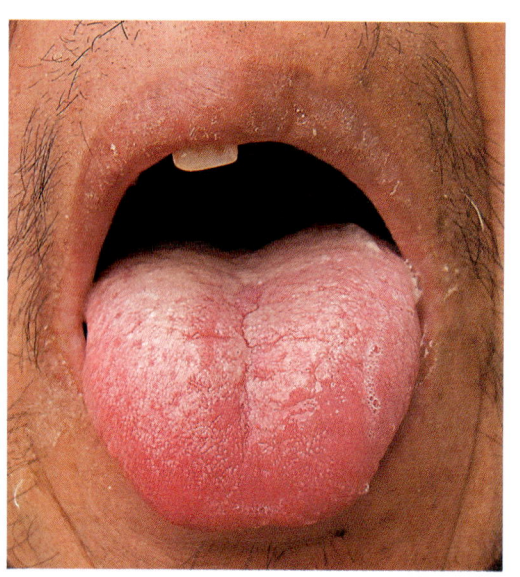

Fig 2.2-161

Patient, Male, 57years,

Case NO.: W56

Red tongue

Fig 2.2-162

Patient, Male, 31years,

Case NO.: W51

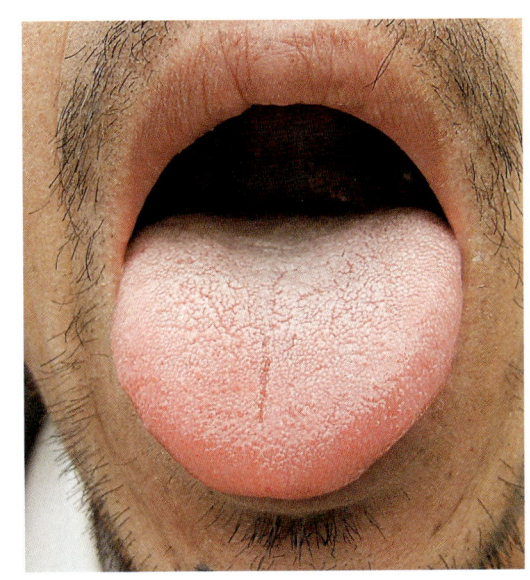

Fig 2.2-163

Patient, Female, 43years,

Case NO.: W256

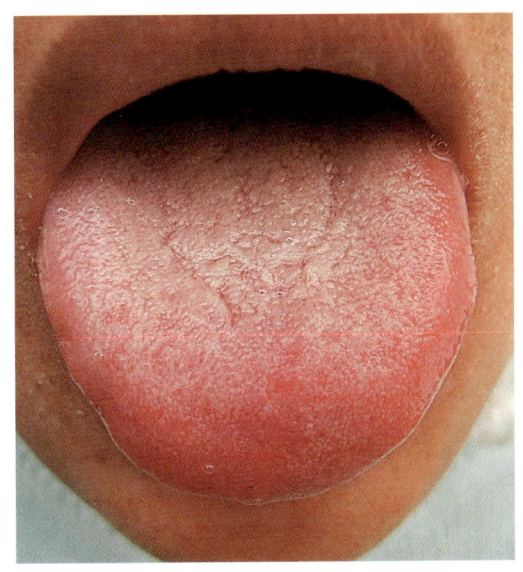

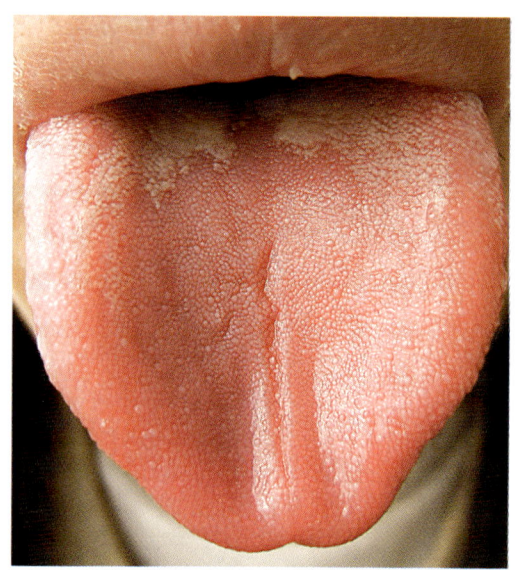

Fig 2.2-164

Patient, Male, 34years,

Case NO.: W203

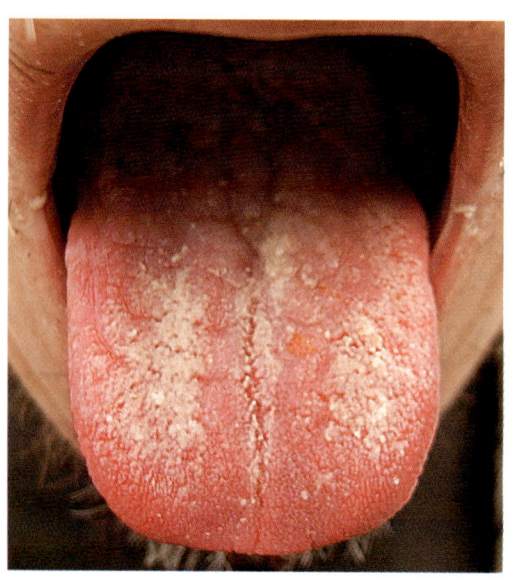

Fig 2.2-165

Patient, Male, 57years,

Case NO.: F130

Fig 2.2-166

Patient, Male, 44years,

Case NO.: W271

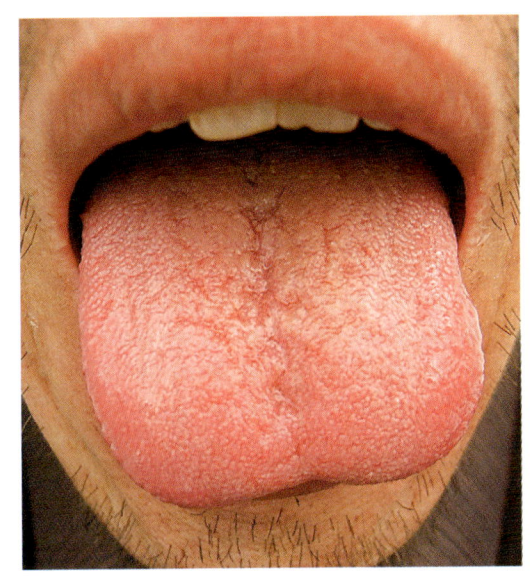

Fig 2.2-167

Patient, Male, 39years,

Case NO.: W594

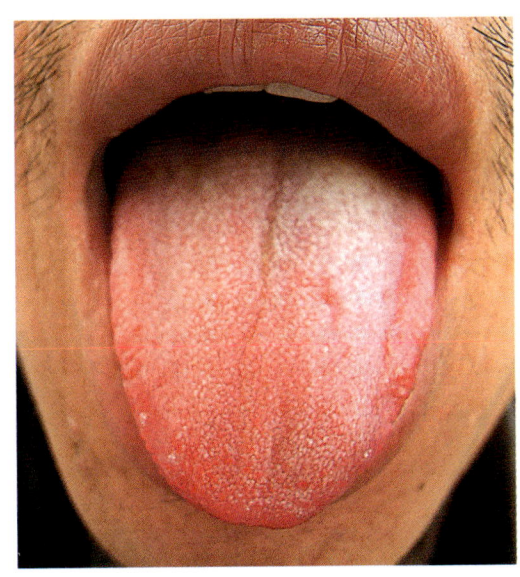

Red tongue

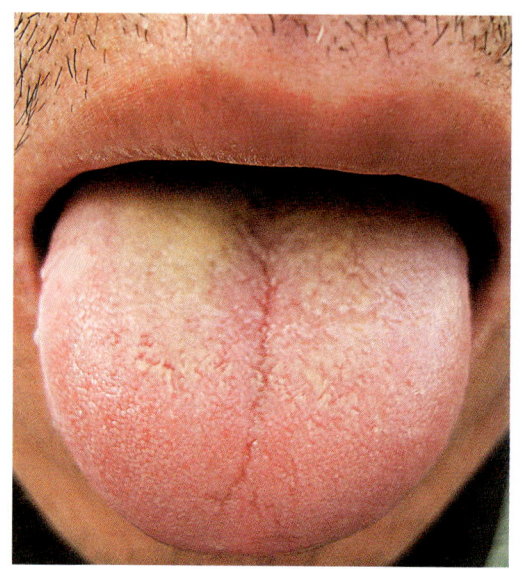

Fig 2.2-168

Patient, Male, 54years,

Case NO.: W615

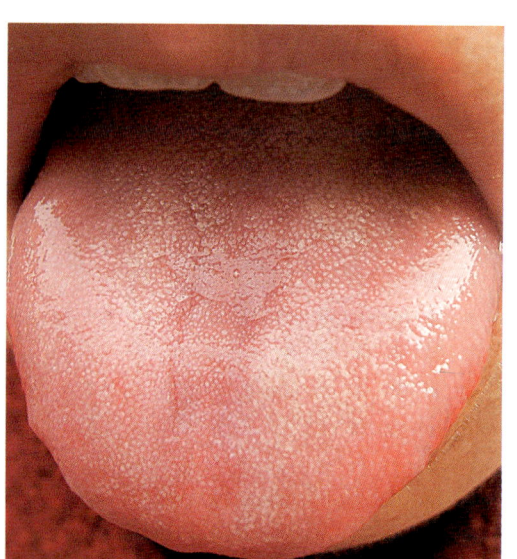

Fig 2.2-169

Patient, Male, 43years,

Case NO.: W465

Fig 2.2-170

Patient, Female, 51years,

Case NO.: W631

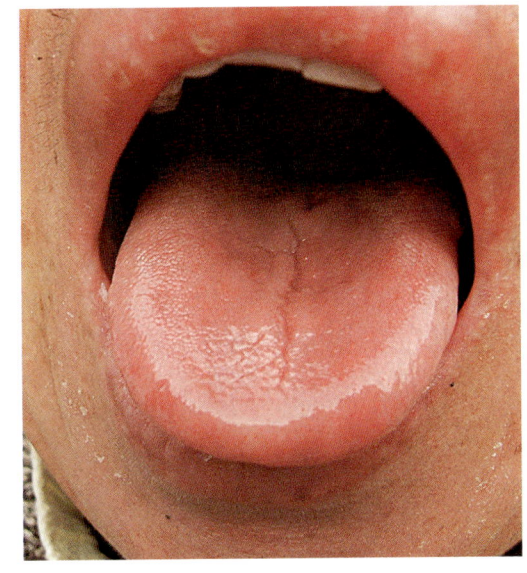

Fig 2.2-171

Patient, Female, 41years,

Case NO.: W674

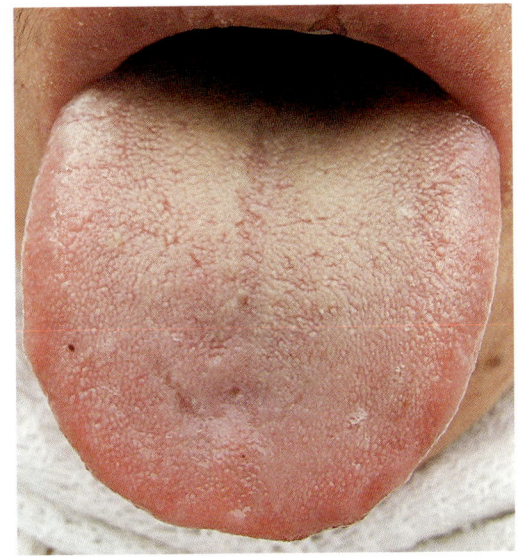

Red tongue

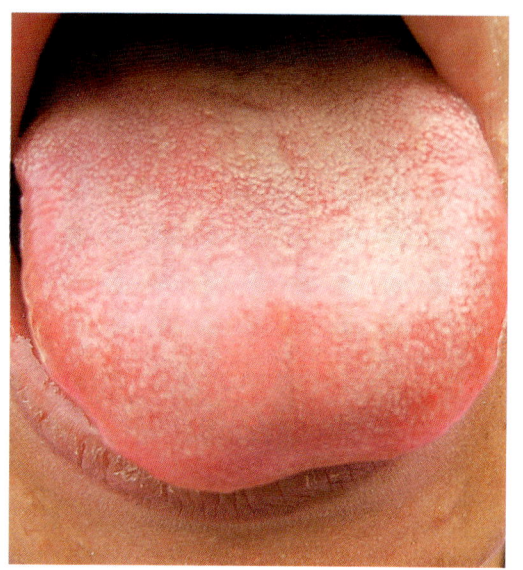

Fig 2.2-172

Patient, Female, 45years,

Case NO.: W308

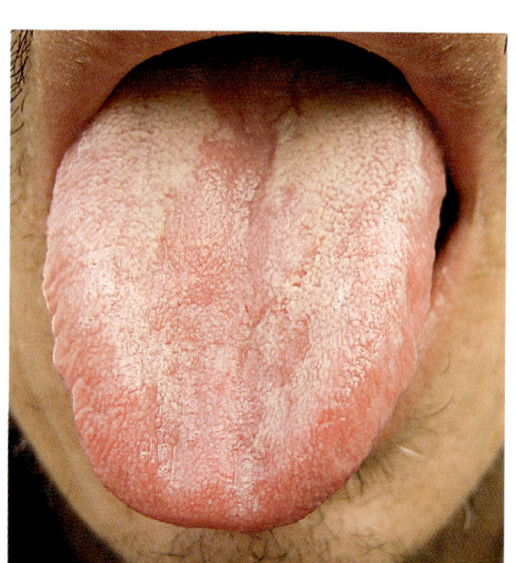

Fig 2.2-173

Patient, Male, 48years,

Case NO.: W312

Fig 2.2-174

Patient, Female, 54years,

Case NO.: F94

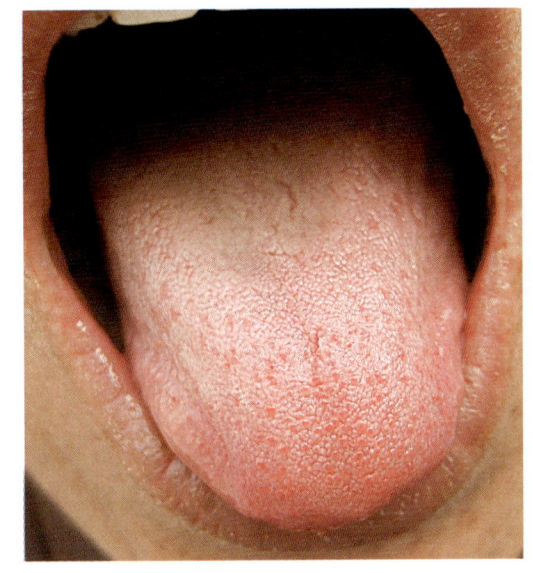

Fig 2.2-175

Patient, Female, 49years,

Case NO.: W356

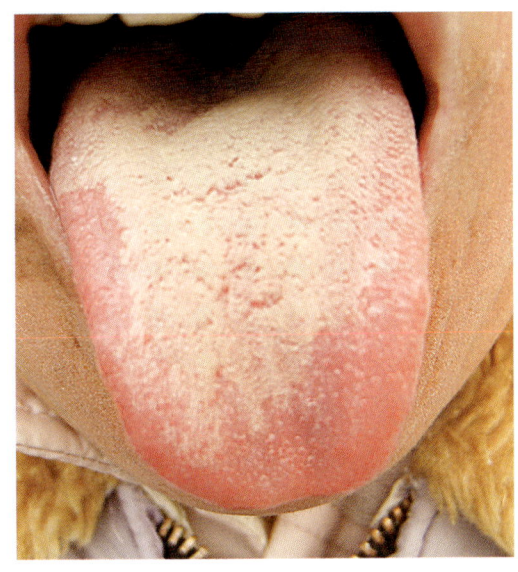

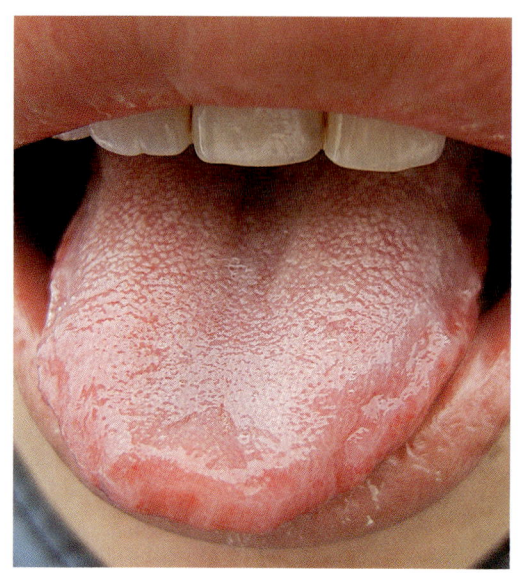

Fig 2.2-176

Patient, Female, 44years,

Case NO.: F244

Red tongue

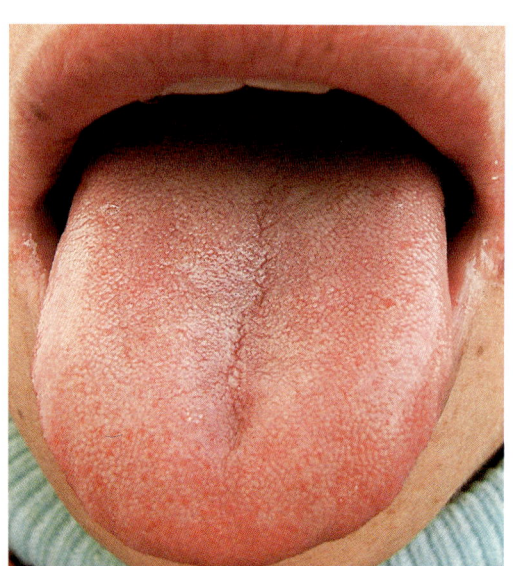

Fig 2.2-177

Patient, Female, 37years,

Case NO.: F264

Fig 2.2-178

Patient, Female, 31years,

Case NO.: W543

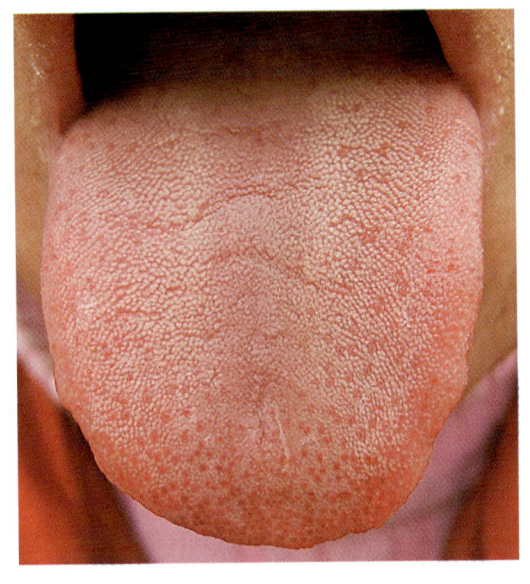

Fig 2.2-179

Patient, Male, 48years,

Case NO.: W742

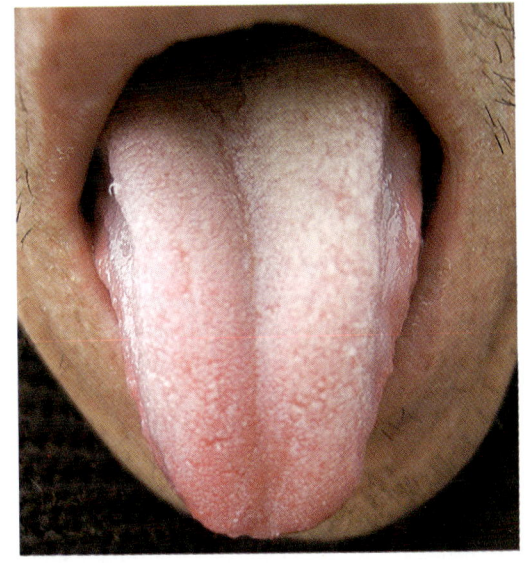

Red tongue

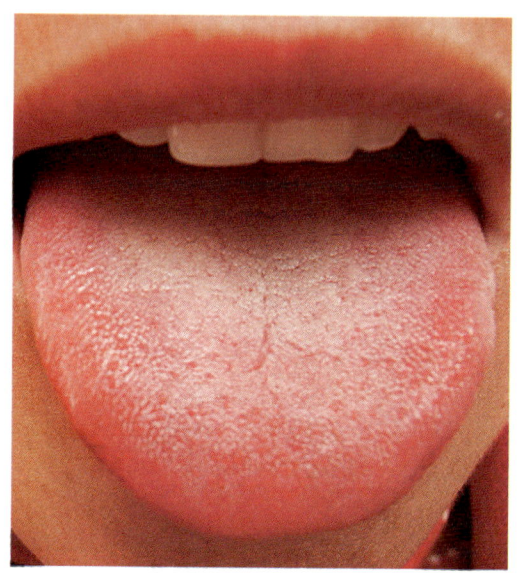

Fig 2.2-180

Patient, Female, 32years,

Case NO.: W554

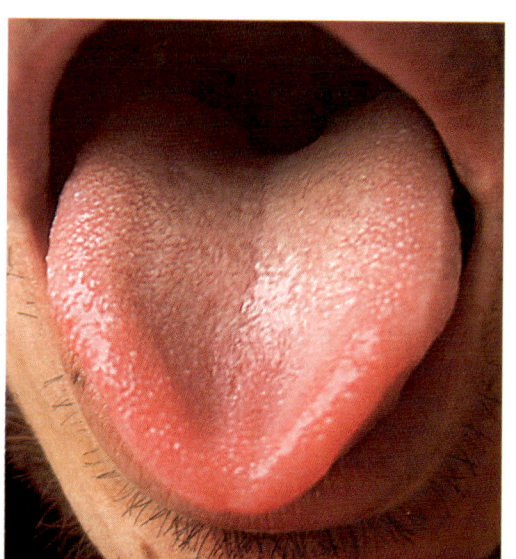

Fig 2.2-181

Patient, Male, 37years,

Case NO.: W419

Fig 2.2-182

Patient, Male, 45years,

Case NO.: F216

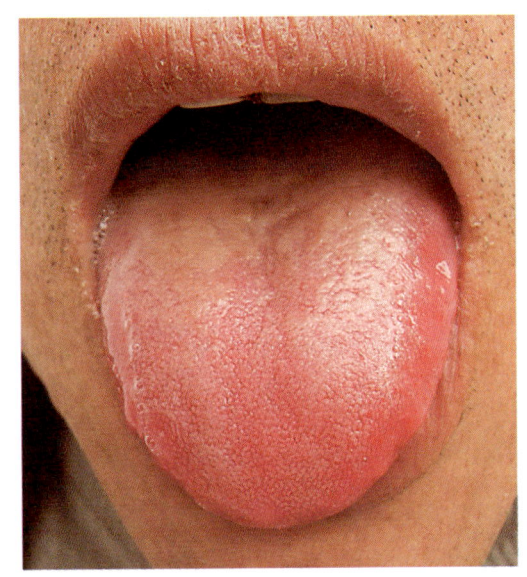

Fig 2.2-183

Patient, Male, 43years,

Case NO.: F151

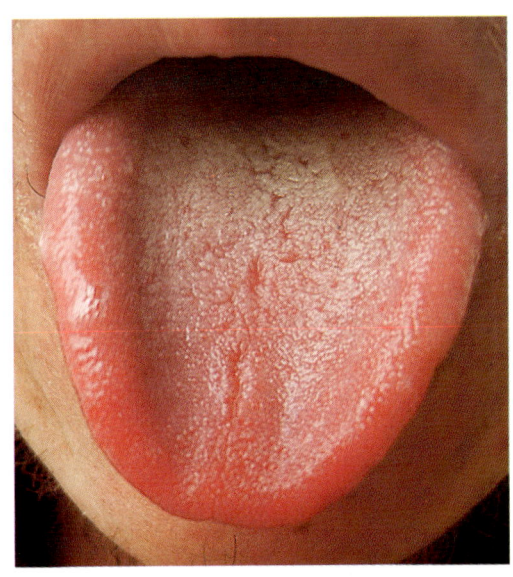

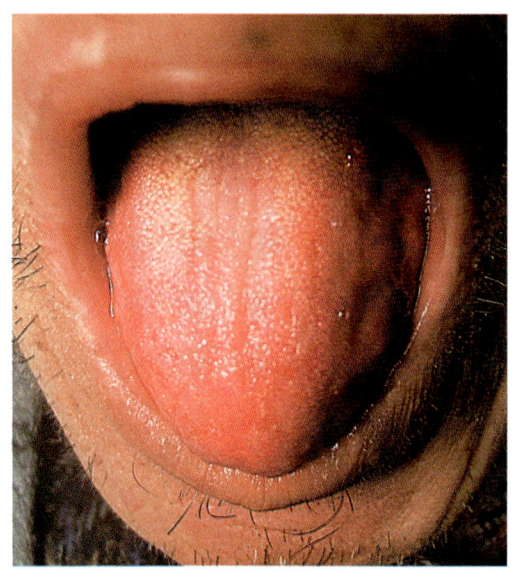

Fig 2.2-184

Patient, Male, 61years,

Case NO.: W620

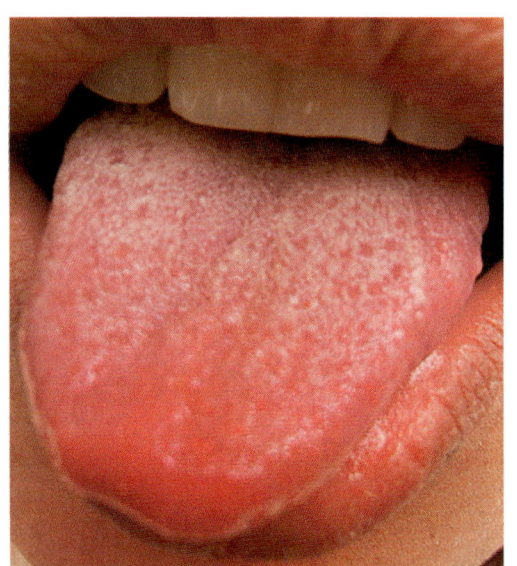

Fig 2.2-185

Patient, Male, 35years,

Case NO.: F297

Fig 2.2-186

Patient, Male, 41years,

Case NO.: F175

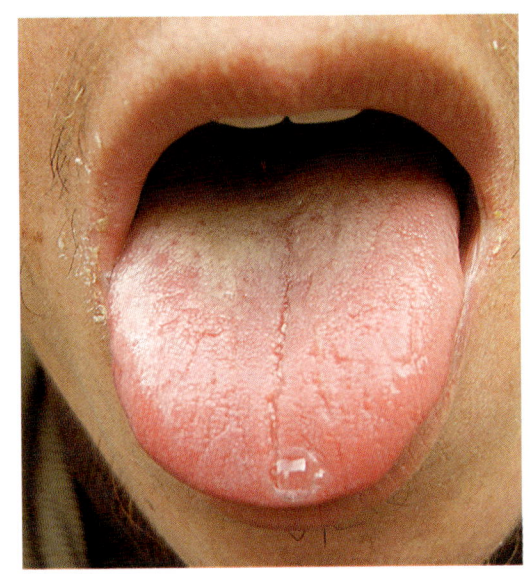

Fig 2.2-187

Patient, Male, 41years,

Case NO.: F154

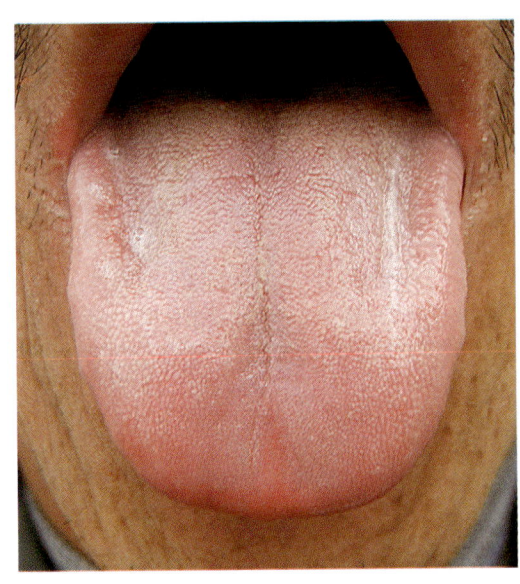

Red tongue

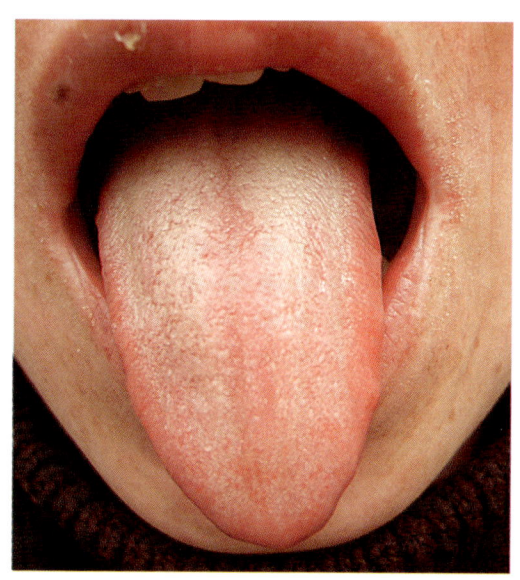

Fig 2.2-188

Patient, Female, 39years,

Case NO.: F203

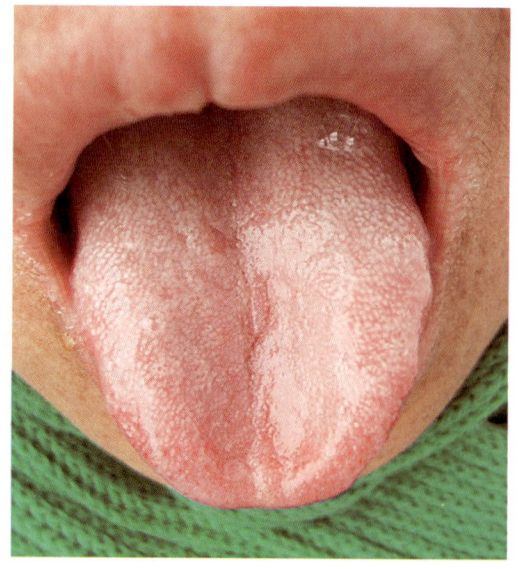

Fig 2.2-189

Patient, Female, 49years,

Case NO.: F360

Fig 2.2-190

Patient, Female, 41years,

Case NO.: W219

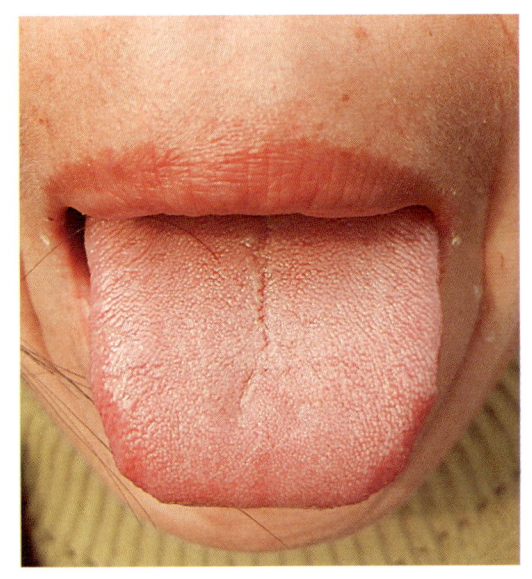

Fig 2.2-191

Patient, Female, 39years,

Case NO.: W209

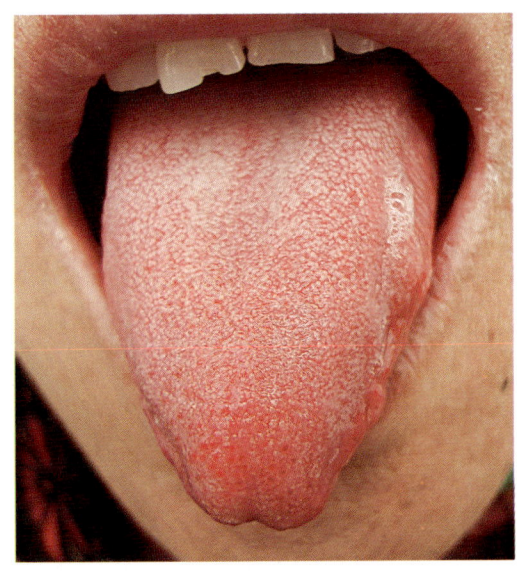

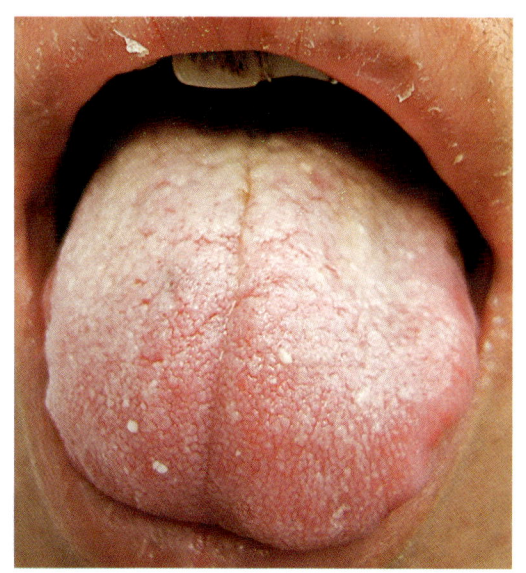

Fig 2.2-192

Patient, Female, 35years,

Case NO.: 304

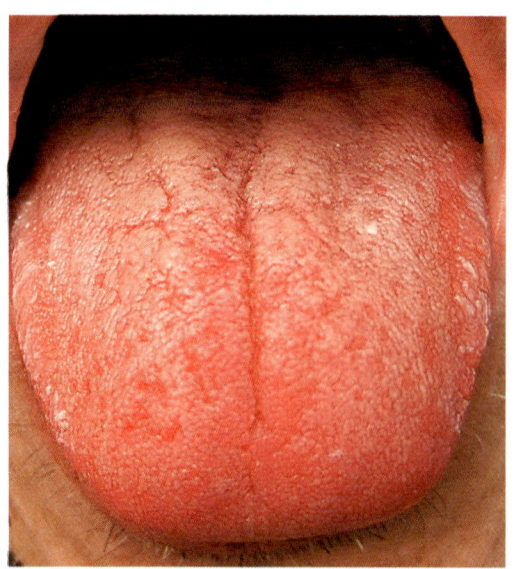

Fig 2.2-193

Patient, Male, 42years,

Case NO.: W353

Fig 2.2-194

Patient, Female, 51years,

Case NO.: W502

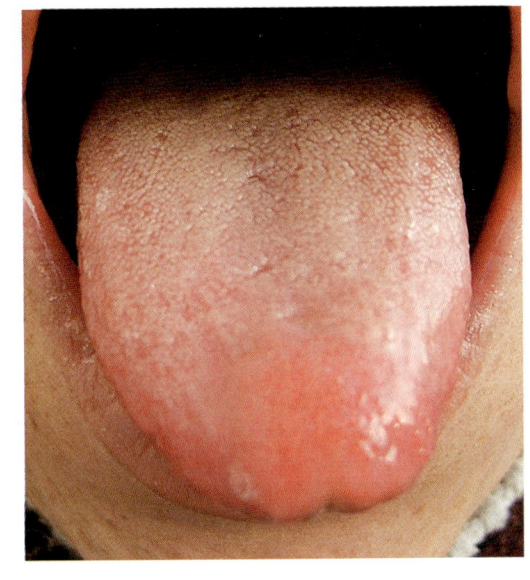

Fig 2.2-195

Patient, Male, 41years,

Case NO.: W78

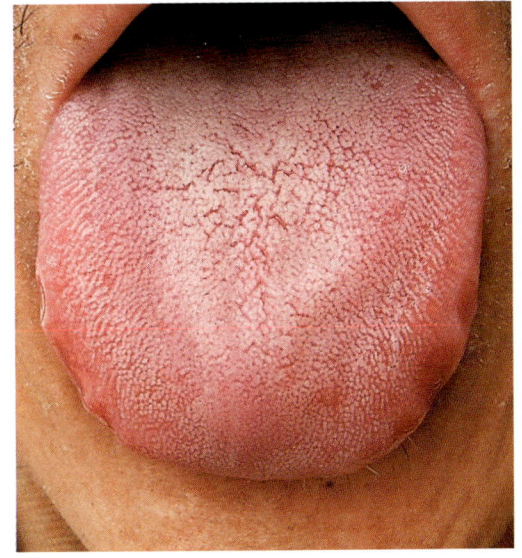

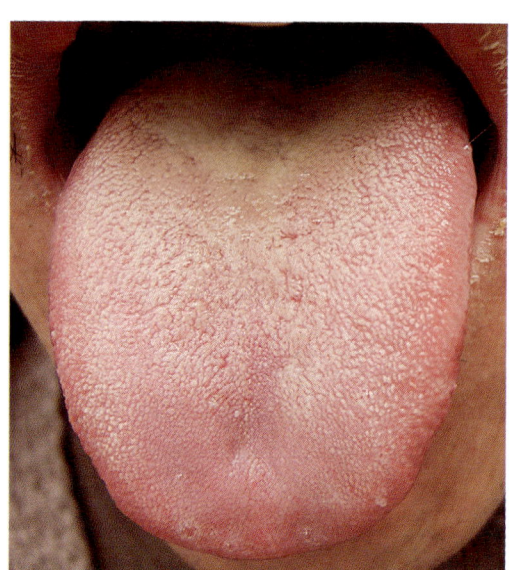

Fig 2.2-196

Patient, Male, 39years,

Case NO.: F179

Red tongue

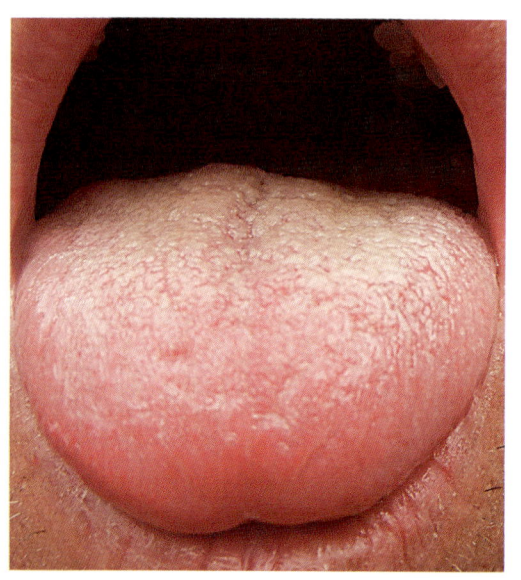

Fig 2.2-197

Patient, Male, 48years,

Case NO.: F159

Fig 2.2-198

Patient, Male, 51years,

Case NO.: F170

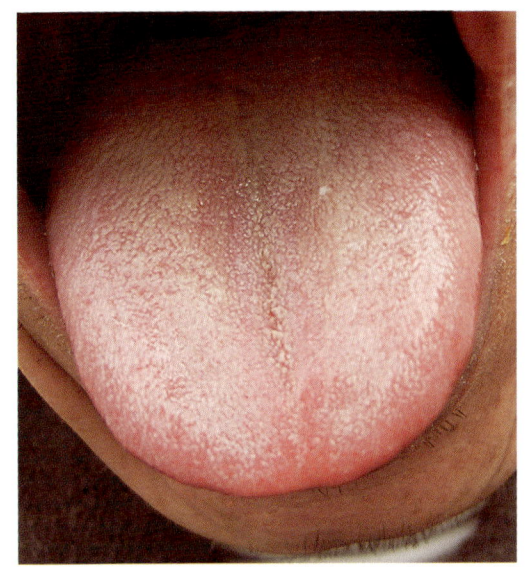

Fig 2.2-199

Patient, Male, 53years,

Case NO.: W669

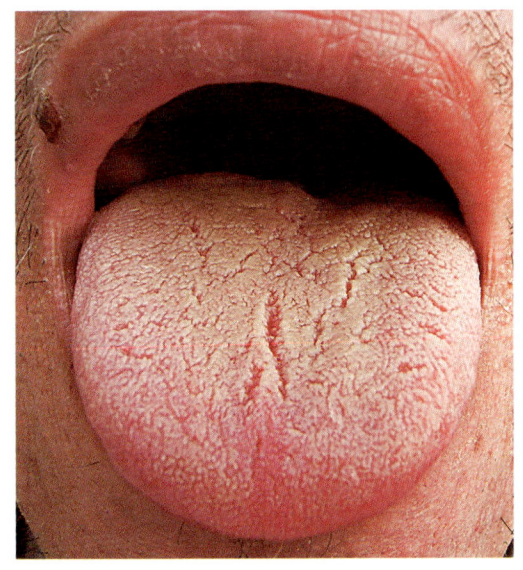

Red tongue

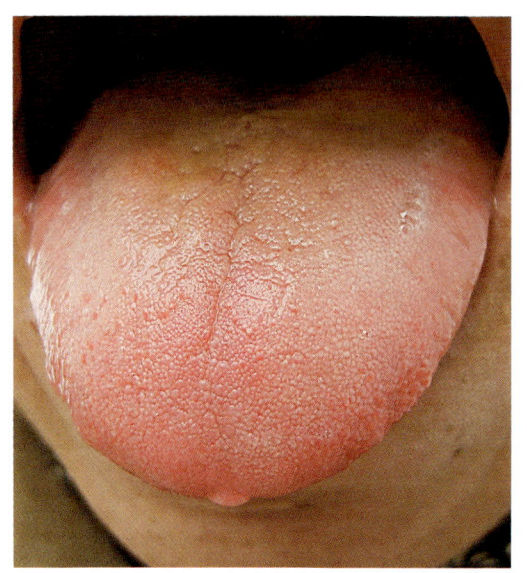

Fig 2.2-200

Patient, Female, 37years,

Case NO.: W106

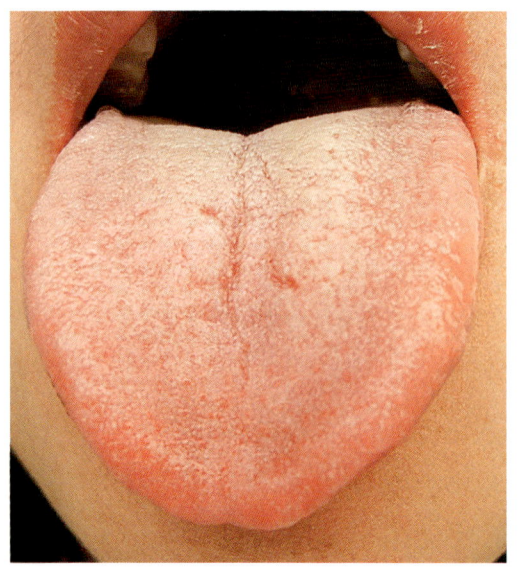

Fig 2.2-201

Patient, Female, 37years,

Case NO.: W250

Fig 2.2-202

Patient, Male, 58years,

Case NO.: W506

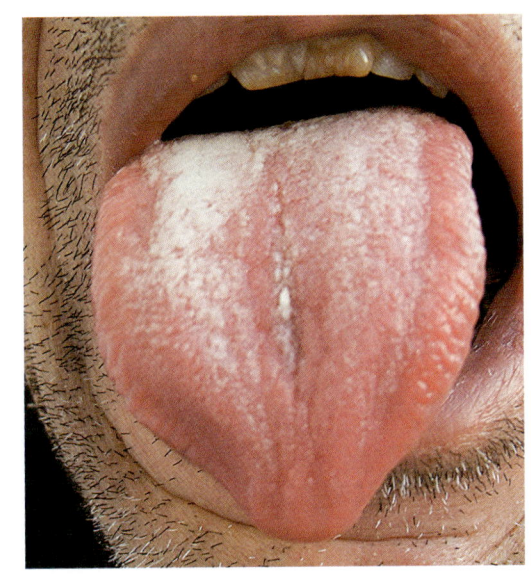

Fig 2.2-203

Patient, Male, 50years,

Case NO.: F343

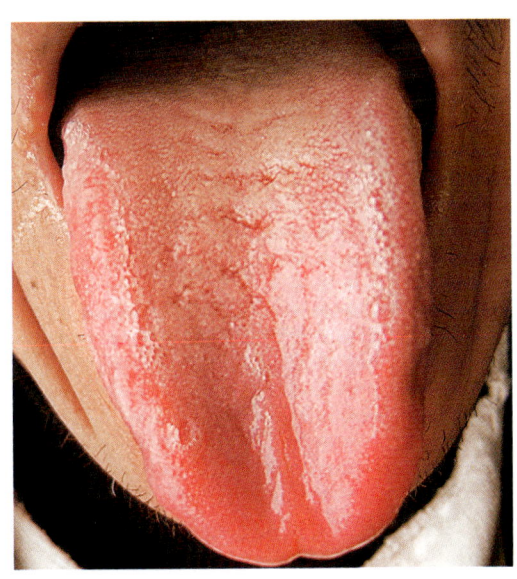

Red tongue

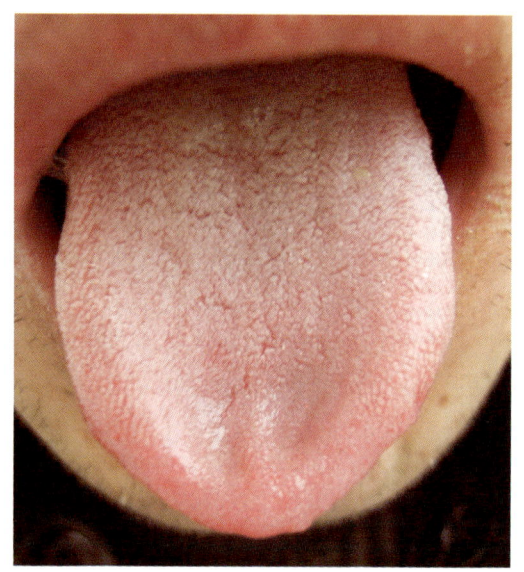

Fig 2.2-204

Patient, Male, 38years,

Case NO.: F283

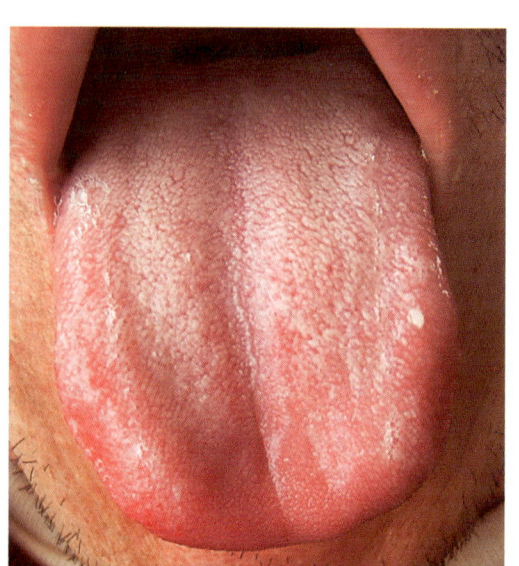

Fig 2.2-205

Patient, Male, 37years,

Case NO.: F315

Fig 2.2-206

Patient, Male, 41years,

Case NO.: F160

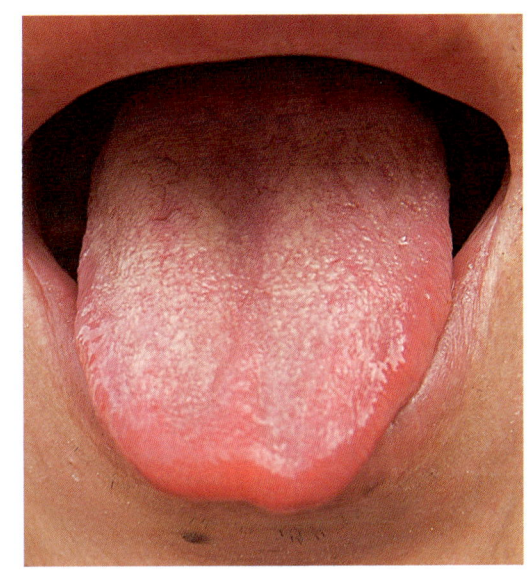

Fig 2.2-207

Patient, Female, 55years,

Case NO.: F260

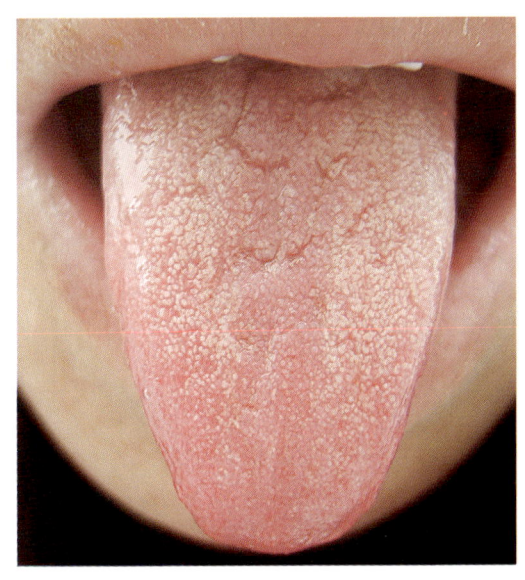

Red tongue

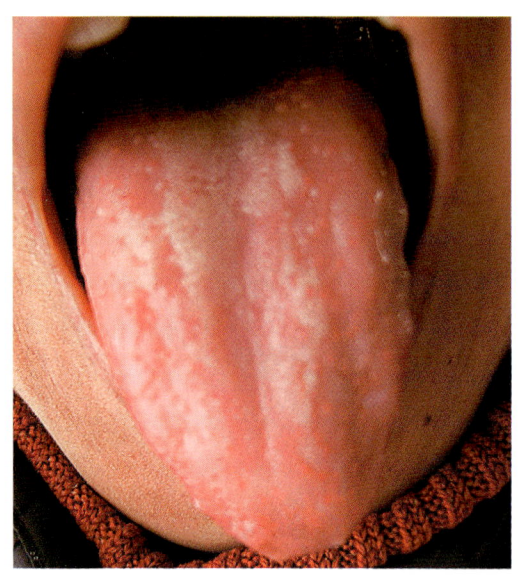

Fig 2.2-208

Patient, Female, 40years,

Case NO.: F303

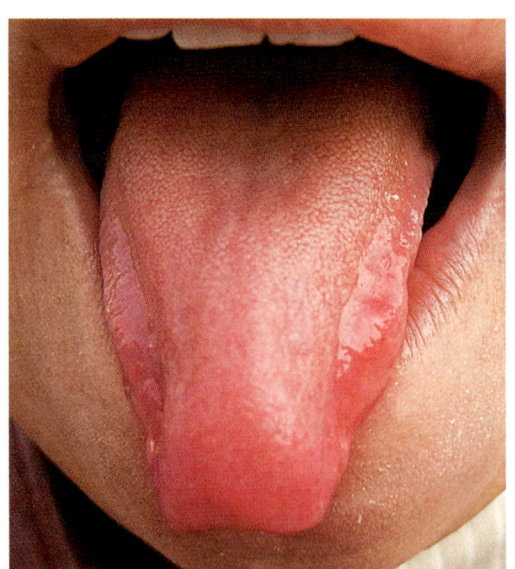

Fig 2.2-209

Patient, Female, 46years,

Case NO.: F211

Fig 2.2-210

Patient, Female, 52years,

Case NO.: W513

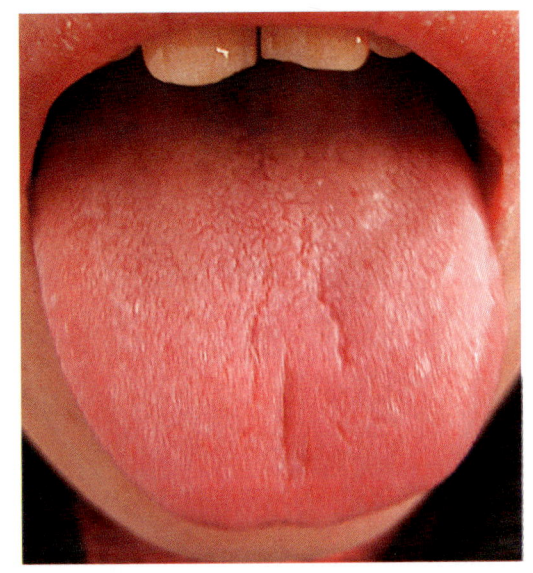

Fig 2.2-211

Patient, Female, 57years,

Case NO.: W55

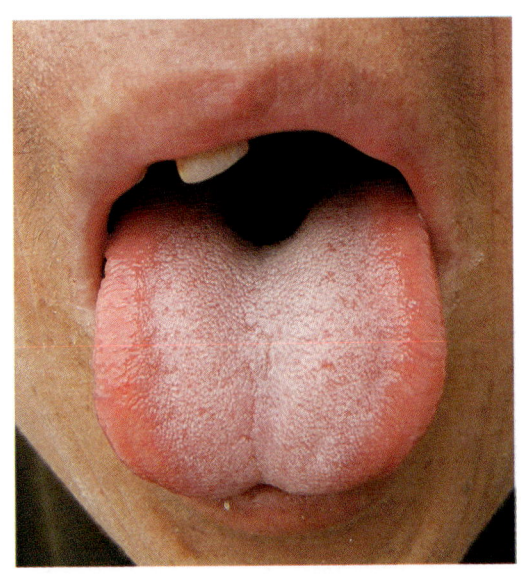

Red tongue

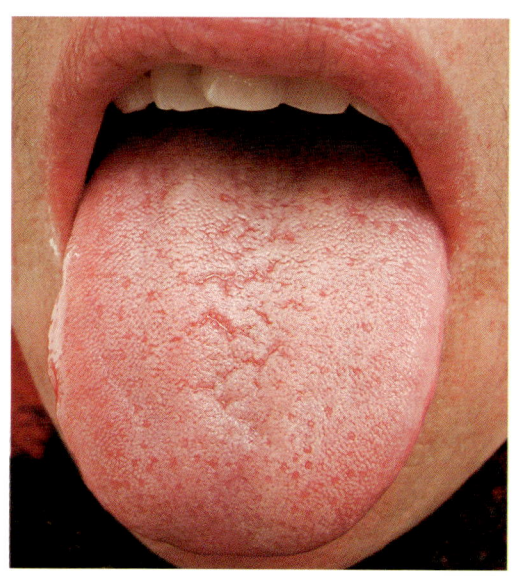

Fig 2.2-212

Patient, Female, 45years,

Case NO.: F220

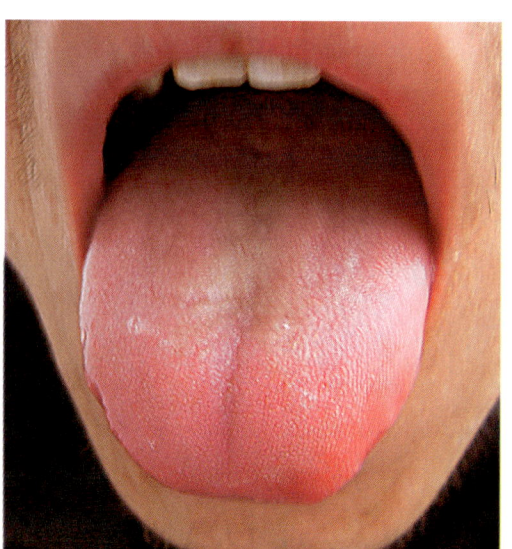

Fig 2.2-213

Patient, Male, 34years,

Case NO.: F298

Fig 2.2-214

Patient, Female, 49years,

Case NO.: F224

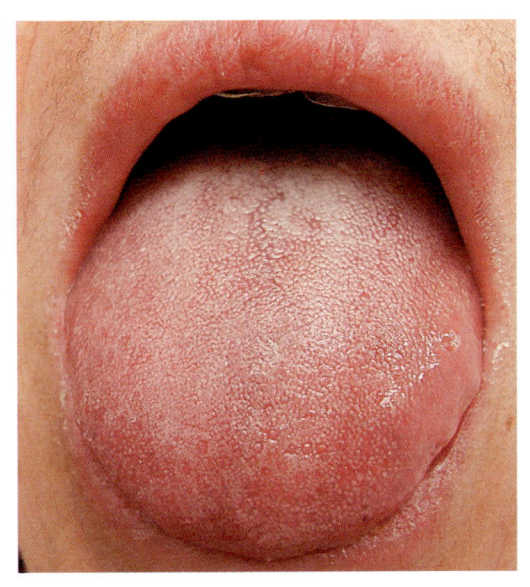

Fig 2.2-215

Patient, Female, 43years,

Case NO.: W536

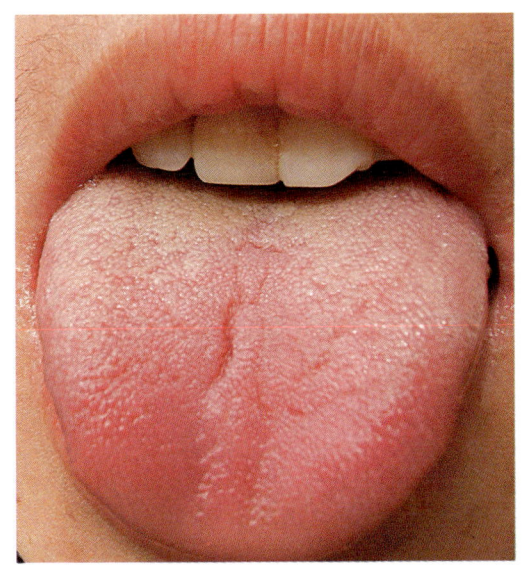

Red tongue

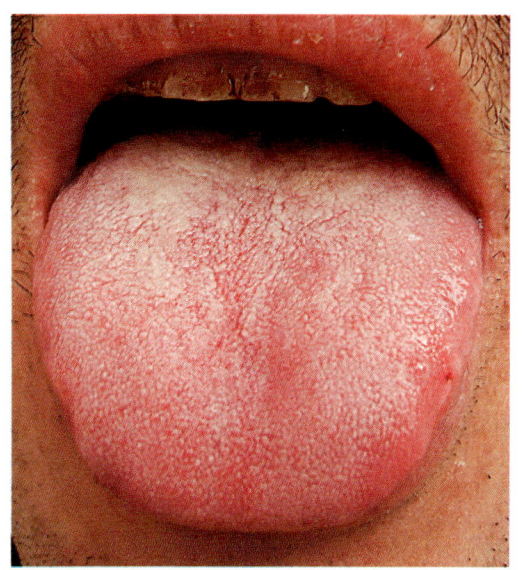

Fig 2.2-216

Patient, Female, 43years,

Case NO.: W368

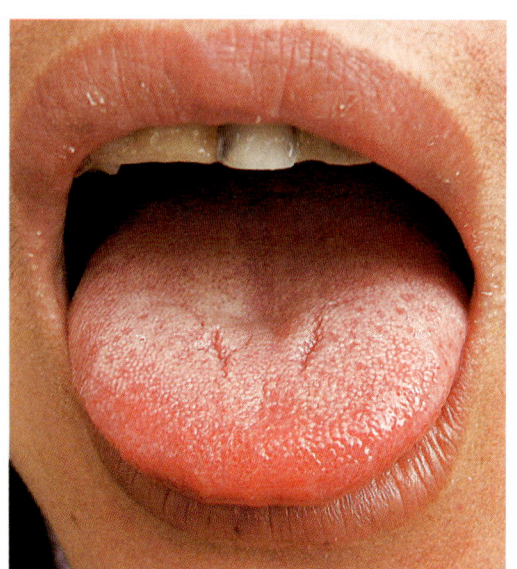

Fig 2.2-217

Patient, Female, 39years,

Case NO.: W528

Fig 2.2-218

Patient, Male, 48years,

Case NO.: W583

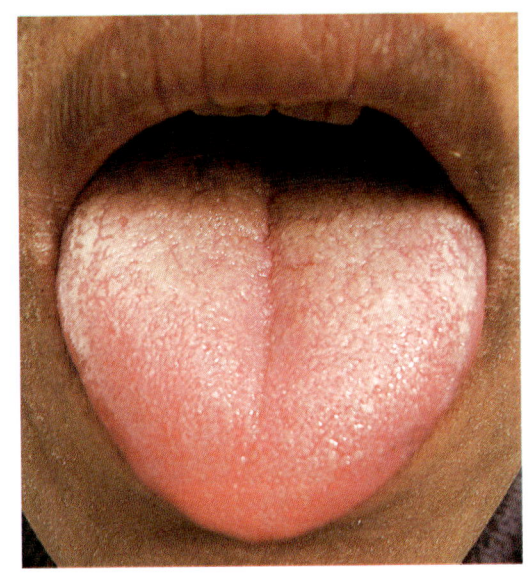

Fig 2.2-219

Patient, Female, 41years,

Case NO.: W612

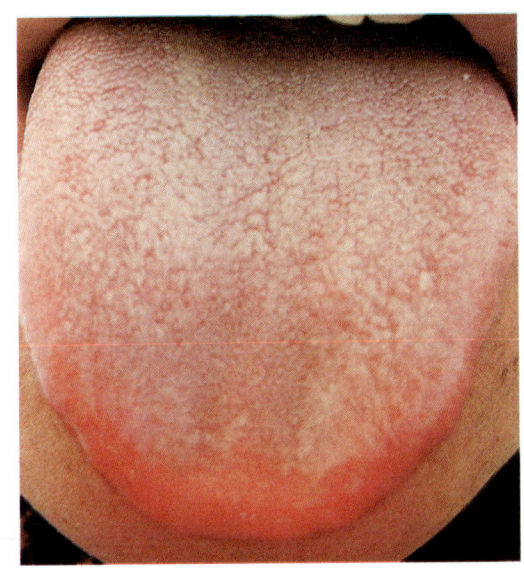

Red tongue

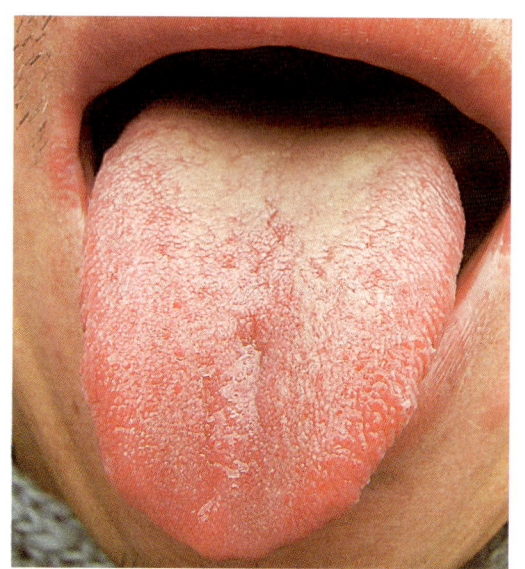

Fig 2.2-220

Patient, Male, 36years,

Case NO.: W670

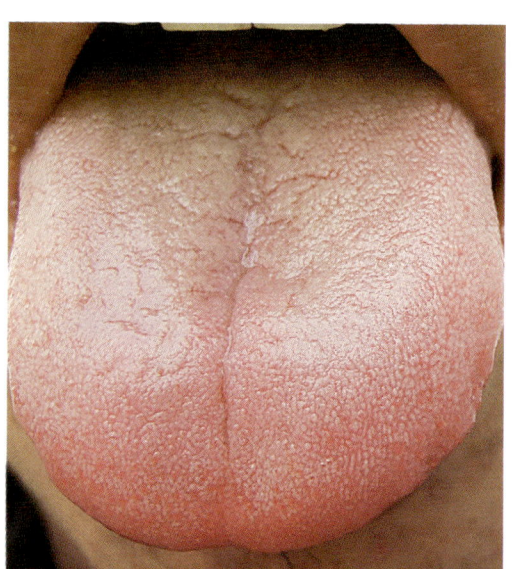

Fig 2.2-221

Patient, Male, 52years,

Case NO.: W178

Fig 2.2-222

Patient, Female, 41years,

Case NO.: F9

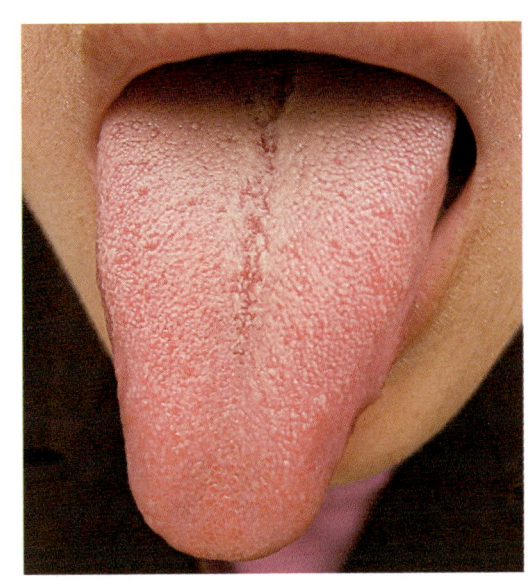

Fig 2.2-223

Patient, Female, 8years,

Case NO.: W296

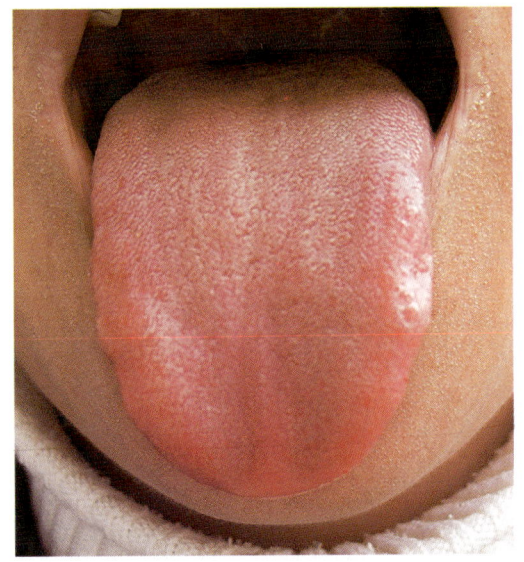

Red tongue

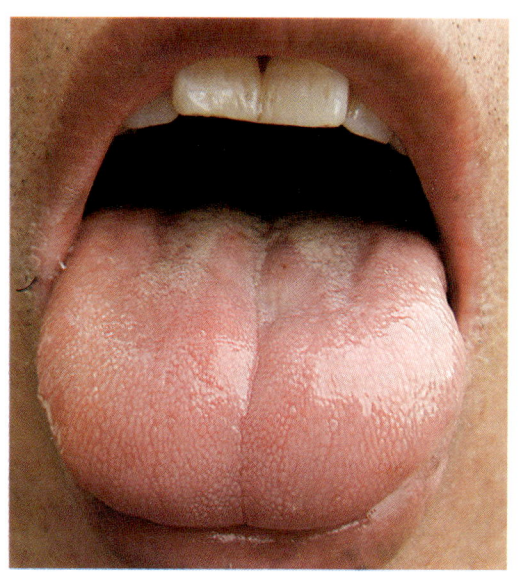

Fig 2.2-224

Patient, Male, 44years,

Case NO.: W118

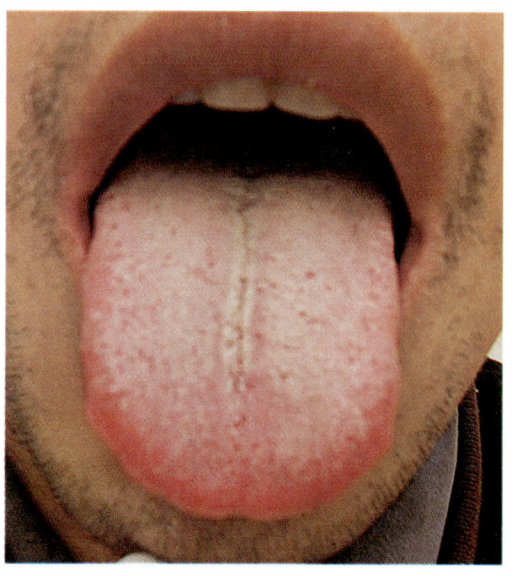

Fig 2.2-225

Patient, Male, 34years,

Case NO.: 313

Fig 2.2-226

Patient, Female, 29years,

Case NO.: F36

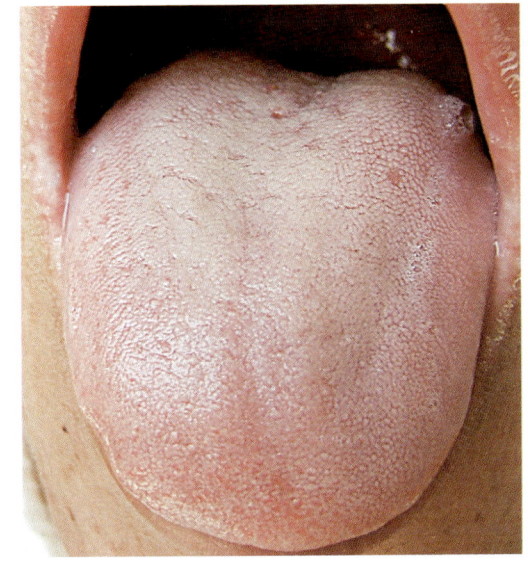

Fig 2.2-227

Patient, Male, 57years,

Case NO.: W33

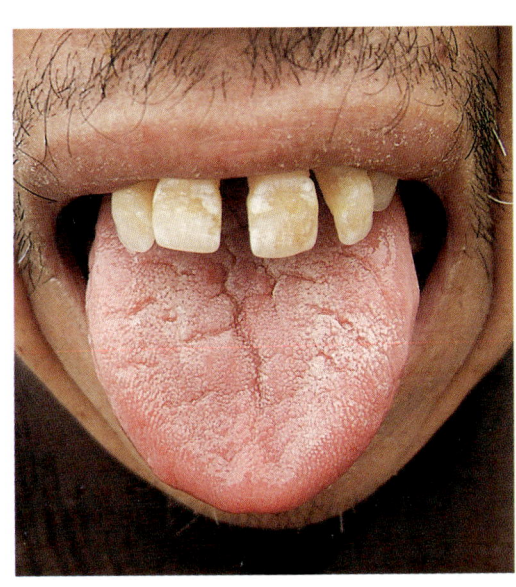

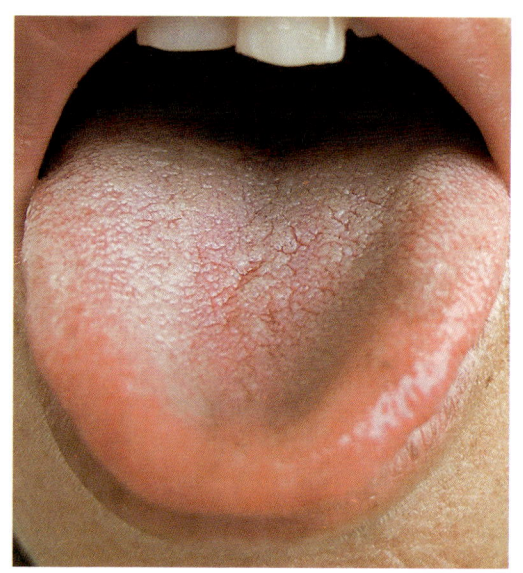

Fig 2.2-228

Patient, Female, 50years,

Case NO.: F66

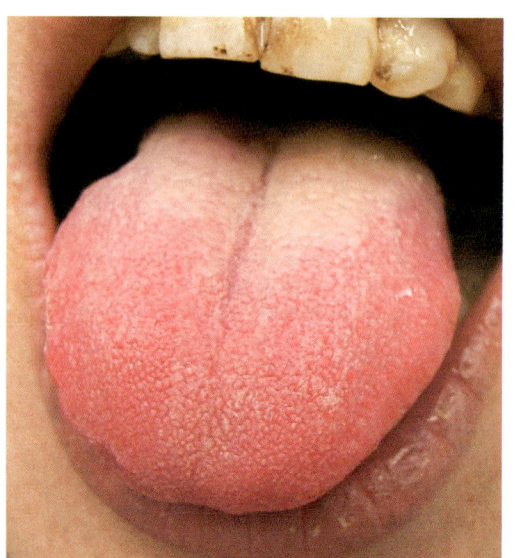

Fig 2.2-229

Patient, Male, 36years,

Case NO.: W578

Fig 2.2-230

Patient, Male, 50years,

Case NO.: W79

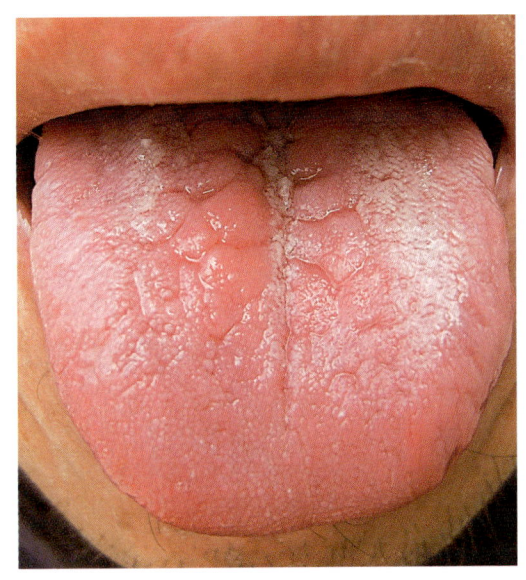

Fig 2.2-231

Patient, Male, 35years,

Case NO.: W84

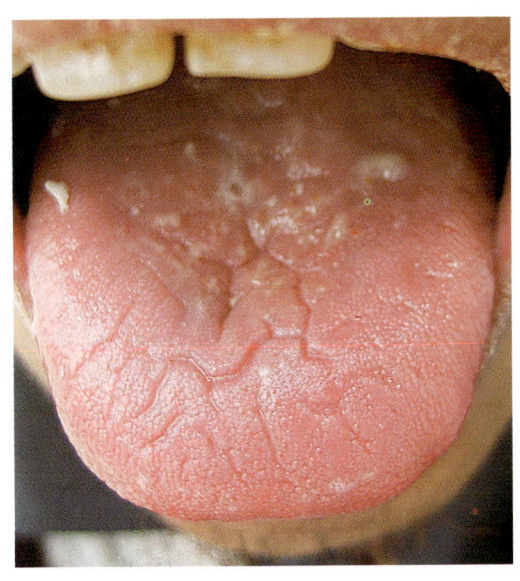

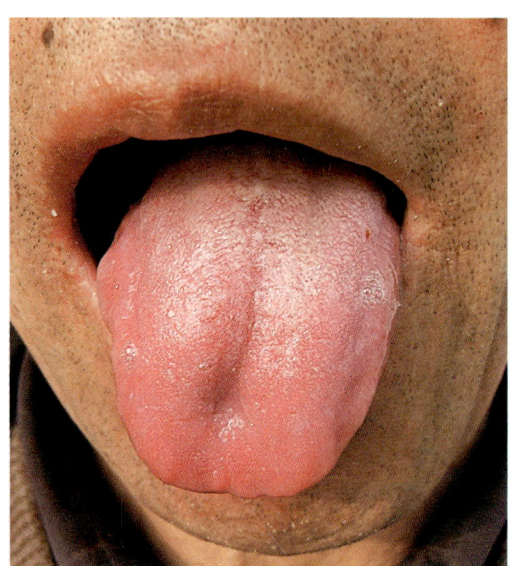

Fig 2.2-232

Patient, Male, 55years,

Case NO.: W218

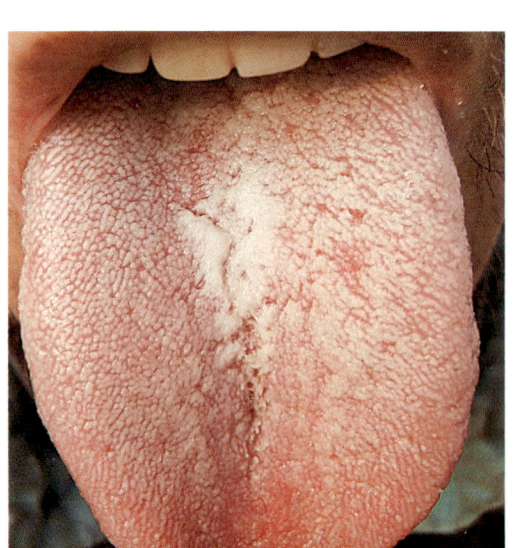

Fig 2.2-233

Patient, Male, 58years,

Case NO.: W231

Fig 2.2-234

Patient, Female, 43years,

Case NO.: W196

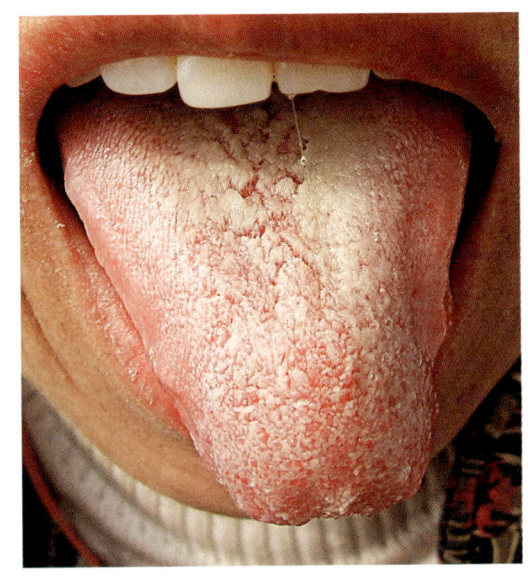

Fig 2.2-235

Patient, Female, 44years,

Case NO.: F52

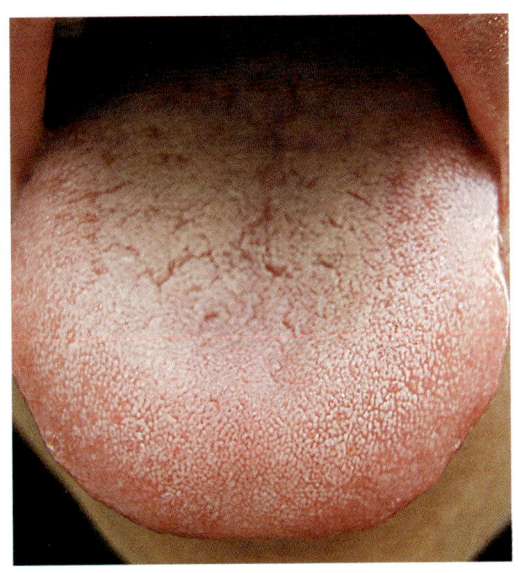

Red tongue

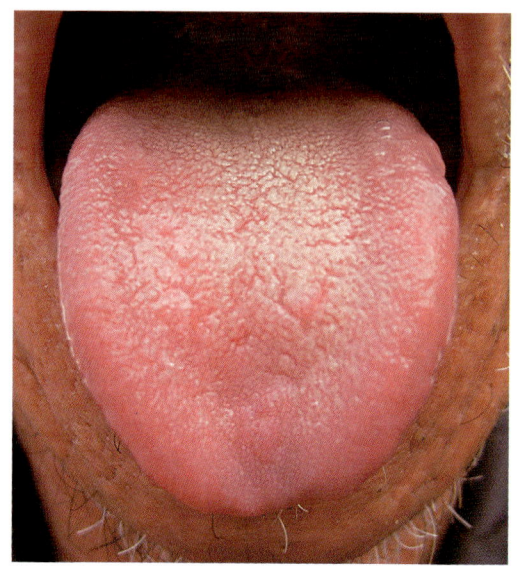

Fig 2.2-236

Patient, Male, 61years,

Case NO.: W358

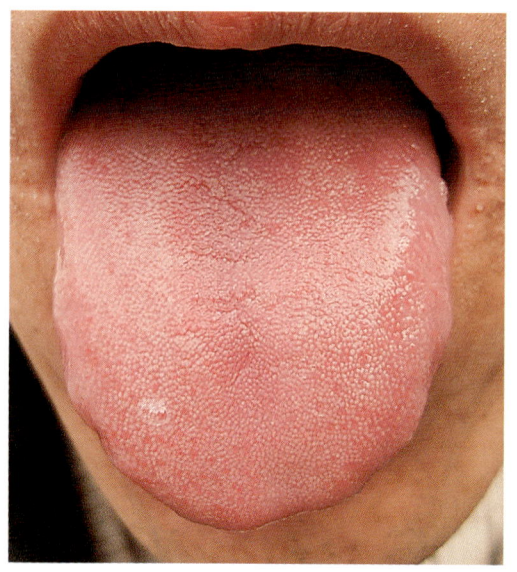

Fig 2.2-237

Patient, Male, 34years,

Case NO.: W374

Fig 2.2-238

Patient, Male, 43years,

Case NO.: F128

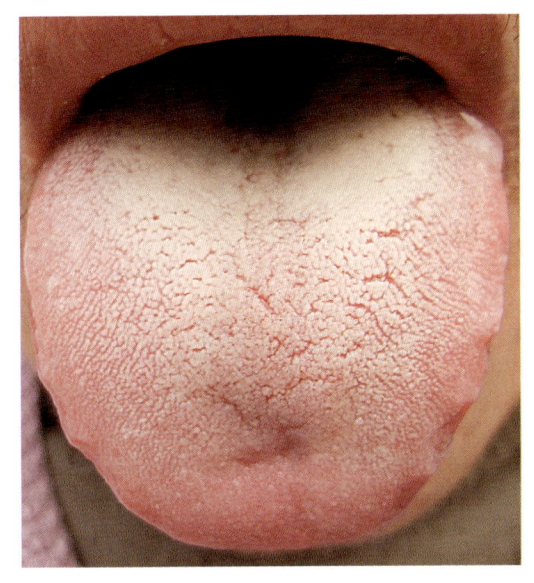

Fig 2.2-239

Patient, Female, 35years,

Case NO.: W348

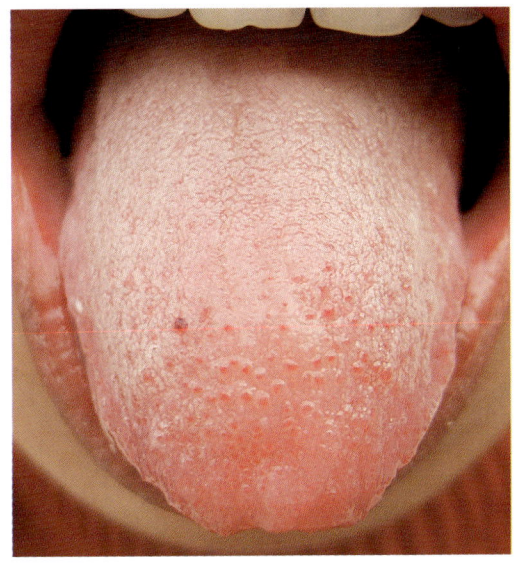

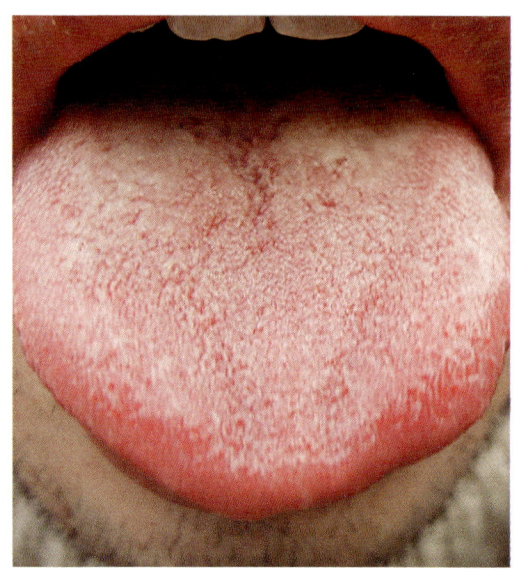

Fig 2.2-240

Patient, Male, 36years,

Case NO.: W375

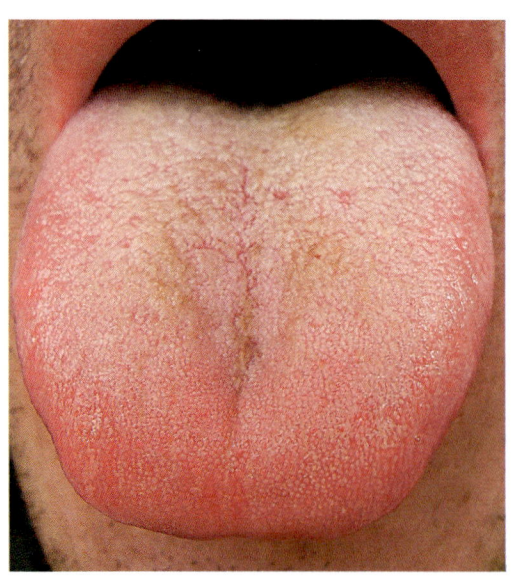

Fig 2.2-241

Patient, Male, 34years,

Case NO.: W534

Fig 2.2-242

Patient, Female, 41years,

Case NO.: W575

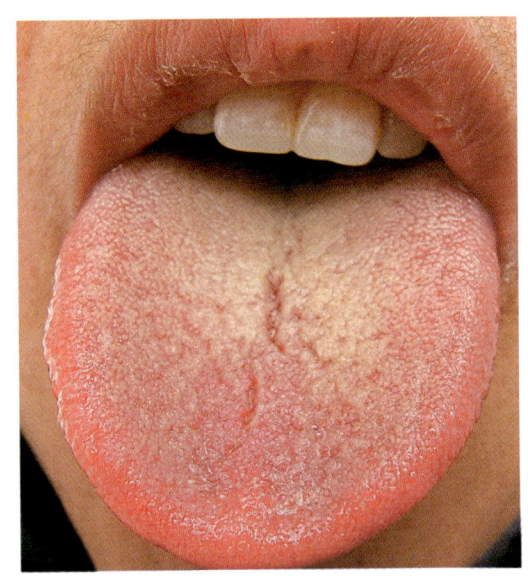

Fig 2.2-243

Patient, Female, 59years,

Case NO.: W606

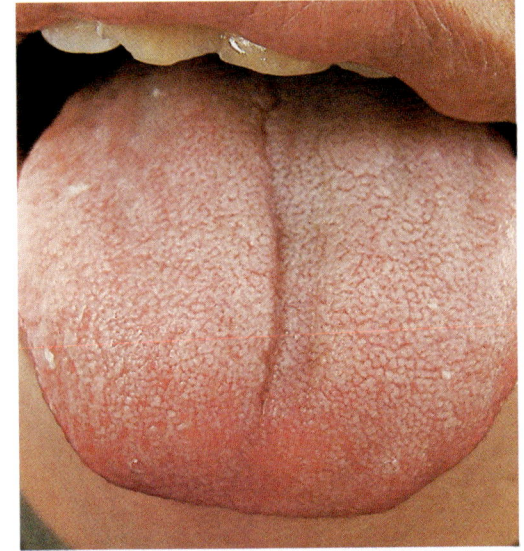

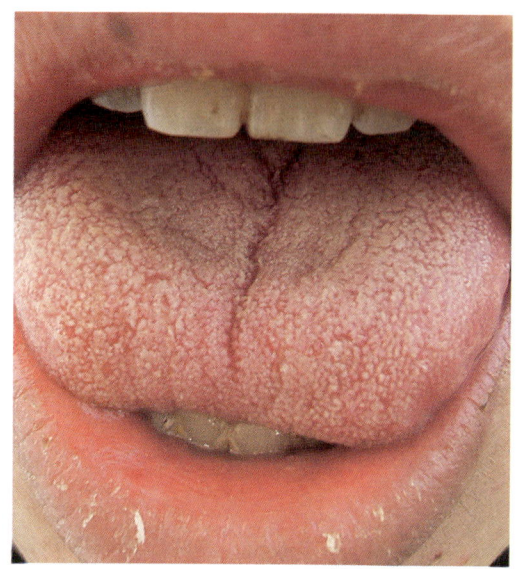

Fig 2.2-244

Patient, Male, 37years,

Case NO.: W598

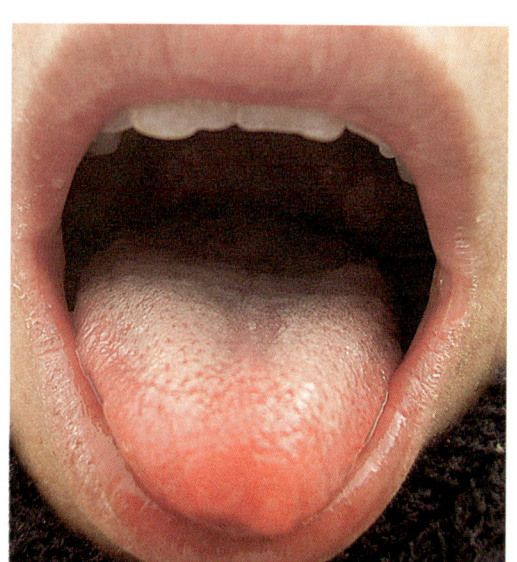

Fig 2.2-245

Patient, Female, 48years,

Case NO.: W635

Fig 2.2-246

Patient, Male, 44years,

Case NO.: W664

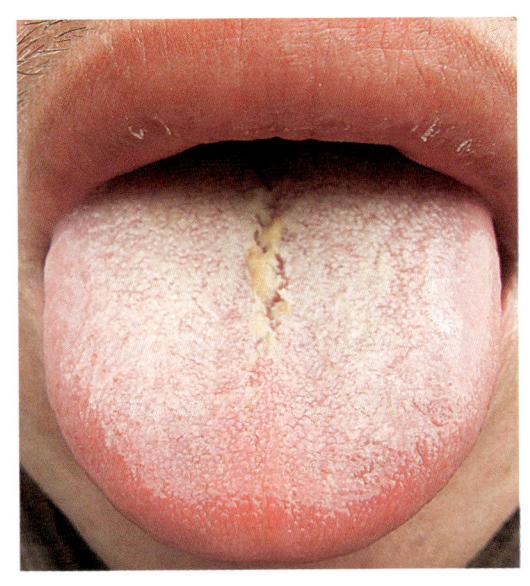

Fig 2.2-247

Patient, Male, 56years,

Case NO.: W652

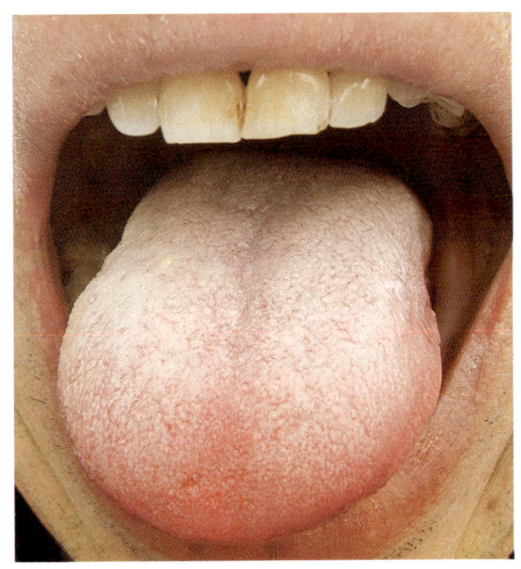

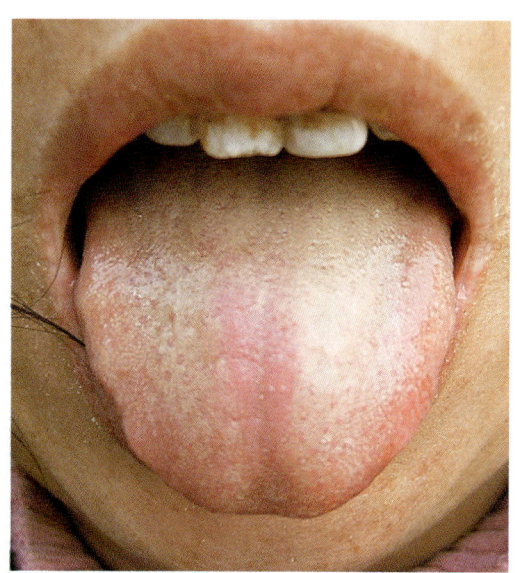

Fig 2.2-248

Patient, Female, 44years,

Case NO.: F212

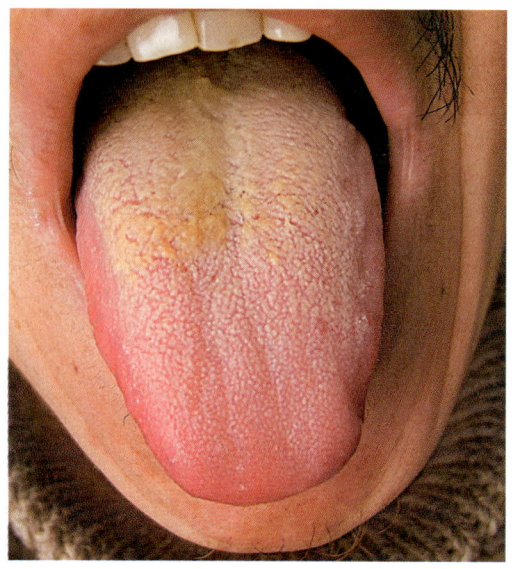

Fig 2.2-249

Patient, Male, 40years,

Case NO.: F725

Fig 2.2-250

Patient, Female, 43years,

Case NO.: W539

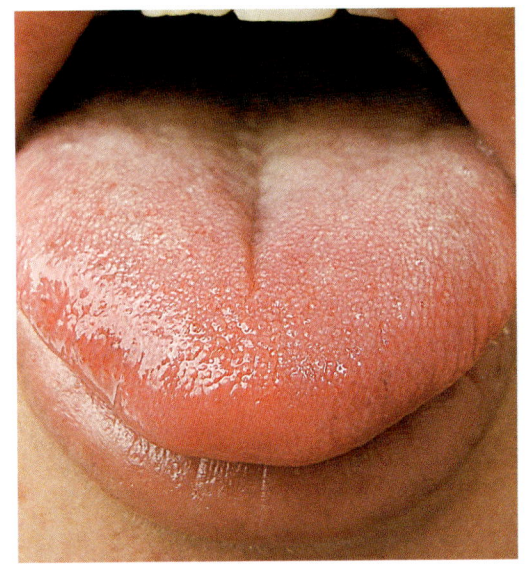

Fig 2.2-251

Patient, Male, 52years,

Case NO.: W531

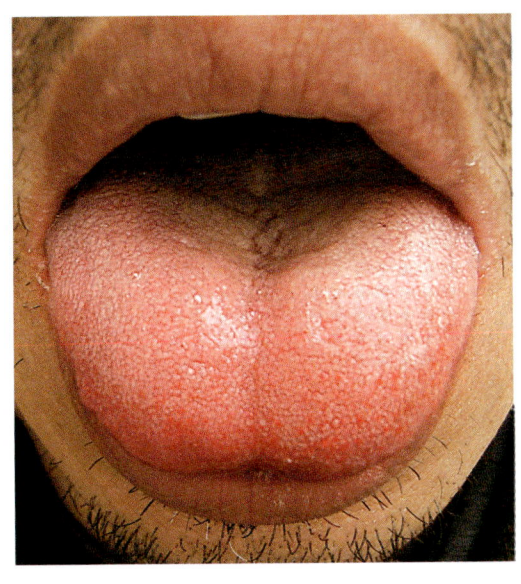

Red tongue

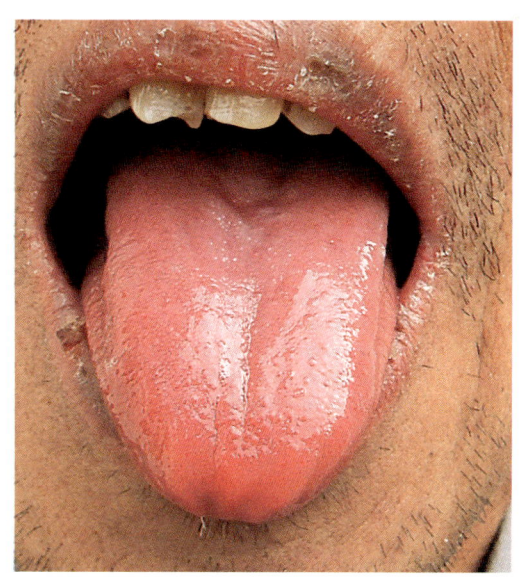

Fig 2.2-252

Patient, Male, 50years,

Case NO.: W530

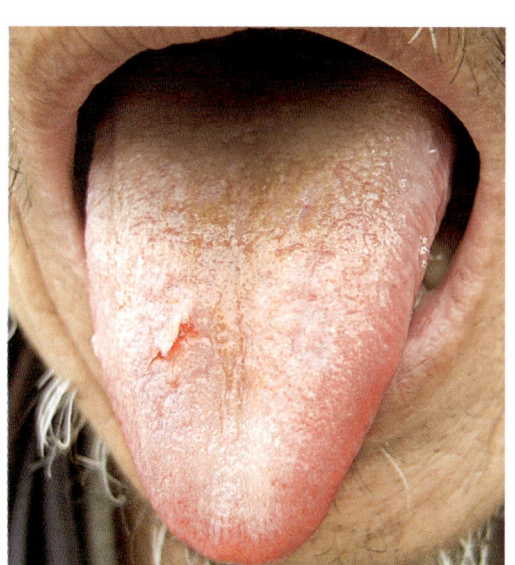

Fig 2.2-253

Patient, Male, 62years,

Case NO.: W397

Fig 2.2-254

Patient, Female, 38years,

Case NO.: W401

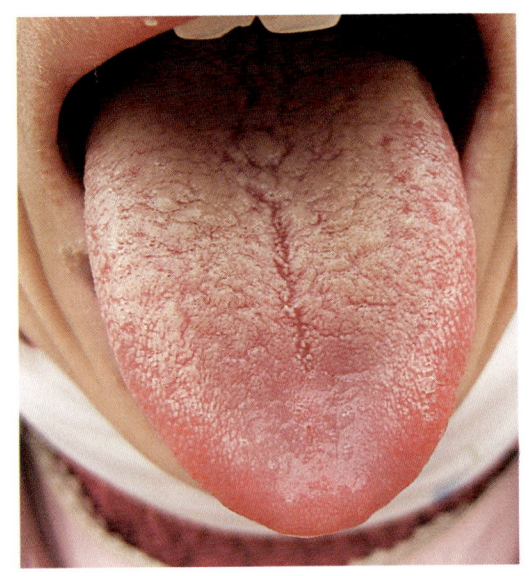

Fig 2.2-255

Patient ,Male, 29years,

Case NO.: F113

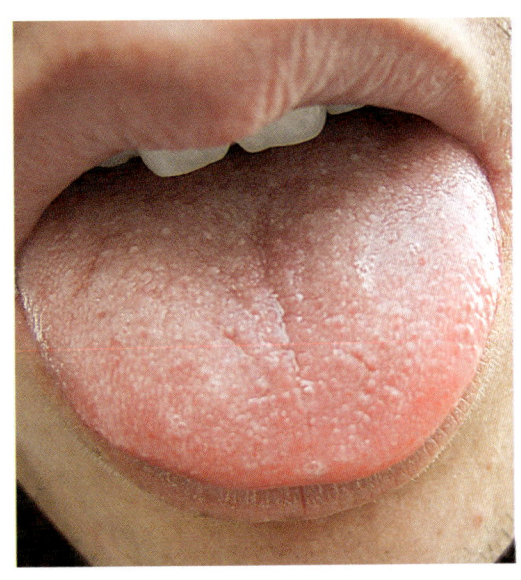

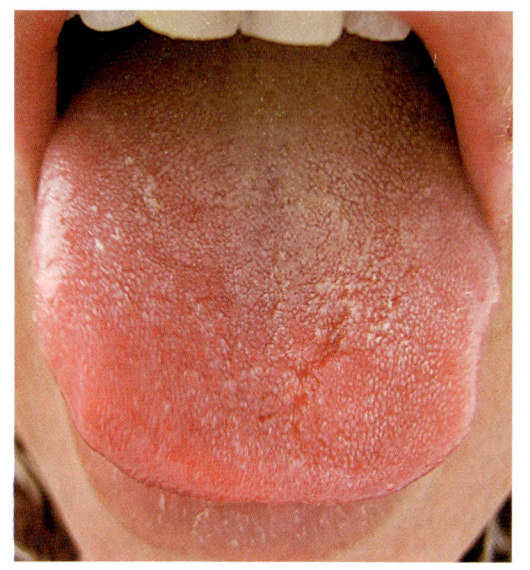

Fig 2.2-256

Patient, Female, 36years,

Case NO.: W723

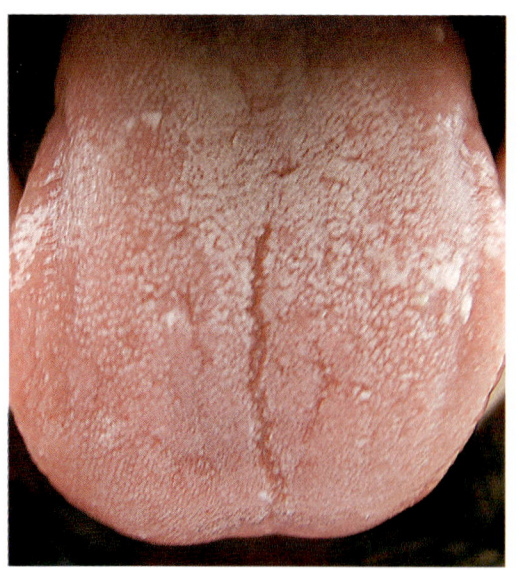

Fig 2.2-257

Patient, Female, 59years,

Case NO.: W700

Fig 2.2-258

Patient, Male, 46years,

Case NO.: F278

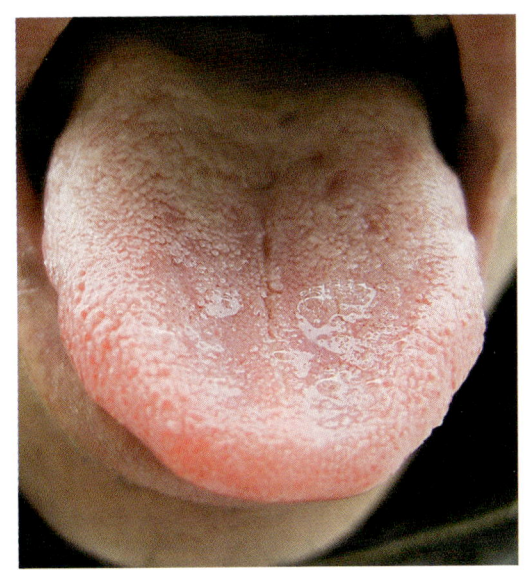

Fig 2.2-259

Patient, Female, 59years,

Case NO.: F249

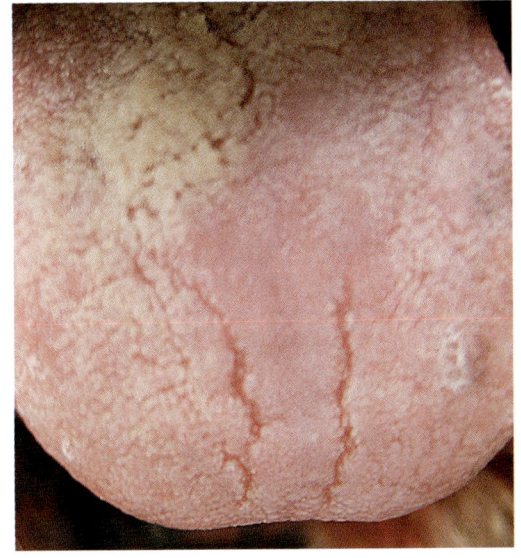

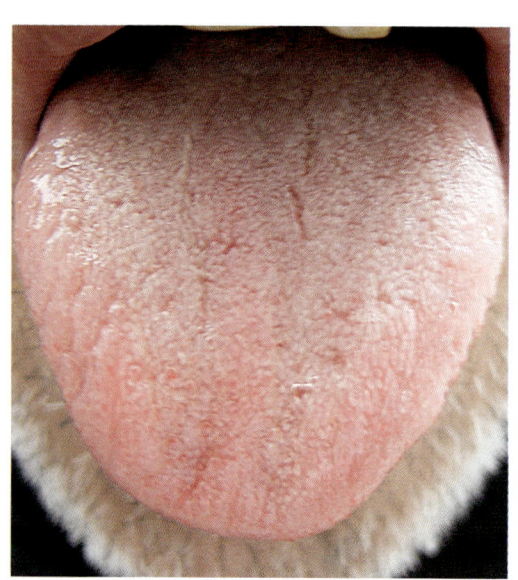

Fig 2.2-260

Patient, Male, 62years,

Case NO.: F268

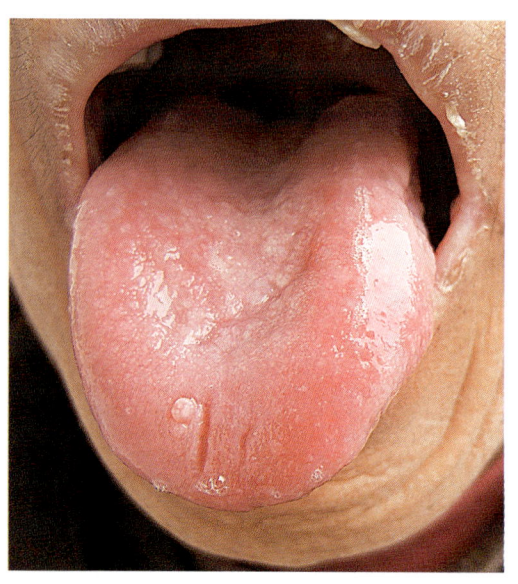

Fig 2.2-261

Patient, Female, 70years,

Case NO.: F284

1.4 Crimson tongue

AIDS stage

Fig 2.2-262

Patient, Male, 39years,

Case NO.: F217

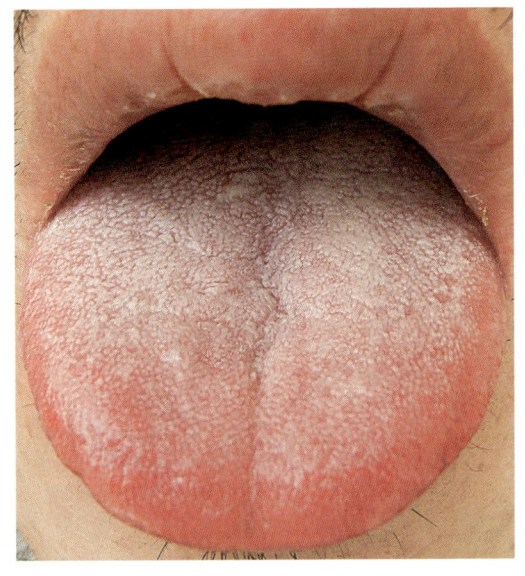

Fig 2.2-263

Patient, Male, 42years,

Case NO.: W629

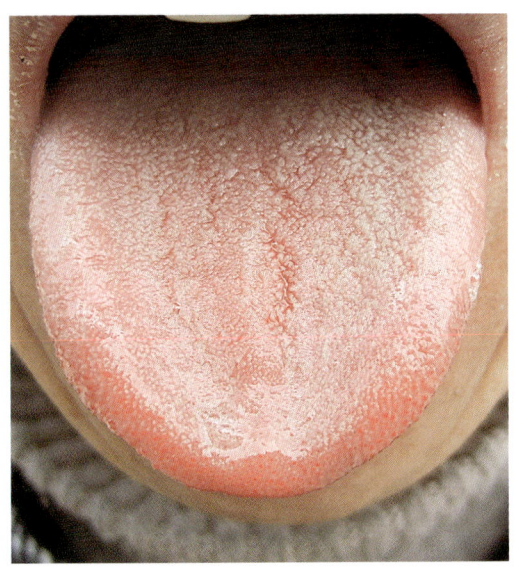

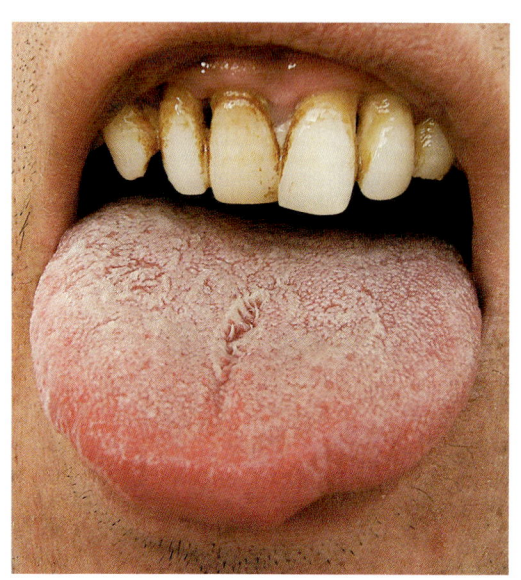

Fig 2.2-264

Patient, Male, 37years,

Case NO.: F235

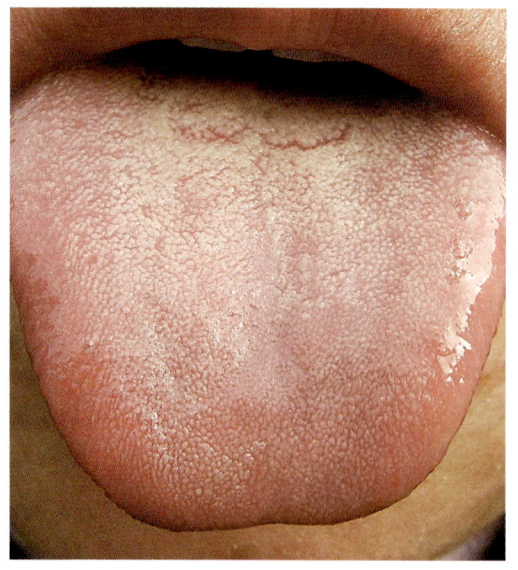

Fig 2.2-265

Patient, Female, 48years,

Case NO.: W642

Fig 2.2-266

Patient, Female, 34years,

Case NO.: W602

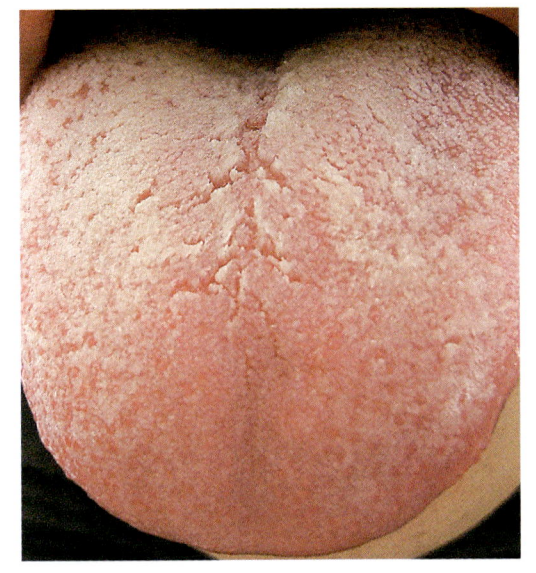

Fig 2.2-267

Patient, Female, 51years,

Case NO.: W660

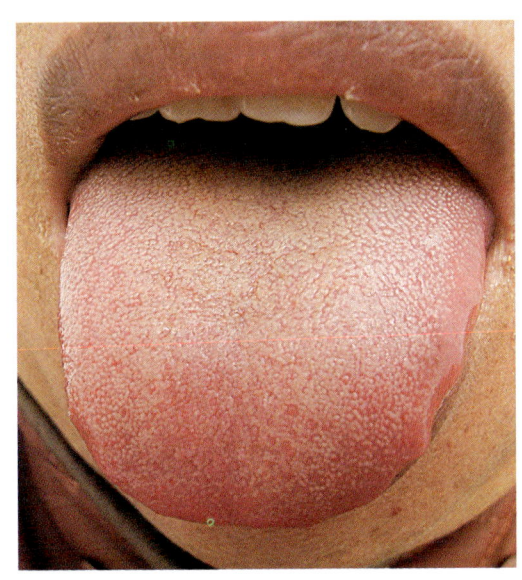

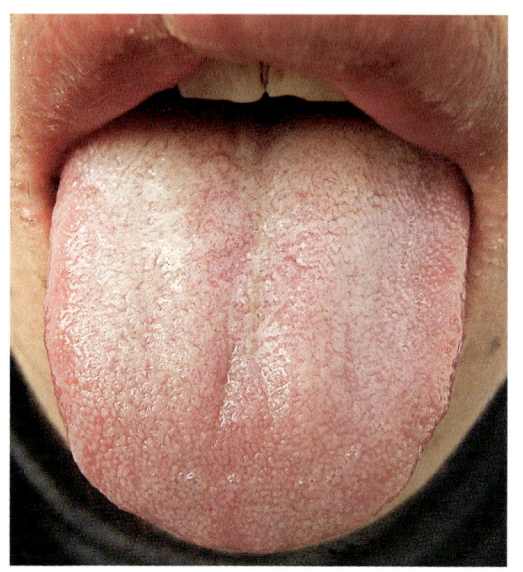

Fig 2.2-268

Patient, Male, 34years,

Case NO.: W617

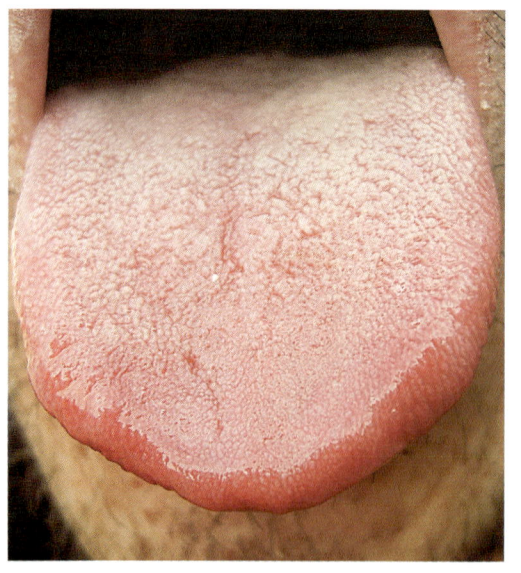

Fig 2.2-269

Patient, Male, 43years,

Case NO.: W683

Fig 2.2-270

Patient, Female, 53years,

Case NO.: W527

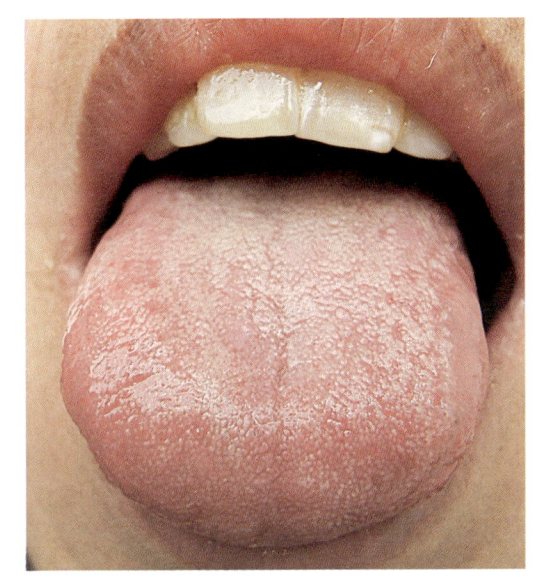

Fig 2.2-271

Patient, Female, 44years,

Case NO.: W551

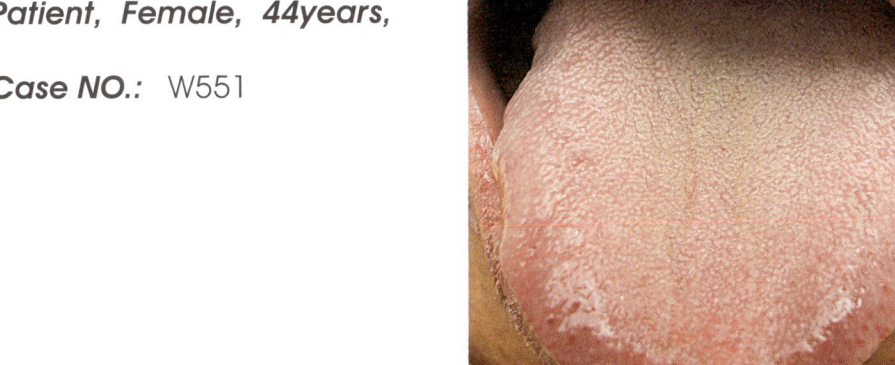

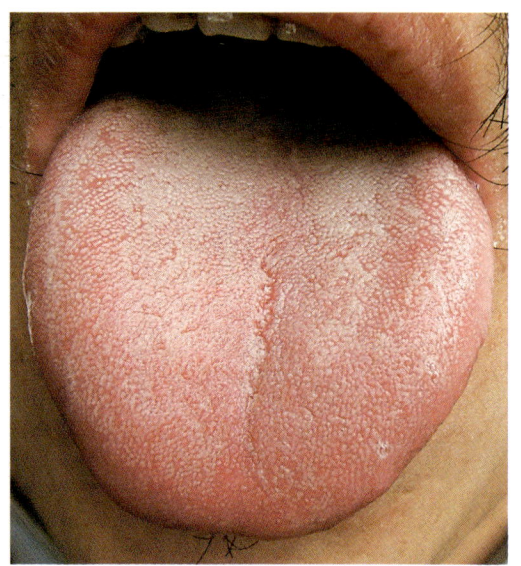

Fig 2.2-272

Patient, Male, 42years,

Case NO.: W635

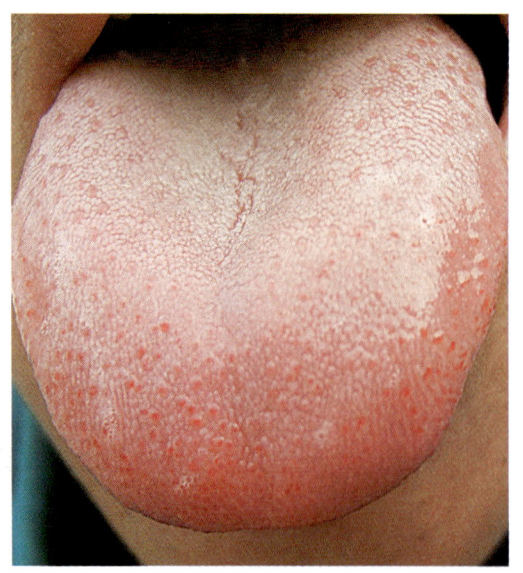

Fig 2.2-273

Patient, Female, 42years,

Case NO.: W380

Fig 2.2-274

Patient, Male, 43years,

Case NO.: W385

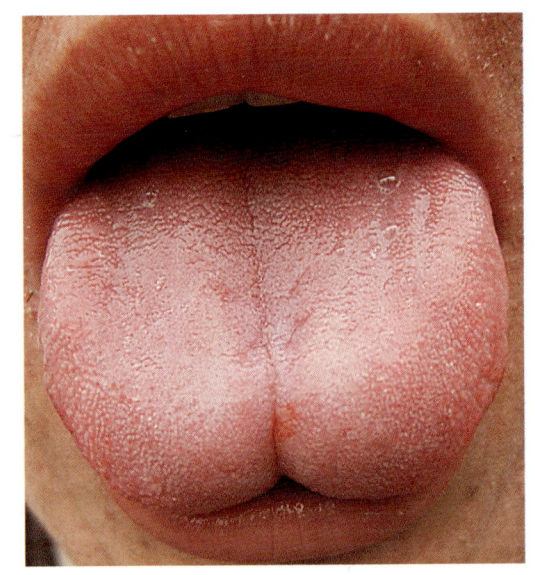

Fig 2.2-275

Patient, Female, 43years,

Case NO.: W564

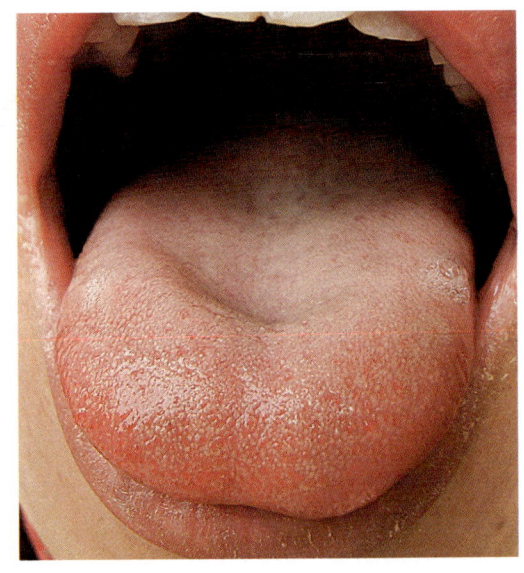

Crimson tongue

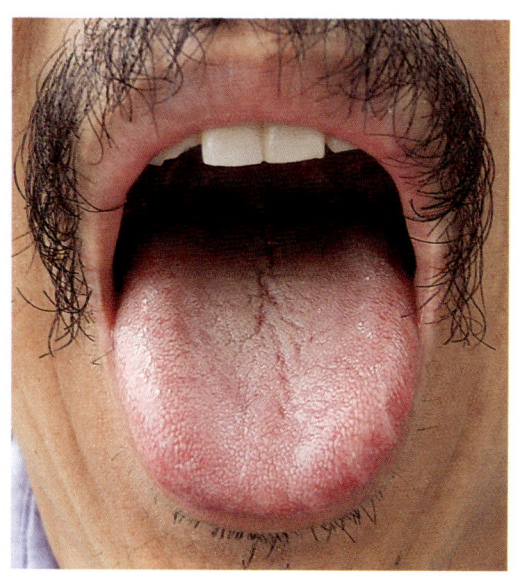

Fig 2.2-276

Patient, Male, 43years,

Case NO.: W9

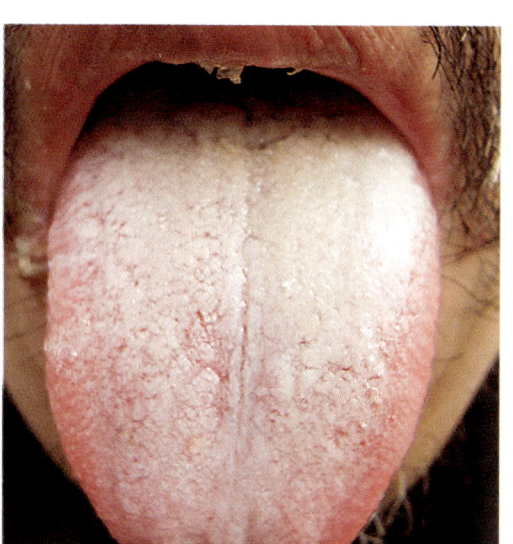

Fig 2.2-277

Patient, Male, 55years,

Case NO.: W622

Fig 2.2-278

Patient, Female, 59years,

Case NO.: F102

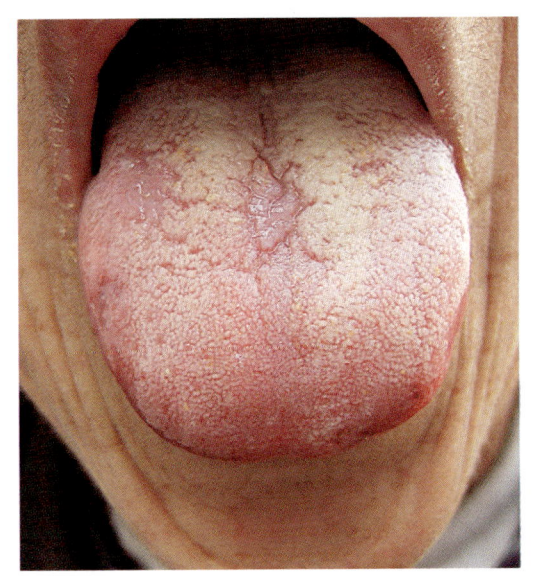

Fig 2.2-279

Patient, Male, 40years,

Case NO.: W96

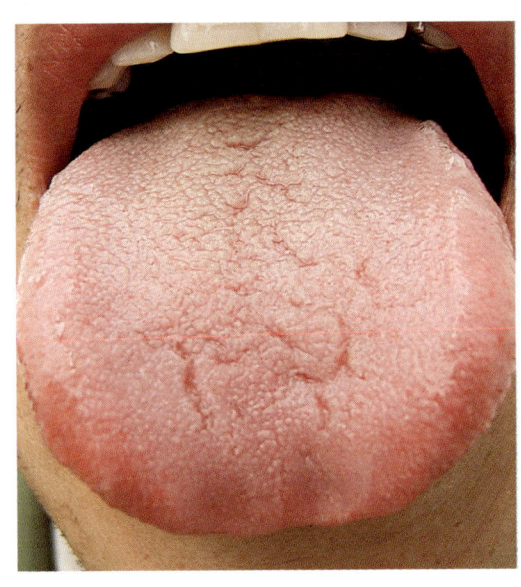

Crimson tongue

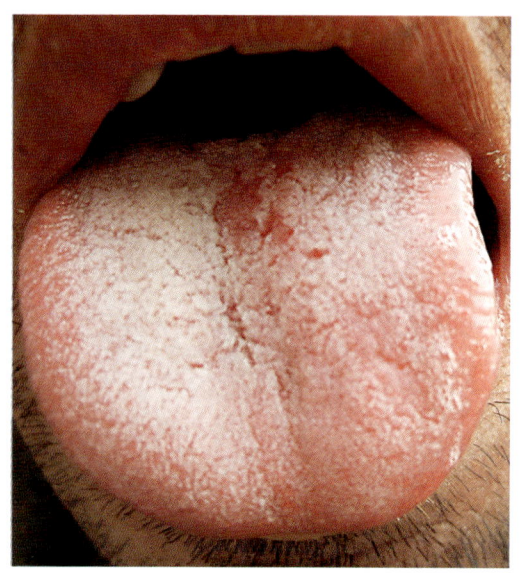

Fig 2.2-280

Patient, Male, 51years,

Case NO.: F109

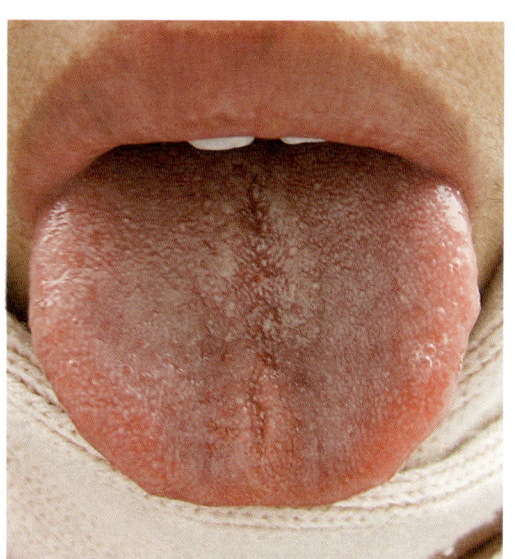

Fig 2.2-281

Patient, Female, 35years,

Case NO.: F265

Fig 2.2-282

Patient, Female, 48years,

Case NO.: W11

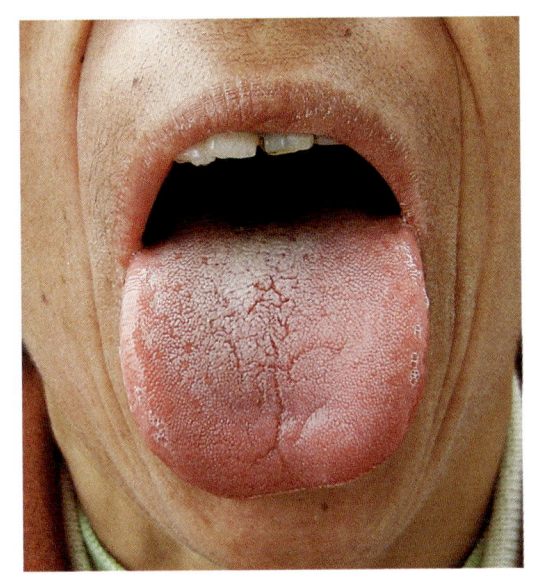

Fig 2.2-283

Patient, Female, 43years,

Case NO.: F1

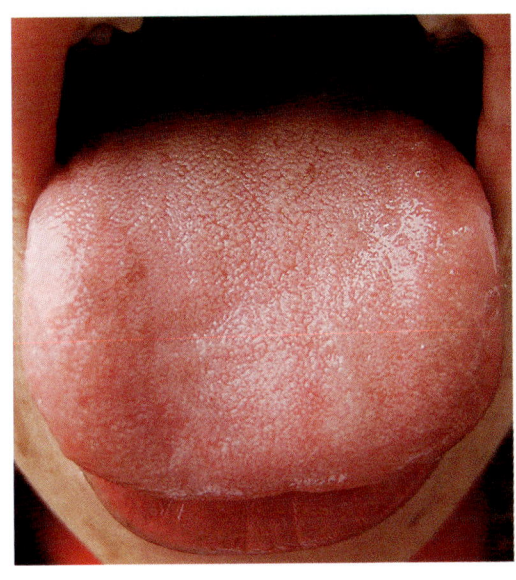

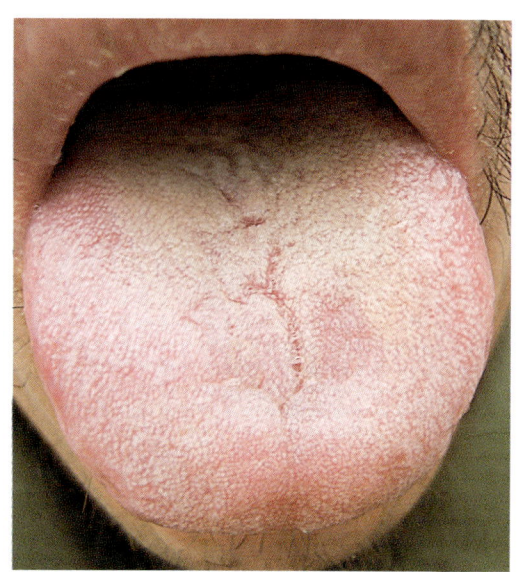

Fig 2.2-284

Patient, Male, 42years,

Case NO.: W395

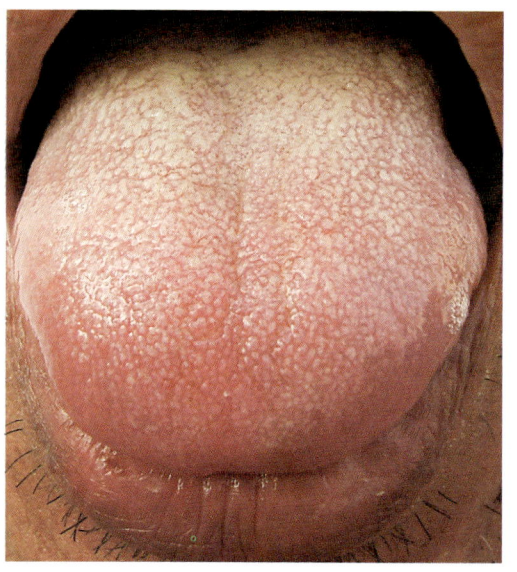

Fig 2.2-285

Patient, Male, 50years,

Case NO.: W611

Fig 2.2-286

Patient, Female, 38years,

Case NO.: W654

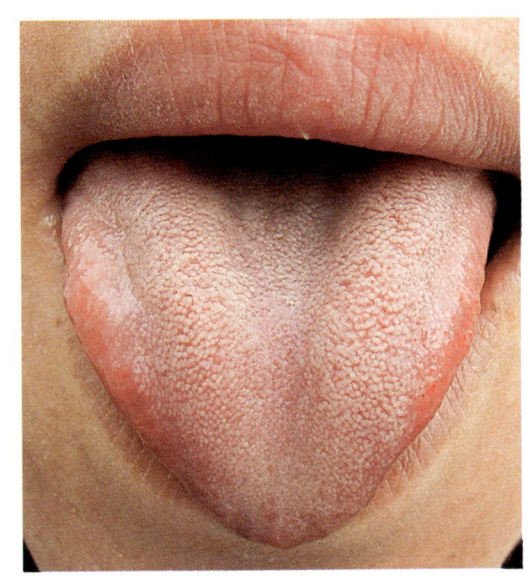

Fig 2.2-287

Patient, Female, 41years,

Case NO.: F213

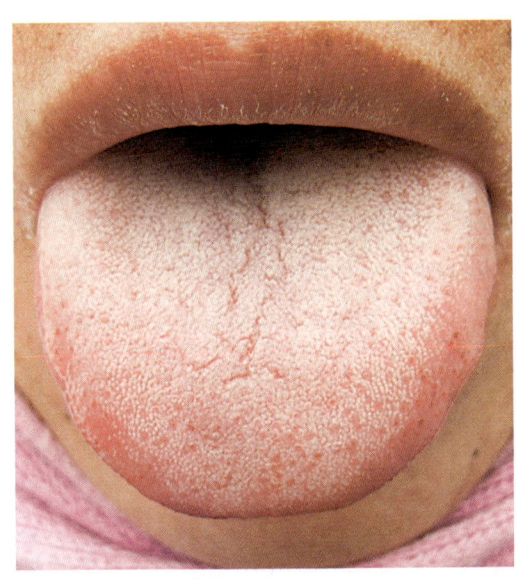

Crimson tongue

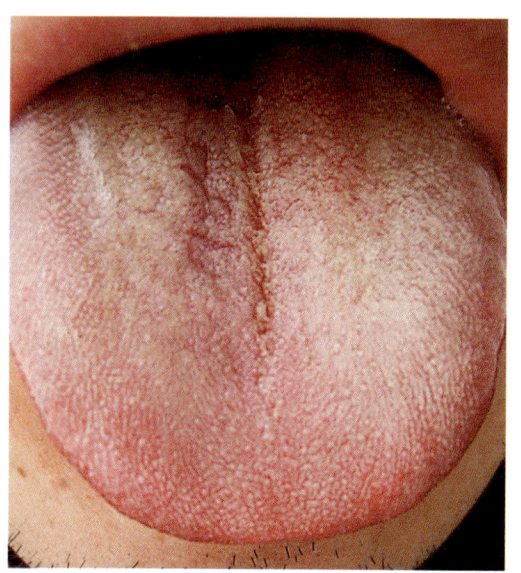

Fig 2.2-288

Patient, Male, 32years,

Case NO.: W739

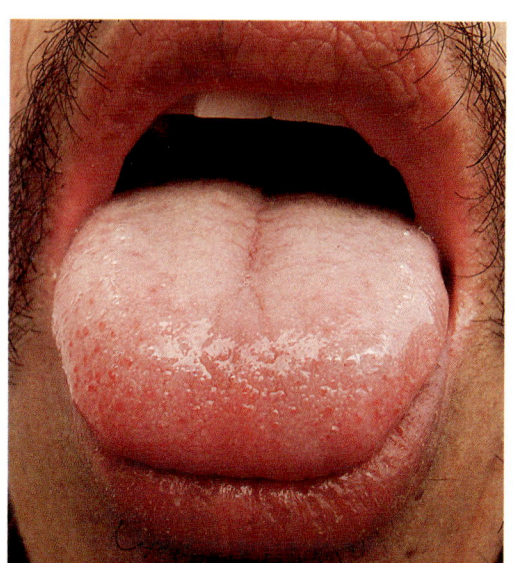

Fig 2.2-289

Patient, Male, 48years,

Case NO.: W591

Fig 2.2-290

Patient, Male, 54years,

Case NO.: F201

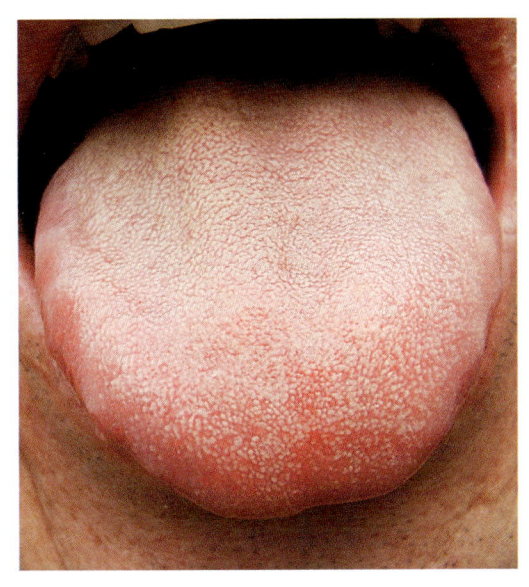

Fig 2.2-291

Patient, Male, 62years,

Case NO.: F268

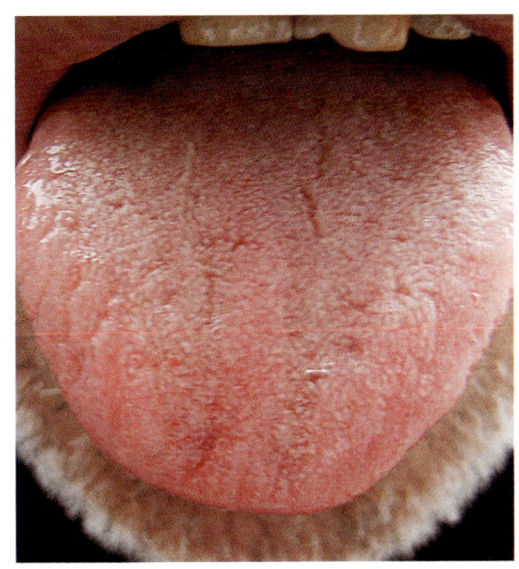

Crimson tongue

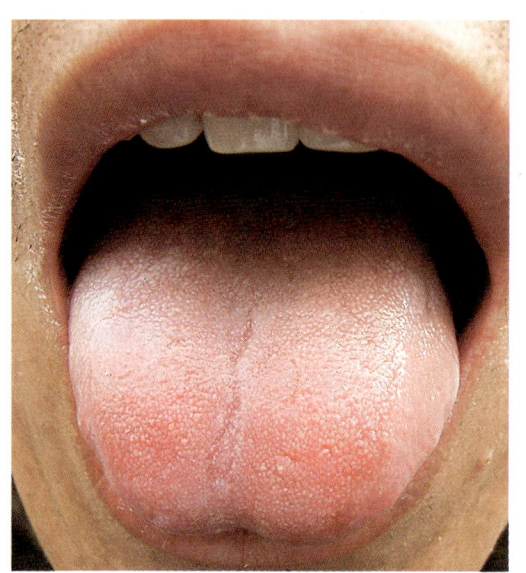

Fig 2.2-292

Patient, Male, 43years,

Case NO.: W465

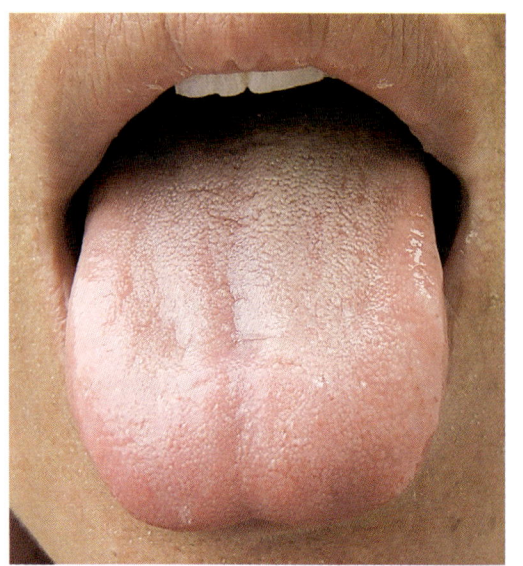

Fig 2.2-293

Patient, Female, 41years,

Case NO.: W16

Fig 2.2-294

Patient, Male, 43years,

Case NO.: W300

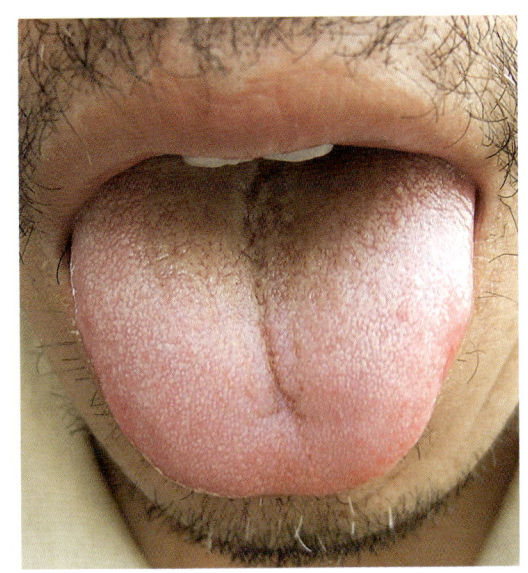

Fig 2.2-295

Patient, Female, 40years,

Case NO.: F301

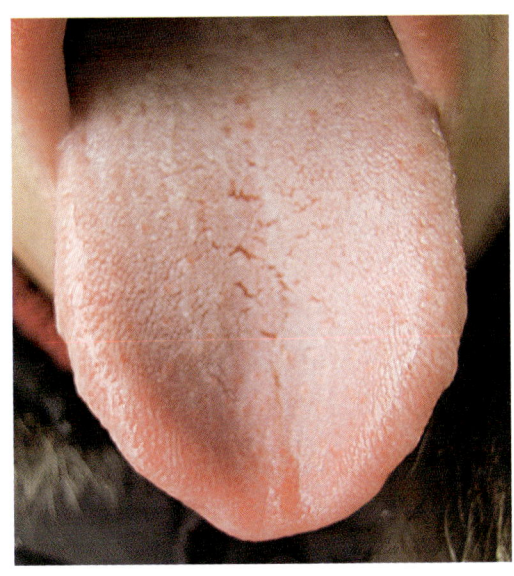

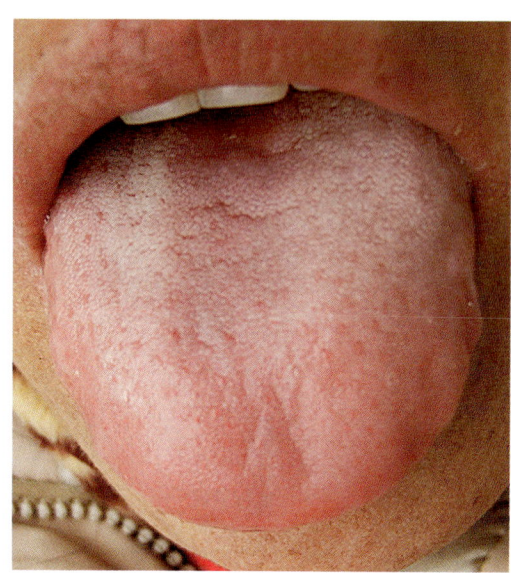

Fig 2.2-296

Patient, Female, 48years,

Case NO.: W738

1.5 Petechial tongue

AIDS stage

Fig 2.2-297

Patient, Female, 54years,

Case NO.: F253

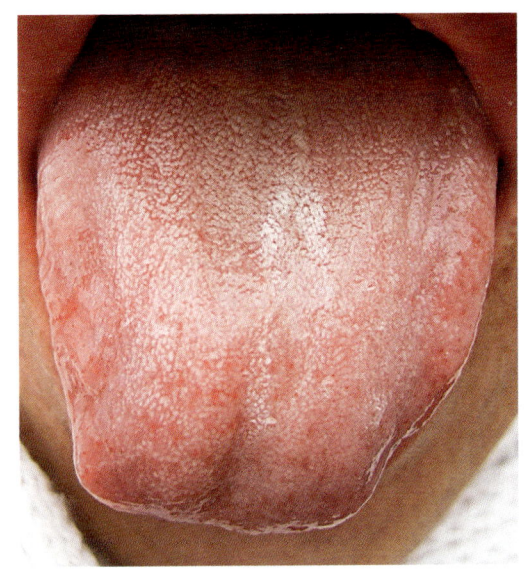

Fig 2.2-298

Patient, Female, 58years,

Case NO.: F218

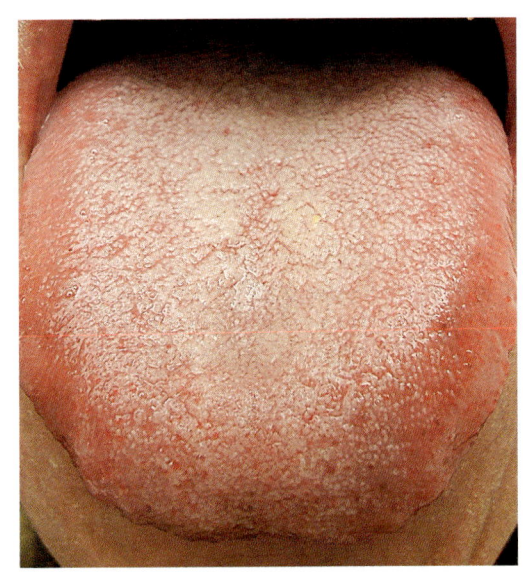

Petechial tongue

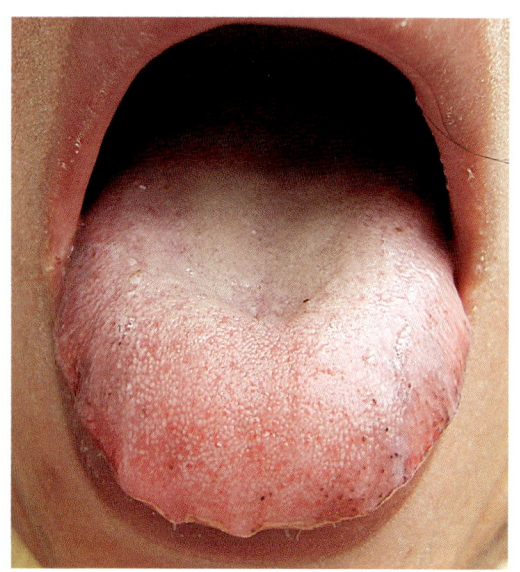

Fig 2.2-299

Patient, Female, 36years,

Case NO.: F65

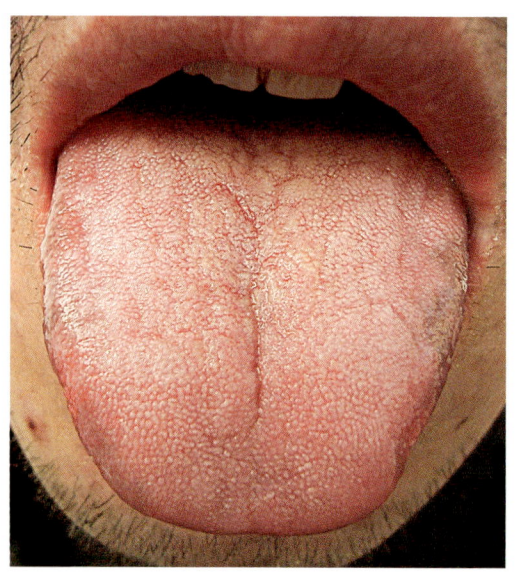

Fig 2.2-300

Patient, Male, 38years,

Case NO.: W618

Fig 2.2-301

Patient, Female, 42years,

Case NO.: F241

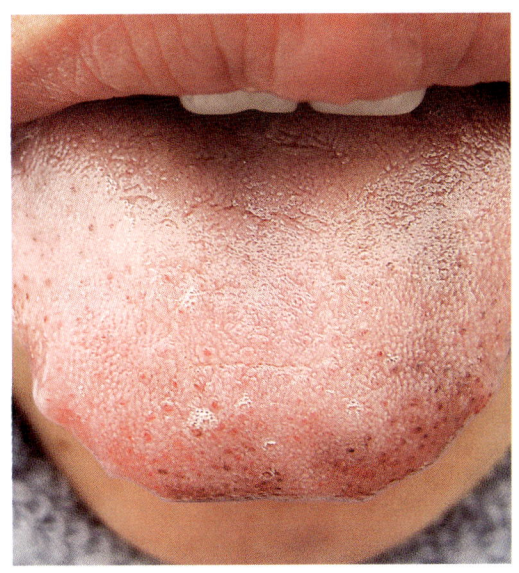

2. *Tongue Shape*

2.1 Cracked tongue
AIDS stage

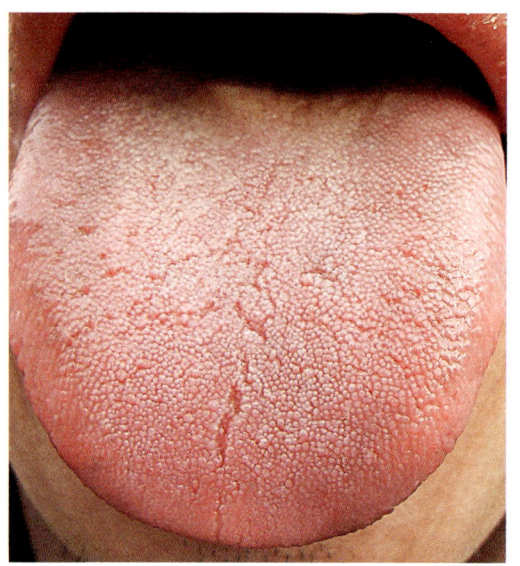

Fig 2.2-302

Patient, Male, 44years,

Case NO.: W644

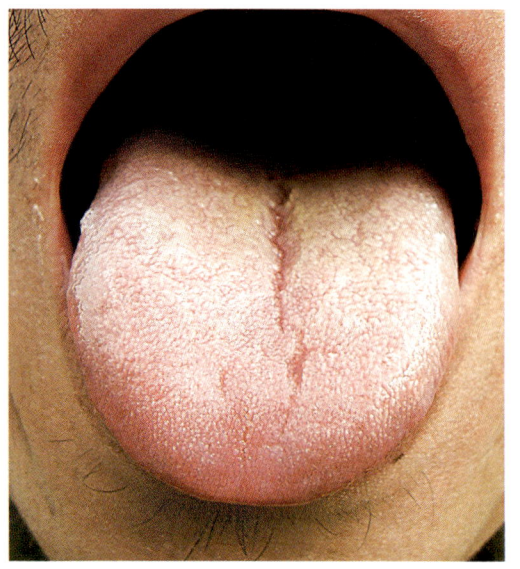

Fig 2.2-303

Patient, Male, 47years,

Case NO.: W658

Fig 2.2-304

Patient, Male, 37years,

Case NO.: W619

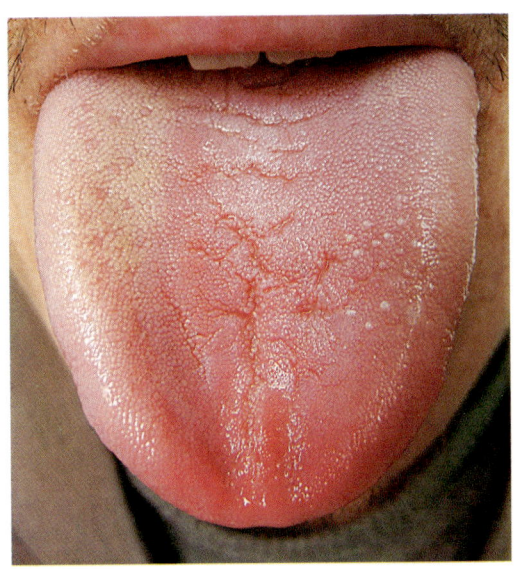

2.2 Tooth-marked tongue

AIDS stage

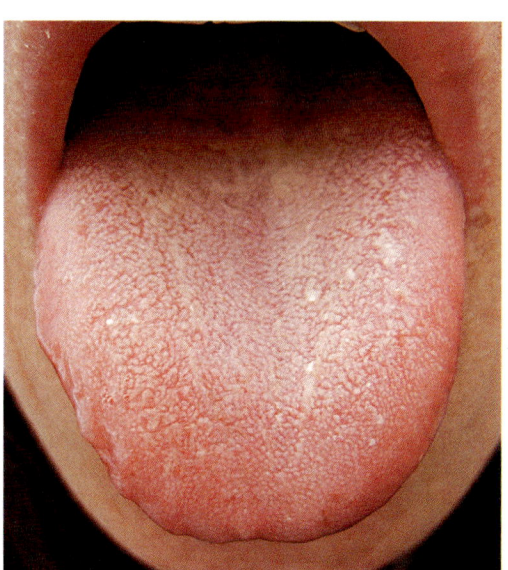

Fig 2.2-305

Patient, Female, 63years,

Case NO.: F252

³. *Tongue Coating*

3.1 Thick-yellow tongue coating
AIDS stage

Fig 2.2-306

Patient, Male, 47years,

Case NO.: W263

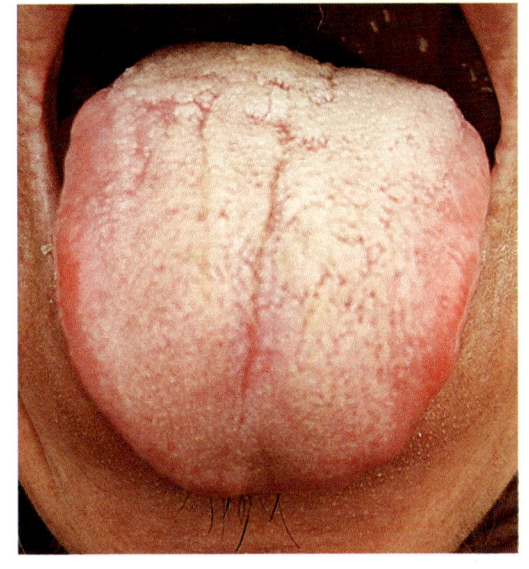

Fig 2.2-307

Patient, Female, 34years,

Case NO.: W257

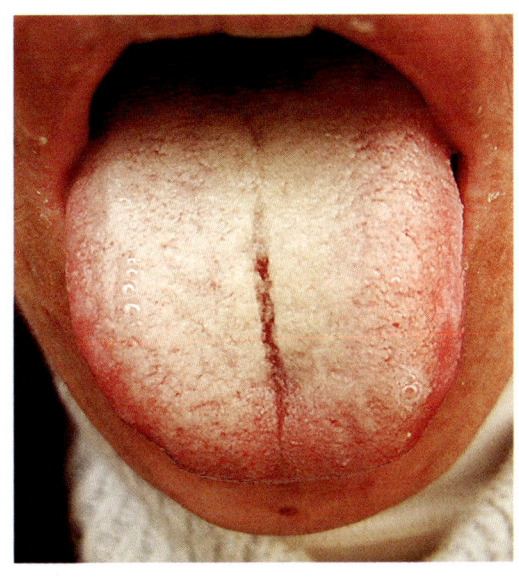

Thick-yellow tongue coating

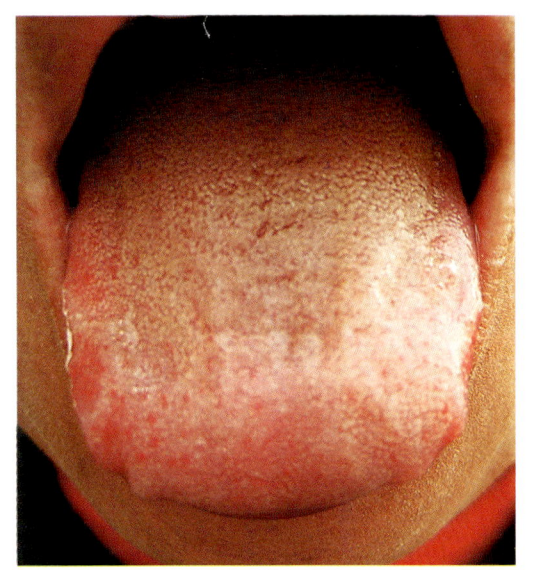

Fig 2.2-308

Patient, Female, 41years,

Case NO.: F51

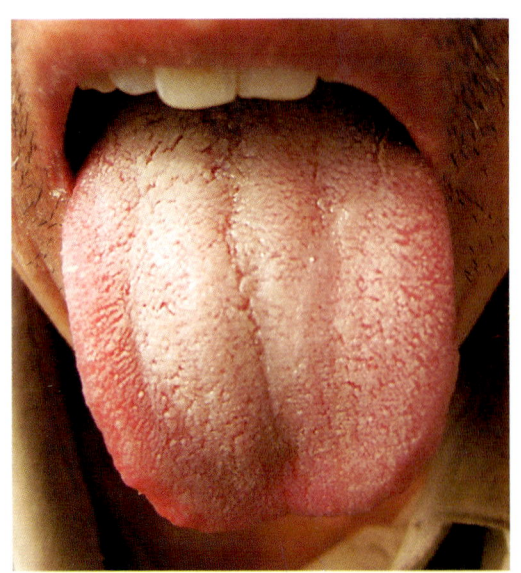

Fig 2.2-309

Patient, Male, 49years,

Case NO.: W207

Fig 2.2-310

Patient, Female, 51years,

Case NO.: W141

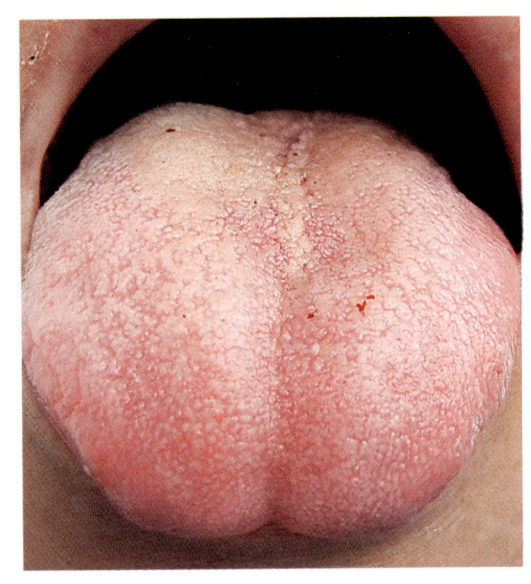

Fig 2.2-311

Patient, Male, 35years,

Case NO.: F310

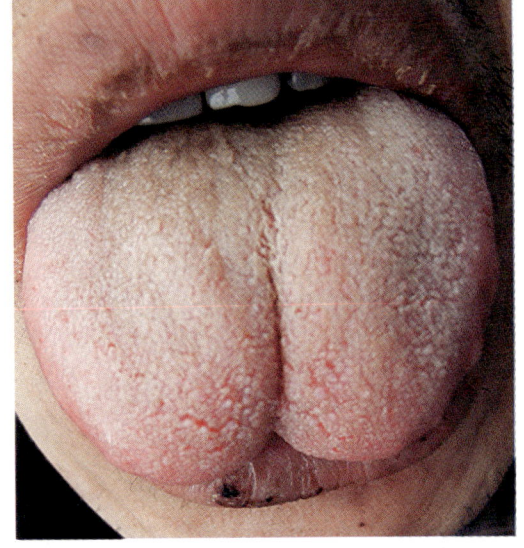

Thick-yellow tongue coating

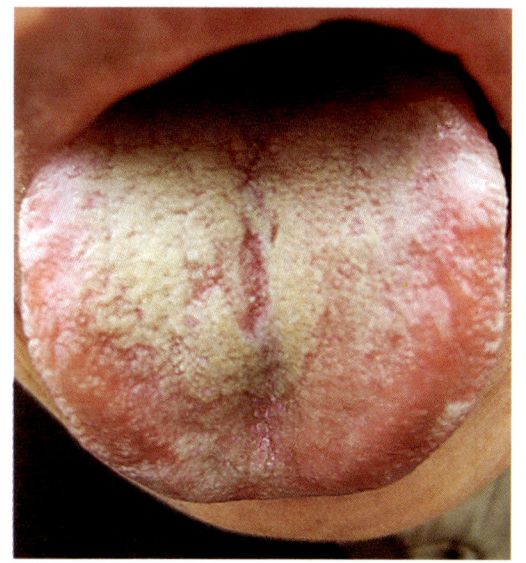

Fig 2.2-312

Patient, Female, 48years,

Case NO.: W383

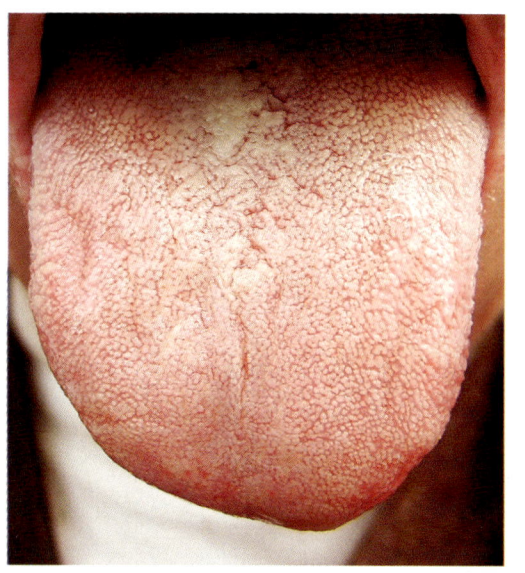

Fig 2.2-313

Patient, Male, 47years,

Case NO.: W273

3.2 Thin-yellow tongue coating

AIDS stage

Fig 2.2-314

Patient, Male, 38years,

Case NO.: F157

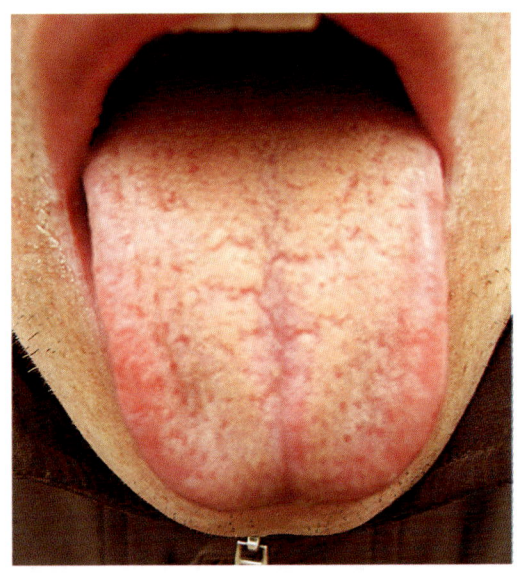

3.3 Thick-white tongue coating

AIDS stage

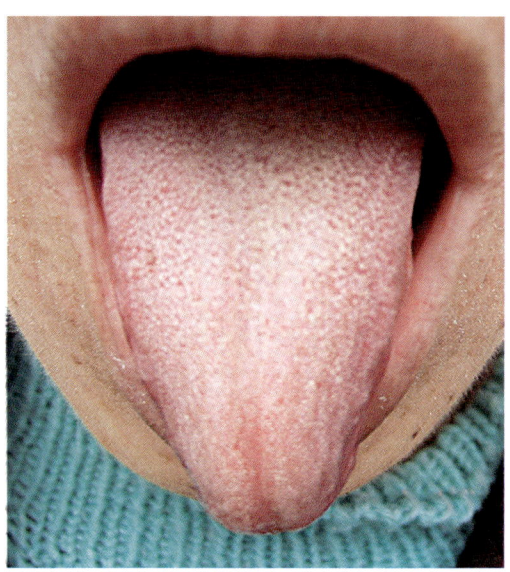

Fig 2.2-315

Patient, Female, 53years,

Case NO.: F5

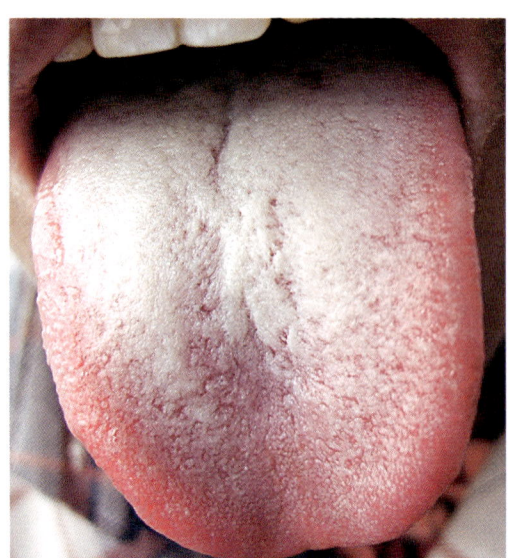

Fig 2.2-316

Patient, Female, 40years,

Case NO.: W188

3.4 Greasy tongue coating

AIDS stage

Fig 2.2-317

Patient, Female, 42years,

Case NO.: W229

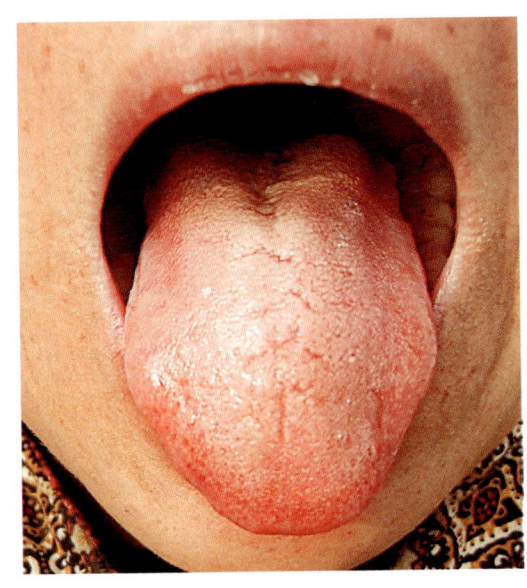

Fig 2.2-318

Patient, Male, 43years,

Case NO.: F300

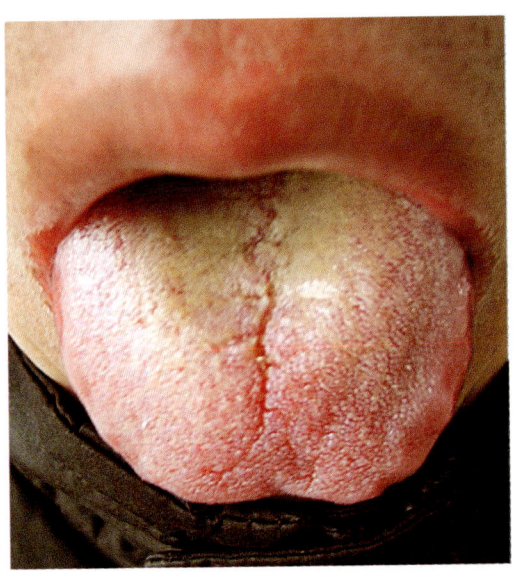

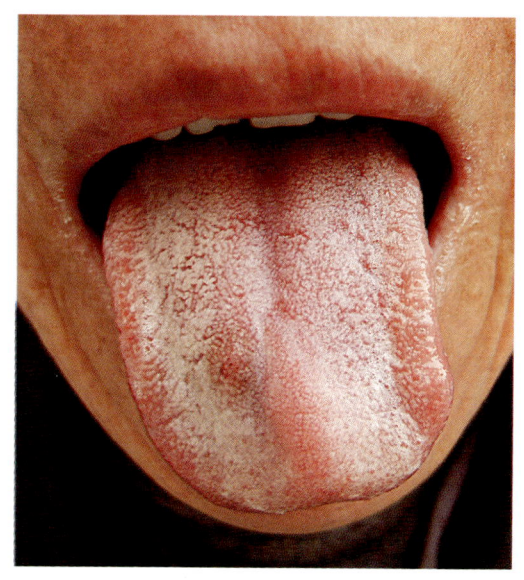

Fig 2.2-319

Patient, Female, 61years,

Case NO.: F47

Greasy tongue coating

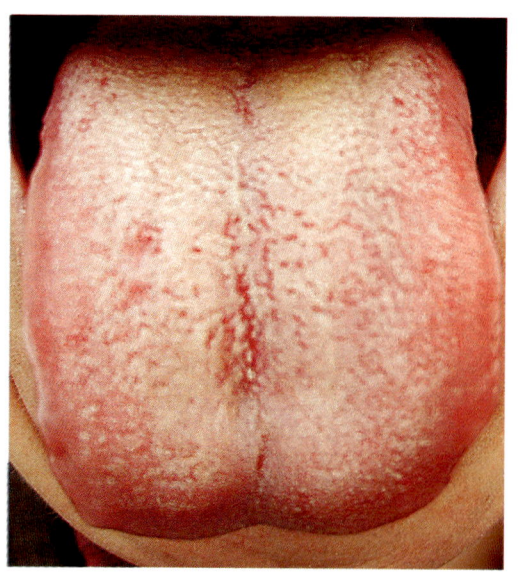

Fig 2.2-320

Patient, Female, 44years,

Case NO.: W254

3.5 Slippery and greasy tongue coating

AIDS stage

Fig 2.2-321

Patient, Male, 44years,

Case NO.: W623

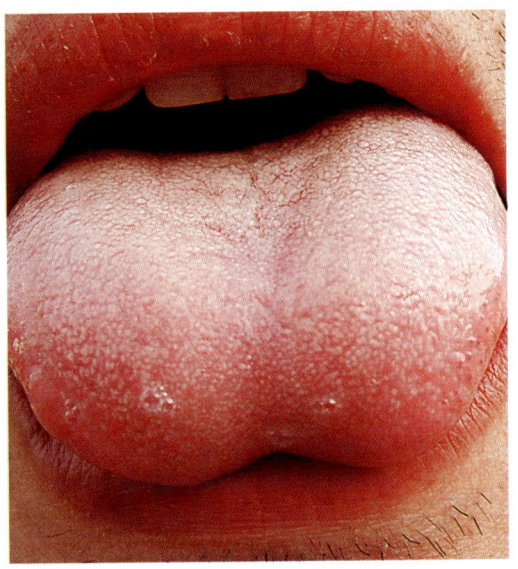

CHAPTER THREE
HIV/AIDS PATIENT'S TONGUE ANALYSIS

Tongue manifestations can objectively and accurately reflect pathological changes in patients. An analysis of the features of tongue manifestations will help to better understand the syndromes affecting AIDS patients and improve differential diagnosis. It also helps the patients to have a better understanding of the disease and its progression. From September 2005 to June 2006, a syndrome investigation was conducted and tongue information was collected from 1284 HIV/AIDS cases. The results of the analysis are summarized below.

1. General Information

Among the 1284 HIV/AIDS cases, there are 620 males and 664 females with a ratio of 1:1.07. The patients range in age from 18 to 65 with an average of 43 years. Marital status includes, 34 unmarried, 1129 married, 9 divorced, 111 bereaved of spouse, and 1 unidentified. Educational status includes 389 illiterate, 493 with primary school education, 363 with junior high school and 39 with senior high school education. The nationalities consist of 1275 Chinese and 9 Hui minority. The asymptomatic stage of HIV infection makes up 634 cases and there are 650 active AIDS patients in the analysis.

2. Differentiation

2.1 Patients in the asymptomatic stage of HIV infection

Of this group of patients 69.98% are in a state of deficiency complicated by excess. These patients show a progressive decline in their health due to a number of syndromes including internal accumulation of damp-heat with spleen qi deficiency, internal accumulation of damp-heat with spleen and lung qi deficiency, internal accumulation of damp-heat with qi and yin deficiency, and stagnant liver qi with spleen qi deficiency. Of the remainder of the group, 12.98% belong to an excess syndrome chiefly characterized by internal accumulation of damp-heat, and 17.03% belong to a deficiency syndrome characterized by a deficiency of spleen qi, spleen and lung qi, qi and yin, or qi and blood.

2.2 AIDS patients

Of this group of patients, 82.43% are in a state of deficiency complicated by excess. These patients show a progressive decline in their health due to a number of syndromes including internal accumulation of damp-heat with spleen qi deficiency, internal accumulation of damp-heat with spleen and lung qi deficiency, excessive accumulation of damp-heat evil with spleen qi deficiency, and internal accumulation of damp-heat with qi and yin deficiency. Of the remainder of the group, 5.27% belong to an excess syndrome chiefly characterized by internal accumulation of damp-heat, and 12.30% belong to a deficiency syndrome characterized by a deficiency of spleen qi, spleen and lung qi, qi and yin, or qi and blood.

3. Collection and Analysis of Tongue Pictures

All the pictures were carefully taken in natural light with a Fuji fine-810 digital camera by professional photographers. The analysis was made by five professors and associate professors in AIDS study, and Chinese Medicine Diagnostics according to tongue colorimeter and *Zhong Yi Zhen Fa Tu Pu (Illustrated Diagnostic Methods in Traditional Chinese Medicine)*.

4. Inspection of Tongue Manifestations

4.1 Tongue color

Table 1 Color Distribution and Comparison in HIV/AIDS Patients

Color	Asymptomatic stage of HIV infection		AIDS		P	χ^2
	Cases	Frequency	Cases	Frequency		
Pale	32	5.05%	54	8.31%	0.019	5.459
Crimson	293	46.21%	332	51.08%	0.359	0.081
Dark	91	14.35%	106	16.31%	0.331	0.994

The above table indicates that the crimson tongue makes up the greatest part of both the asymptomatic stage of HIV infection and AIDS resulting in 46.21% and 51.08% respectively. Dark and pale tongues make up 14.35% and 16.31%, and 5.05% and 8.31% respectively. Frequency of colors in the asymptomatic stage and AIDS stage were compared using χ^2 test, with the results being $P > 0.05$ and suggesting no statistical significance.

4.2 Morphological tongue description

Table 2 Morphological Distribution and Comparison in HIV/AIDS Patients

Morphological description	Asymptomatic stage of HIV infection		AIDS		P	χ^2
	Cases	Frequency	Cases	Frequency		
Thin	52	8.20%	73	11.23%	0.067	3.351
Swollen	99	15.62%	151	23.23%	0.001	11.872
Tooth-marked	57	8.99%	83	12.77%	0.030	4.717
Cracked	33	5.21%	47	7.23%	0.133	2.254

This table indicates that swollen tongues make up 15.62% and 23.23%, and tooth-marked tongues make up 8.99% and 12.77% respectively. Thin tongues make up 8.20% and 11.23%, and cracked tongues make up 5.21% and 7.23% respectively. A comparison of the frequency of swollen and tooth-marked tongues in both stages was made by means of χ^2 test with ρ=0.001 < 0.01 and ρ=0.03 < 0.05 which is indicative of statistical significance.

4.3 Color of coating

Table 3 Comparison of Coating Color in HIV/AIDS Patients

Color	Asymptomatic stage of HIV infection		AIDS		P	χ^2
	Cases	Frequency	Cases	Frequency		
White	347	54.73%	304	46.77%	0.004	8.141
Yellow	203	32.02%	276	42.46%	0.000	14.964
Dark grey	3	0.47%	8	1.23%	0.141	2.169
White-yellow-mixed	84	13.25%	81	12.46%	0.673	0.178

The above table shows that a white coating makes up the greatest percentage resulting in 54.73% and 46.77% of the cases, and a yellow coating makes up 32.02% and 42.46% of cases in each stage respectively. A white-yellow-mixed tongue coating makes up 13.25% and 12.46% of cases, and a dark grey coating makes up 0.47% and 1.23% of cases respectively. The frequency of white and yellow coatings was compared using χ^2 test with $P=0.004 < 0.01$ and $P=0.000 < 0.001$ resulting in a suggestion of marked statistical significance.

4.4 Quality of coating

Table 4 Quality of Coating and Comparison in HIV/AIDS Patients

Quality	Asymptomatic stage of HIV infection		AIDS		P	χ^2
	Cases	Frequency	Cases	Frequency		
Thick	227	35.80%	288	44.31%	0.002	9.661
Moist	37	5.84%	58	8.92%	0.035	4.464
Greasy	281	44.32%	303	46.62%	0.409	0.681
Peeled	25	3.94%	34	5.23%	0.271	1.214

The above table shows that a thick coating with 35.80% and 44.31%, and a greasy coating with 44.32% and 46.62% take the lead both in the asymptomatic stage of HIV infection and AIDS respectively. Moist coatings make up 5.84% and 8.92%, and peeled coatings make up 3.94% and 5.23% respectively. The frequency of thick and moist coatings was compared by means of χ^2 test with $P=0.002 < 0.01$ and $P=0.035 < 0.05$ suggesting statistical significance.

5. Discussion

As a modern day disease, AIDS is not recorded in ancient Chinese medical literature. However, as a highly infectious and epidemic disease with some common clinical manifestations, AIDS is identical to the disease of pestilence in Chinese medicine.

As one of the diagnostic methods in Chinese medicine, tongue manifestations objectively and accurately reflect the condition of patients, thus offering clues for the etiology and pathogenesis of AIDS and providing a method of syndrome differentiation. The analysis conducted reveals crimson tongues represent 46.21% and 51.08% respectively in the two stages without statistical significance when compared. The crimson tongue is typical of heat syndromes, which implies the predominant pathogen of AIDS is heat evil. Yellow and dark grey as well as white-yellow-mixed coatings, which are also signs of heat syndromes, make up 45.74% and 56.15%. This also shows the pathogenic nature of heat in AIDS. In terms of the morphological analysis, the tongues appear mostly swollen and tooth-marked which are signs of damp accumulation. In terms of the texture of the coating, greasy, thick, and moist coatings, which are indicative of dampness, constitute the majority of cases suggesting the pathogenic nature of dampness in AIDS. When compared with the asymptomatic stage, the AIDS stage has a statistically significant greater amount of swollen and tooth-marked tongues, and thick and moist tongue coatings which suggests the progressive trend of dampness accumulation as the disease advances. Pale, thin, cracked, peeled, and dark features also indicate HIV/AIDS has the characteristics of consuming qi and impairing yin giving rise to stagnation or stasis. Such tongue manifestations typical of preponderant heat and dampness evils causing stagnation/stasis and impairing qi and yin are consistent with the clinical pattern differentiation.

CHAPTER FOUR
COMMON SYNDROMES
OF HIV/AIDS
IN CHINESE MEDICINE

Chinese Medicine holds that syndromes are the mirror of the true nature of diseases. In the course of illness, syndrome is a group of facts inclusive of symptoms, signs, tongue manifestations, and pulse conditions, which are the base and core for differential treatment as well as the premise to and proof of prescription. The clinical syndromes of HIV/AIDS are quite complicated. HIV/AIDS patients surveyed are classified into two categories-one in the category of deficiency syndrome and the other excess, mostly being concurrent. The survey of those patients reveals the characteristics of syndrome distribution, which are illustrated in Table 1 to Table 3.

Table 1 Statistical Summary of AIDS Syndrome Frequency Distribution

Excess syndrome	Deficiency syndrome									Total
	Regualr	Failure of lung's defensive capacity	Deficiency of spleen qi	Deficiency of qi and yin	Deficiency of qi and blood	Qi deficiency of lung and spleen	Yin deficiency of liver and kidney	Yin deficiency of lung and kidney	Yang deficiency of spleen and kidney	
Regualr	24	2	60	18	14	58	11	2	12	201
Wind-heat invasion	6	7	1	4	0	5	1	0	2	26
Wind-cold invasion	2	16	1	4	3	18	1	1	2	48
Internal accumulation of damp-heat	63	14	193	63	32	122	21	7	8	523
Toxic accumulation of damp-heat	10	1	38	21	11	31	3	2	2	119
Retention of phlegm-heat in the lung	3	2	8	9	5	30	2	2	1	62
Pathogenic accumulation in skin	15	7	19	11	17	25	6	4	3	107
Stagnation of liver qi	8	5	27	10	1	15	9	0	4	79
Stagnation of qi and phlegm	4	0	4	3	1	4	0	0	2	18
Phlegm mingling with blood stasis	1	1	3	2	1	4	2	0	1	15
Total	136	55	354	145	85	312	56	18	37	1198

Table 2 Syndrome Frequency Distribution in the Stage of Asymptomatic Infection with HIV

Excess syndrome	Regualr	Failure of lung's defensive capacity	Deficiency of spleen qi	Deficiency of qi and yin	Deficiency of qi and blood	Qi deficiency of lung and spleen	Yin deficiency of liver and kidney	Yin deficiency of lung and kidney	Yang deficiency of spleen and kidney	Total
Regualr	24	2	43	11	10	26	5	1	3	125
Wind-heat invasion	5	3	0	2	0	0	1	0	0	11
Wind-cold	0	11	1	4	1	10	0	0	0	27
Internal accumulation of damp-heat	50	9	108	35	15	45	14	4	3	283
Toxic accumulation of damp-heat	6	0	8	5	0	5	1	1	0	26
Retention of phlegm-heat in the lung	3	1	3	5	1	11	2	0	0	26
Pathogenic accumulation in skin	7	0	9	2	7	6	1	2	1	35
Stagnation of liver qi	4	3	18	7	0	6	5	0	1	44
Stagnation of qi and phlegm	2	1	3	1	0	1	0	0	0	8
Phlegm mingling with blood stasis	0	0	0	2	4	1	1	0	0	4
Total	101	30	193	74	38	111	30	8	7	589

Common syndromes

Table 3 Syndrome Frequency Distribution in the Stage of AIDS

Excess syndrome	Deficiency syndrome									Total
	Regular	Failure of lung's defensive capacity	Deficiency of spleen qi	Deficiency of qi and yin	Deficiency of qi and blood	Qi deficiency of lung and spleen	Yin deficiency of liver and kidney	Yin deficiency of lung and kidney	Yang deficiency of spleen and kidney	
Regualr	2	0	17	8	4	32	6	1	9	79
Wind-heat invasion	1	4	1	2	0	5	0	0	1	14
Wind-cold invasion	1	6	0	0	2	8	1	1	2	21
Internal accumulation of damp-heat	12	4	85	28	16	77	7	3	6	238
Toxic accumulation of damp-heat	4	1	30	16	11	26	2	1	2	93
Retention of phlegm-heat in the lung	0	1	5	4	4	19	0	2	1	36
Pathogenic accumulation in skin	8	7	10	9	10	19	5	2	2	72
Stagnation of liver qi	4	0	9	2	1	9	4	0	3	32
Stagnation of qi and phlegm	2	0	1	2	1	3	0	0	2	11
Phlegm mingling with blood stasis	1	0	3	0	1	3	0	0	1	9
Total	35	23	161	71	50	201	25	10	29	605

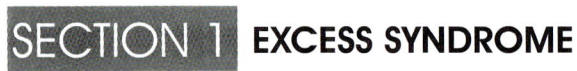

SECTION 1 EXCESS SYNDROME

1. Internal accumulation of damp-heat:

Syndrome marked by internal accumulation of damp-heat obstructing *qi fen*.

Clinical manifestations: recessive fever (i.e. fever not felt initially until after a rather long time), chest distress, epigastric fullness and oppression, thirst yet not for drinking, halitosis, heaviness of limbs, poor appetite, loose stool, yellow urine, viscous and foul leucorrhea; red tongue with thick/ yellow and greasy coating or with yellow and white coating, soft rapid pulse or slippery rapid pulse.

2. Stagnation of liver qi:

Syndrome marked by failure of the liver in dispersion leading to qi stagnation.

Clinical manifestations: emotional depression, frequent sighs, fullness or migratory pain in the chest, hypochondria or lower abdomen, dysphoria,_menoxenia, distending pain of breast, thin and white coating, wiry or taut pulse.

3. Pathogenic accumulation in skin:

Including eruptions caused by wind-heat, heat accumulation in the liver channel, dampness retention due to deficiency of the spleen, and qi stagnation and blood stasis. Herpes (infection caused by AIDS complicated herpes zoster virus) is observed in the latter three syndromes.

3.1 Eruptions caused by wind-heat:

Syndrome marked by skin eruptions caused by wind-heat attack.

Clinical manifestations: millet-like red or white eruptions over skin, itchy skin, red tip and margins of the tongue, floating and rapid pulse.

3.2 Heat accumulation in the liver channel:

Syndrome marked by herpes caused by failure of the liver in dispersion due to heat accumulation in the liver channel.

Clinical manifestations: burning and prickly lesions of the skin in scarlet color, tight vesicle wall, with stinging pain, bitter taste and dry throat, irritability, dry stool or yellow urine, red tongue with thin/thick yellow coating, wiry, slippery and rapid pulse.

3.3 Dampness retention due to deficiency of the spleen:

Syndrome marked by herpes caused by retention of damp heat in zhongjiao (the middle warmer) due to deficient spleen qi.
Clinical manifestations: light-colored herpes with loose vesicle wall, poor appetite and abdominal distension, loose stool, pale tongue with white or white and greasy coating, deep and slow or slippery pulse.

3.4 Qi stagnation and blood stasis:

Syndrome caused by stagnation of qi and obstructed flow of blood.
Clinical manifestations: constant pain for months or longer and dark color in the local area of skin rashes even after disappearance, dark-colored tongue with white coating, wiry and thready pulse.

4. Wind-cold invasion:

Syndrome marked by stagnated defensive qi due to wind-cold attacking the superficies.
Clinical manifestations: aversion to cold, fever, stuffy and runny nose, cough with thin sputum, headache, body pain, anhidrosis, thin white coating, floating and tense pulse.

5. Toxic accumulation of damp-heat:

Syndrome caused by heat evil retaining in the qifen as the result of interaction of dampness and heat.
Clinical manifestations: fever; skin ulceration, itchy and painful ulceration and swelling of throat, mouth, tongue, eyes, urethra and anus with secretions, recurrent, bitter taste and sticky mouth, auricular and nasal ulceration with secretions, diarrhea, thick and sticky leukorrhea,

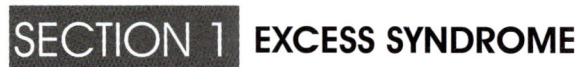

bright yellow coloration of the sclera and skin, scanty dark urine, crimson tongue with thick yellow, or yellow and white, or greasy coating, or with white scales, or granules or powder, soft rapid or slippery rapid pulse.

6. Retention of phlegm-heat in the lung:

Syndrome marked by failure of the lung's capacity for ascending and descending due to retention of phlegm-heat in the lung.

Clinical manifestations: yellowish sticky sputum, asthmatic breath, fever, thirst, restlessness, sore throat, chest distress and pain, sputum with blood, scanty dark urine, red tongue with yellow and greasy coating, slippery and rapid pulse.

7. Wind-heat invasion:

Syndrome marked by functional disorder of the lung due to wind heat attacking the lung.

Clinical manifestations: fever, slight aversion to wind and cold, swelling and pain of the throat, headache, cough, hypohidrosis, slight thirst, red tip and margins of tongue, thin and white coating with little moisture, floating and rapid pulse.

8. Stagnation of qi and phlegm:

Syndrome marked by phlegm obstructing channels and collaterals due to qi stagnation.

Clinical manifestations: scrofula or nodule in neck, nape and groin, fullness and migratory pain in the chest, hypochondrium, gastric cavity and abdomen; skin numbness, emotional depression, feeling of a foreign body obstructing the throat, white and sticky sputum, reddish tongue with white and greasy coating, wiry and slippery pulse.

9. Phlegm mingling with blood stasis:

Syndrome caused by obstruction of collaterals by phlegm and blood stasis.

Clinical manifestations: lump or pricking pain in local areas; numbness of limbs, moving difficulty or hemiplegia; chest distress with much sputum, amenorrhea, dysmenorrhea or menstruation with blood clot, or prickly breast; dark purple or petechial tongue, white greasy or white slippery coating, deep and uneven pulse.

390

10. Deficiency of spleen qi:

Syndrome marked by dysfunction of the spleen in transportation and transformation due to deficiency of spleen qi.

Clinical manifestations: loose stool, lassitude, poor appetite, epigastric fullness, abdominal distension, lingering abdominal pain, gradual emaciation, weight loss, short breath, spontaneous perspiration, sallow complexion, swollen and pale tongue with white coating, feeble pulse.

11. Qi Deficiency of the lung and spleen:

Feeble condition marked by failure of the lung in purifying and descending function and failure of the spleen in transformation and transportation due to qi deficiency of the lung and spleen.

Clinical manifestations: short breath, lassitude, gasp on movement or prolonged coughing in low voice, clear sputum, spontaneous perspiration, susceptibility to colds, poor appetite, epigastric distension, loose stool, listlessness, soreness of limbs, even swollen face and limbs, pale tongue with white or white slippery coating, feeble pulse.

12. Deficiency of qi and yin:

Syndrome marked by simultaneous presence of qi deficiency and yin deficiency.

Clinical manifestations: listlessness and lassitude, short breath, no desire to speak, spontaneous perspiration and night sweating, feverish palms and soles, emaciation, weight loss, dry cough with scanty sputum, dry feeling in the mouth and throat, dizziness, scanty urine and constipation; red or light red tongue with scanty saliva, or fissured tongue, scanty dry or peeled coating, feeble rapid pulse, or feeble, thready rapid pulse.

13. Deficiency of qi and blood:

Syndrome marked by simultaneous presence of qi deficiency and blood deficiency.

Clinical manifestations: pale or sallow complexion, lassitude and fatigue, dizziness, pale lips and nails, short breath, spontaneous perspiration, susceptibility to colds, palpitation and

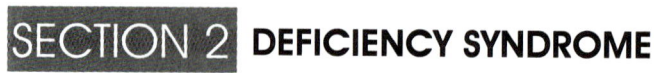

insomnia, numbness of limbs, pale tongue, thready and weak pulse.

14. Failure of lung's defensive capacity:

Syndrome marked by deficiency and failure of the lung qi to protect the body against exogenous invasion.

Clinical manifestations: susceptibility to colds, slight aversion to wind and cold, spontaneous perspiration, short breath, listlessness, no desire to speak, pale tongue with white coating, feeble pulse.

15. Yin deficiency of kidney and liver:

Syndrome marked by insufficient yin fluid of kidney and liver.

Clinical manifestations: soreness and weakness of the loins and knees, hectic fever, night sweating, feverish sensation in the "five centers" (palms, soles and chest), dizziness, tinnitus, extreme emaciation (rackabones), low fever, flushed cheeks, tremor of hands and feet, blurred vision, scanty menstrual blood or amenorrhea; red or crimson tongue with scanty coating, thready and rapid pulse.

16. Yin deficiency of lung and kidney:

Syndrome marked by insufficient yin fluid of lung and kidney.

Clinical manifestations: cough with scanty sputum or dry cough, dry mouth and throat, soreness and weakness of the loins and knees, flushed cheeks and night sweating, emaciation, sputum mingled with blood, hoarseness, osteopyrexia and hectic fever; red tongue with scanty coating, thready rapid pulse.

17. Yang deficiency of spleen and kidney:

Syndrome marked by dysfunction of spleen and kidney due to yang deficiency.

Clinical manifestations: cold limbs and body, bright-white complexion, chronic diarrhea and dysentery, sore and cold feeling in the loins and knees, clear and profuse urine, frequent nocturnal urination, emaciation and listlessness, cold and painful abdomen, stool with the

Common
syndromes

indigested food, poor appetite, epigastric and abdominal distension, facial and limb dropsy, gomphiasis, gingival atrophy; infertility due to cold in the uterus, thin leucorrhea; impotence and seminal emission or immature ejaculation and infertility, pale and swollen tongue with teeth imprints on the margins, white coating, deep, slow and weak pulse.

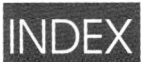

图书在版编目（ＣＩＰ）数据

艾滋病舌诊图谱／彭勃等编译．－北京：人民卫生
出版社，2006.10
ISBN 7-117-08042-6

I.艾　　II.彭　　III.艾滋病－舌诊－图谱
IV.①R241.25-64　②R512.910.4-64

中国版本图书馆CIP数据核字（2006）第117544号

艾滋病舌诊图谱

编　　译：彭勃 等
出版发行：人民卫生出版社
地　　址：中国北京市丰台区方庄芳群园 3 区 3 号楼
邮　　编：100078
网　　址：http://www.pmph.com
E - mail：pmph @ pmph.com
发　　行：zzg@pmph.com.cn
购书热线：+8610-6761-7350（电话及传真）
开　　本：787×1092　1/16
版　　次：2006 年　月第 1 版　2006 年　月第 1 版第 1 次印刷
标准书号：ISBN 7-117-08042-6／R・8043